Radiology of Iatrogenic Disorders

Series Editor:
Morton A. Meyers, M.D.

Iatrogenic Thoracic Complications

Edited by
Peter G. Herman, M.D.
Professor of Radiology
Harvard Medical School;
Director
Division of Thoracic Radiology
Brigham and Women's Hospital

With 256 Illustrations

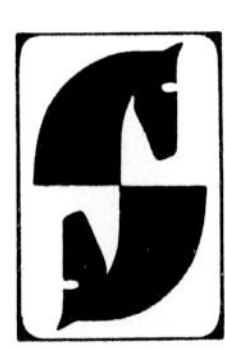

Springer-Verlag
New York Heidelberg Berlin

Series Editor
Morton A. Meyers, M.D.
Professor and Chairman
Department of Radiology
School of Medicine
State University of New York at Stony Brook
Stony Brook, New York 11794 U.S.A.

Volume Editor
Peter G. Herman, M.D.
Professor of Radiology
Harvard Medical School;
Director, Division of Thoracic Radiology
Brigham and Women's Hospital
75 Francis Street
Boston, Massachusetts 02115

Sponsoring Editor: Marie D. Low
Production: Berta Steiner

Library of Congress Cataloging in Publication Data
Main entry under title:
Iatrogenic thoracic complications.

  (Radiology of iatrogenic disorders)
  Bibliography: p.
  Includes index.
  1. Chest—Radiography. 2. Chest—Diseases—
Diagnosis. 3. Iatrogenic diseases. I. Herman, Peter G.
II. Title. [DNLM: 1. Thoracic diseases—Complications.
2. Thoracic radiography. 3. Iatrogenic disease.
4. Postoperative diseases—Complications. WF 970 I11]
RC941.I27   1983   617′.5407572   82-19465

Typeset by Kingsport Press, Kingsport, Tennessee
Printed and bound by Halliday Lithograph, West Hanover, Massachusetts
Printed in the United States of America.

9 8 7 6 5 4 3 2 1

ISBN 0-387-**90729**-7 Springer-Verlag New York Heidelberg Berlin
ISBN 3-540-**90729**-7 Springer-Verlag Berlin Heidelberg New York

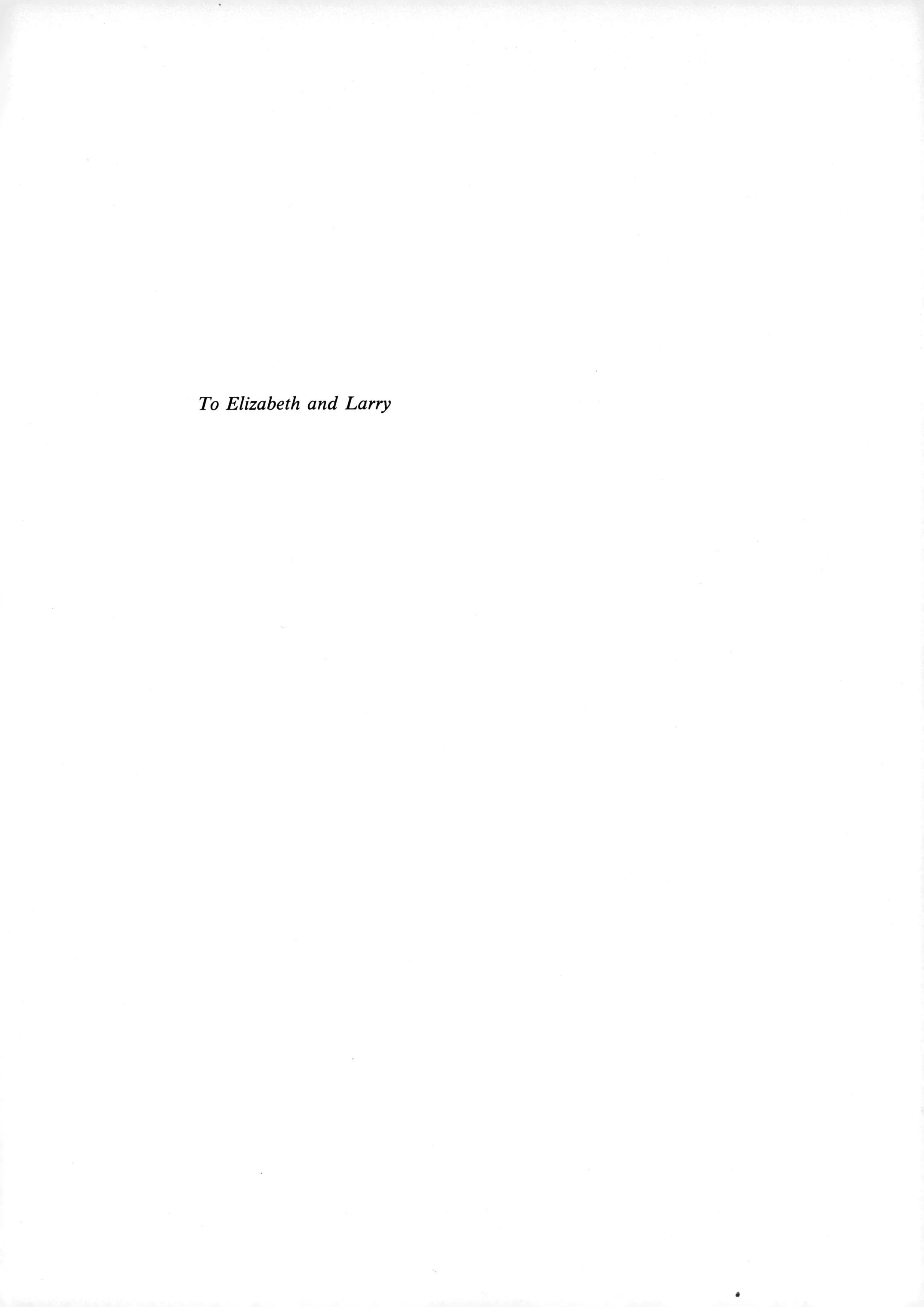

To Elizabeth and Larry

Contents

Series Editor's Foreword

The purpose of this series of volumes is to present a comprehensive view of the complications that result from the use of acceptable diagnostic and therapeutic procedures. Individual volumes will deal with iatrogenic complications involving (1) the alimentary system, (2) the urinary system, (3) the respiratory and cardiac systems, (4) the skeletal system and (5) the pediatric patient.

The term *iatrogenic,* derived from two Greek words, means physician-induced. Originally, it applied only to psychiatric disorders generated in the patient by autosuggestion, based on misinterpretation of the doctor's attitude and comments. As clinically used, it now pertains to the inadvertent side-effects and complications created in the course of diagnosis and treatment. The classic categories of disease have included: (1) congenital and developmental, (2) traumatic, (3) infectious and inflammatory, (4) metabolic, (5) neoplastic, and (6) degenerative. To these must be added, however, iatrogenic disorders—a major, although generally unacknowledged, source of illness. While great advances in medical care in both diagnosis and therapy have been accomplished in the past few decades, many are at times associated with certain side-effects and risks which may result in distress equal to or greater than the basic condition. Iatrogenic complications, which may be referred to as "diseases of medical progress," have become a new dimension in the causation of human disease.

A highly accurate index of the overall incidence of iatrogenic illnesses is difficult to establish, but there is little doubt that it approaches epidemic proportions in certain instances. The literature indicates that paramount causes include drugs and hospital-associated risks:

• Every year in the United States, up to one and a half million people—between 3 and 5 percent of all hospital admissions—are admitted primarily because of drug reactions. Once in the hospital, between 18 and 30 percent of all patients have a drug reaction. The length of their stay is about doubled as a result.[1-3]

• In one study of a general medical unit over a twelve-month period, one-quarter of the 67 deaths in the unit were due to adverse drug reactions.[3] In acutely ill hospitalized patients, the drug-related death rate has been recently reported to be nearly one per thousand.[4]

• Hospital-acquired infections occur in about one in 20 patients and there is approximately 25 percent excess mortality among patients with nosocomial bloodstream infections. About one-third of all infections seen in hospital practice are nosocomial in origin.[5] The incidence of postoperative wound infections is about 7.4 percent.[6]

• It has been reported that one out of every five patients admitted to the medical service of a typical university teaching hospital suffers an iatrogenic episode, which is classified as moderate or severe in 40 percent. Over one-fourth of the episodes result from diagnostic and therapeutic procedures.[7]

• Of all patients admitted to a multidisciplinary intensive care unit in one recent study,[8] over 12 percent were admitted because of iatrogenic disease. Potentially avoidable therapeutic and technical errors accounted for half of these; the remaining adverse reactions that were determined to be unpreventable represent the risk-benefit ratio of a treatment compared with the natural history of the illness. Furthermore, once in a medical-surgical intensive care unit, patients are subject to often harmful adverse occurrences.[9]

• Ten percent of hospital deaths are associated with a diagnostic or therapeutic procedure which is considered a contributing, precipitating or primary cause of obitus.[10]

This series is not intended to support or encourage any concept of diagnostic or therapeutic nihilism. Rather, it is intended to assess and detail the broad spectrum of the mechanisms and effects of complications experienced in order to further refine clinical practice. Undue conservatism would effectively prohibit the meaningful application of any diagnostic or therapeutic method, virtually any of which carries a potential risk to the patient. Many inherent complications of medical and surgical techniques can be controlled only to an irreducible minimum, despite the exercise of utmost care and skill. In this series, areas of practical clinical concern are addressed rather than topics of pure academic interest. Radiologic documentation is often critical to uncover or confirm the presence and to evaluate the extent of many iatrogenic complications. The large number of illustrations used in each volume attest to the aim of fully employing the power of visual instruction.

Oscar Wilde's wry statement that "experience is the name men give to their mistakes" is beneficial only if physicians continue to be open-minded and to learn from each other. It is a medical axiom that advances introduce new problems which, in turn, generate solutions and further advances. Lewis Thomas[11] affirms that "Mistakes are at the very base of human thought . . . What is needed, for progress to be made, is the move based on the error." This series is designed in the hope that iatrogenic illnesses may be minimized, or appropriately anticipated and promptly recognized and managed, so that the prime injunction of clinical medicine can be further fulfilled: "Physician, do no harm."

Morton A. Meyers, M.D.

References

1. Wade N: Drug regulation: FDA replies to charges by economists and industry. Science 179:775–777, 1973
2. Seidl LG, Thornton GF, Smith JW, et al: Studies on the epidemiology of adverse drug reactions. III. Reaction in patients on a general medical service. Bull Johns Hopk Hosp 119:299–315, 1966
3. Ogilvie RI, Reudy J: Adverse drug reactions during hospitalization. Canad Med Assn J 97:1450–1457, 1967
4. Porter J. Jick H: Drug-related deaths among medical inpatients. JAMA 237 No 9:879–881, 1977
5. Hospital Infections. Bennett John V., Brachman Philip S. (eds). Little, Brown and Company, Boston, 1979
6. Altemeier WA: Postsurgical infections. Antibiotics Chemother 21:11–21, 1976
7. McLamb JT, Huntley RR: The hazards of hospitalization. Southern Med J 60:469–472, 1967
8. Trunet P, LeGall J-P, Lhoste F, et al: The role of iatrogenic disease in admissions to intensive care. JAMA 244:2617–2620, 1980
9. Abramson N, Ward K, Grenvik A, et al: Adverse occurrences in intensive care units. JAMA 244:1582–1584, 1980
10. Schimmel EM: The hazards of hospitalization. Ann Intern Med 60:100–116, 1964
11. Thomas L: The Medusa and the Snail. The Viking Press, New York, 1979

Preface

> The ordinary course of a cure is carried on at the expense of life. . . . One step further and we are completely cured.
>
> Michel de Montaigne (1533–1592)
> *Essays,* Book II, Chapter 3

> I owe my reputation to the fact that I use digitalis in doses the textbooks say are dangerous and in cases that the textbooks say are unsuitable.
>
> Karel Frederik Wenckebach (1864–1940)
> *Lancet,* 1937

One has only to scan the current medical journals and new book titles to appreciate the concern of the medical profession to document, prevent, and treat iatrogenic complications. Physicians and philosophers alike have recognized for centuries that the dangers inherent in disease may be surpassed by the risks involved in its diagnosis and treatment. It is generally accepted and certainly not surprising that complications are proportional to the complexity and invasiveness of the various diagnostic and therapeutic interventions. For these reasons, practitioners find it increasingly difficult to estimate accurately the risks and benefits that are part of an intelligent management decision.

Unfortunately, may publications dealing with iatrogenic complications tend to exaggerate the risk side of the risk-benefit relationship. This in turn may promote an attitude that may lead to diagnostic and therapeutic nihilism. In order to present a balanced view, the efficacy of a given diagnostic test or treatment would have to be fully documented, including the risks involved in not performing it. Such data, even if available, would be outside of the scope of this volume. The purpose of this book is to facilitate the decision-making process by providing a concise summary of thoracic iatrogenic complications.

Since this book deals specifically with complications involving the thorax, the rationale of this approach must be explained. One of the unique features of thoracic complications is that they are often detectable only on the chest radiograph. The common thoracic complications which are extensively dealt with in this publication include the drug reactions, malpositions of lines and tubes, pacemakers and cardiac valves, effects of radiation and complications associated with intubation and respiratory care. Awareness of these complications and their recognition on the chest film will often be decisive in patients' care. Needless to say, the role of imaging procedures is by no means exclusive and their findings are meaningful only if they are integrated into the total body of observations. However, the scope of discussions is by no means limited to radiology.

The publication of this book became possible only because leading experts were willing to contribute their work.

I would like to express my particular appreciation to Dr. Morton A. Meyers, who conceived the idea of publishing this series. Springer-Verlag provided splendid editorial support and particularly the help of Berta Steiner and Marie Low has to be recognized. The help of my secretary, Ms. Nancy Harrison, was invaluable.

Peter G. Herman, M.D.

Contributors

Michael A. Bettmann, M.D.
Assistant Professor of Radiology, Harvard Medical School; Cardiovascular Radiologist, Brigham and Women's Hospital, Boston, Massachusetts 02115; Scholar of the James F. Picker Foundation
Chapter 10

John M. Braver, M.D.
Assistant Professor in Radiology, Harvard Medical School; Radiologist, Brigham and Women's Hospital, Boston, Massachusetts 02115
Chapter 9

Solon Cole, M.D.
Radiologist, Hartford Hospital, Hartford, Connecticut 06106
Chapter 6

Robert P. Fortunato, M.D.
Instructor in Radiology, Harvard Medical School; Radiologist, Brigham and Women's Hospital, Boston, Massachusetts 02115
Chapter 4

Jeffrey D. Goldstein, M.D.
Research Fellow in Pathology, Harvard Medical School, Brigham and Women's Hospital, Boston, Massachusetts 02115
Chapter 1

G.B. Clifton Harris, M.D.
Associate Professor of Radiology, Harvard Medical School, Boston, Massachusetts; Associate Radiologist-in-Chief, The Children's Hospital Medical Center, Boston, Massachusetts 02115
Chapter 7

Peter G. Herman, M.D.
Professor of Radiology, Harvard Medical School; Director, Division of Thoracic Radiology, Brigham and Women's Hospital, Boston, Massachusetts 02115
Chapters 1, 3

Cyprus C. Hopkins, M.D.
Assistant Professor of Medicine, Harvard Medical School, Massachusetts General Hospital, Boston, Massachusetts 02114
Chapter 2

Ira J. Isaacson, M.D.
Assistant Professor of Anesthesiology, Emory University School of Medicine, Atlanta, Georgia 30322
Chapter 4

Herman I. Libshitz, M.D.
Professor of Diagnostic Radiology, M.D. Anderson Hospital and Tumor Institute, Texas Medical Center, Houston, Texas 77030
Chapter 8

Gary Mintz, M.D.
Associate Professor of Medicine and Radiology, Thomas Jefferson University Hospital Medical College, Co-Director, Non-Invasive Cardiovascular Laboratory, Hahnemann Medical College and Hospital, Philadelphia, Pennsylvania 19107
Chapter 12

Charles F. O'Cain, M.D.
131 McDowell Street, Asheville, North Carolina 28803
Chapter 5

Gale S. Pasternack, M.D.
Clinical Fellow in Radiology, Harvard Medical School, Brigham and Women's Hospital, Boston, Massachusetts 02115
Chapter 5

James E. Pennington, M.D.
Associate Professor of Medicine, Associate Chief, Infectious Diseases Division, Harvard Medical School, Boston, Massachusetts 02115
Chapter 3

Steven E. Seltzer, M.D.
Assistant Professor of Radiology, Harvard Medical School; Radiologist, Brigham and Women's Hospital, Boston, Massachusetts 02115
Chapter 1

Robert M. Steiner, M.D.
Chief, Cardiac and Pulmonary Radiology, Professor of Radiology,
Thomas Jefferson University Hospital Medical College, Philadelphia,
Pennsylvania 19107
Chapter 12

Charles J. Tegtmeyer, M.D.
Professor of Radiology, Associate Professor of Anatomy, University
of Virginia School of Medicine, Charlottesville, Virginia 22908
Chapter 11

Jack L. Westcott, M.D.
Professor of Radiology, New York Hospital-Cornell Medical Center,
Attending Radiologist, New York Hospital, New York, New York
10021
Chapter 6

1 Iatrogenic Thoracic Complications Induced by Drugs

Steven E. Seltzer, Jeffrey D. Goldstein, and Peter G. Herman

Drug-induced diseases account for 3% to 4% of admissions to a medical service (1), and between 5% and 15% of hospitalized patients suffer adverse drug reactions. This takes into account only those events that are associated with prolonged hospital stay, permanent impairment, or death. Three percent of all hospital deaths may be drug-related. It has been estimated that the financial cost of drug-related complications is $3 billion annually (2). Since many iatrogenic complications induced by drugs are associated with abnormal chest radiographs, the radiologist plays an early and important role in diagnosis.

The classification of a drug-induced pulmonary disease is difficult, since it may be categorized on the basis of radiologic appearance, clinical presentation, or the histopathology of the abnormality. We have decided to organize drug reactions according to their clinical-pathologic presentation. The injuries induced by drugs may involve primarily the thoracic structures, or drug-induced abnormalities originating in other organs secondarily may injure the respiratory system. We will provide a brief description of the general pathogenesis of drug reactions and subsequently discuss specific clinical-pathologic patterns in detail. The difficulty with this classification lies in the fact that some drugs fall into several clinical-pathologic categories. In these cases we assigned the drug reaction to the group that describes the most usual reactions. The various radiologic appearances of thoracic drug reactions will be summarized. The tables included contain information about many commonly used drugs. In this review, occupational or environmental agents are not considered.

Pathogenesis

Drug reactions may induce disease by two general mechanisms (3):

1. *Direct Drug Toxicity*—Lung damage may be secondary to overdose, intolerance, side effects, and idiosyncratic events. Clinically, drug toxicity will resemble the known therapeutic or side effects of the drug.
2. *Drug Hypersensitivity*—In a significant percentage of drug reactions, this mechanism is indeed suspected. Since the immunologic basis of many of these reactions is well understood, a brief summary of the immunologic events is in order.

The molecular size of most drugs is too small to produce an immune response. Drugs most likely act as haptenes and combine with endogenous larger molecules. The haptene-protein complexes activate the lymphocytes. The complex interaction between T and B lymphocytes then eventually will lead to host sensitization (4). Upon reexposure of the sensitized host to antigen, tissue or cell injury will occur. The immunopathologic mechanisms are commonly classified into four types (5):

Type I (immediate hypersensitivity reactions)—Antibodies, usually IgE, are produced against the haptenes, which will bind to mast cells and basophils. The interaction of antigen with cell-bound antibody will result in mast cell degranulation and release of mediators, which in turn are responsible for inflammation.

Type II (cytotoxic reactions)—Antibodies, usually IgM or IgG, react against membrane-bound drug haptenes. In the process complement is fixed, resulting in cellular damage.

Type III (immune complex reactions)—Antibody-antigen complexes are formed. These circulating immune complexes may lodge in the basement membranes of blood vessels in various organs, particularly in the kidneys and the lungs. Subsequently the complement cascade is triggered, leading to tissue damage.

Type IV (delayed hypersensitivity reactions)—This is an essentially cell-mediated immune response. Sensitized T lymphocytes react against locally deposited antigens. Following this interaction, lymphokines will be released. Other cells, particularly macrophages, will be recruited and cellular injury will occur.

Types I and III are the most usual reactions responsible for drug-induced hypersensitivity.

The clinical presentation of hypersensitivity reactions, as opposed to direct drug toxicity, will not resemble the pharmacologic actions of the drug. The time interval between drug administration and the reaction may vary. It usually will be seven to ten days. On occasion, however, reactions may be present within several hours or may develop as late as a number of years later. Clinical syndromes associated with drug hypersensitivity are anaphylaxis, contact dermatitis, serum sickness, urticaria, angioedema, asthma, and eosinophilia. A favorable clinical response to antiallergic therapy is a reasonable indication that the clinical symptoms represented a drug reaction (6–13).

Clinical-Pathologic Patterns

This classification is based on the correlation of the most commonly occurring symptom complexes and pathologic changes. For each pattern, the clinical features, the underlying pathologic changes, and the pathogenesis, if known, will be discussed. The most commonly encountered radiologic findings will be listed. For each category, reactions to commonly used drugs will be briefly described.

Table 1-1 summarizes the radiologic, clinical-pathologic, and immunologic features associated with the administration of commonly used drugs.

Hypersensitivity of the Airways (Asthma)

The drugs associated with acute asthmatic reactions are summarized in Table 1-2 (14).

The clinical presentation includes wheezing and other signs of airway obstruction. Some agents have a direct effect on bronchial innervation—β-adrenergic antagonists like propranolol (15), and parasympathomimetics like neostigmine and bethanechol (16). Other drugs may act through a type I immune response involving IgE. Some of the patients with asthmatic reaction to a drug have actually preexisting asthma or atopy. A recognized syndrome of bronchoconstriction, nasal polyposis, and sinusitis is known to be associated with the administration of aspirin, indomethacin, and tartrazine. Aspirin and some similar antiinflammatory agents very likely cause asthma by inhibiting prostaglandin synthesis (17). Asthma is usually induced by a type I immune reaction, which causes mucous hypersecretion and inspissation, submucosal edema, and eosinophilic infiltration in addition to bronchial smooth muscle constriction. Permanent histologic changes are unlikely to be associated with a short exposure to a drug.

The chest radiograph in asthma is usually unremarkable. During severe attacks, however, increased lung volume and hyperlucent lungs may be noted. Segmental atelectasis secondary to mucous plugging of bronchi may be seen (Fig. 1-1).

Injury of the Lung Parenchyma

Numerous drugs and physical agents are capable of injuring the lung parenchyma. While the damage results in a spectrum of histopathologic abnormalities, a classification of the lung injury distinguishing diffuse alveolar damage, interstitial pneumonitis, intraalveolar fibrosis, and interstitial fibrosis is a useful one.

In *diffuse alveolar damage,* hyaline membranes line the alveolar septa. Type I pneumocytes have disappeared and focal intraalveolar hemorrhage is usually present (Fig. 1-2a). This pattern is often seen with oxygen toxicity and as a reaction to chemotherapeutic agents.

In *interstitial pneumonitis,* chronic inflammatory cells are present in the interstitium and also within alveolar spaces, where they are accompanied by alveolar macrophages. Regenerating, large, atypical type II (granular) pneumocytes are promi-

Table 1-1. Summary of Drug Reactions in the Lungs

Drug or Agent	Clinical-Pathologic Pattern	Roentgenographic Pattern
Aspirin	Asthma	Normal (common) Overexpansion of lungs Regional emphysema Atelectasis
BCNU	Diffuse parenchymal injury	Alveolar and/or interstitial infiltrates
Bleomycin	Diffuse parenchymal injury	Basal symmetric interstitial infiltrate Nodular infiltrate Elevated diaphragms Positive ^{67}Ga scans
Blood	Noncardiac pulmonary edema	Pulmonary edema
Busulfan	Diffuse parenchymal injury Early—Pulmonary edema	Patchy alveolar and interstitial infiltrates
	Late—Pulmonary fibrosis	Interstitial fibrosis and infiltrate Ossification (rare)
Cyclophosphamide	Diffuse parenchymal injury Cardiogenic pulmonary edema (rare)	
Diphenylhydantoin (Dilantin)	Lymph node enlargement	Mediastinal adenopathy
	Diffuse parenchymal injury	Diffuse reticulonodular infiltrate ?Increased bronchovascular markings
		?Interstitial fibrosis
Doxorubicin HCL (Adriamycin)	Pulmonary edema (cardiogenic)	Congestive heart failure
Ganglionic blocking agents (Hexamethonium, Mecamylamine)	Diffuse parenchymal injury	*See* Busulfan
Gold	Lupus-like reaction Vasculitis	*See* Procainamide
Heroin	Noncardiac pulmonary edema	Pulmonary edema
	Pulmonary vascular injury	Angiitis with microaneurysms, indistinct vessels, luminal irregularities, and thrombosis on arteriograms
	Granulomatous reaction	Granulomas
Hydralazine	Lupus-like reaction	*See* Procainamide

(*Continued*)

Table 1-1. (cont.)

Drug or Agent	Clinical-Pathologic Pattern	Roentgenographic Pattern
Iodides	Acute anaphylaxis (Vasculitis) (Iodism)	Pulmonary edema
Iodinated oils	Pulmonary embolism	Diffuse stippling
	Lipoid pneumonia	Confluent opacities
Methotrexate	Diffuse parenchymal injury	Pleural effusion Pulmonary fibrosis Interstitial and/or alveolar infiltrate
	Pulmonary infiltrates with eosinophilia	Peripheral migratory alveolar infiltrates
Methysergide	Pulmonary fibrosis	Pleural effusion Local fibrosis simulating masses Diffuse ground-glass haze
Mineral oil	Granulomatous reaction	Fibrosis Interstitial infiltrate Mass lesion Rosettes of oil-filled acini
Nitrofurantoin	Acute—Pulmonary infiltrates with eosinophilia or pulmonary edema	Pleural effusion Patchy interstitial basilar infiltrates Pulmonary edema
	Chronic—Pulmonary fibrosis, desquamative interstitial pneumonitis (rare)	Diffuse interstitial fibrosis
Oxygen	Diffuse parenchymal injury	Acute—Diffuse patchy infiltrates Chronic—Pulmonary fibrosis
Para-aminosalicylic acid (PAS)	Pulmonary infiltrates with eosinophilia	Peripheral migratory alveolar infiltrates
Penicillin	Pulmonary infiltrates with eosinophilia	Pleural effusion Pneumonic infiltrates accentuated in periphery, migratory, persistent
	Vasculitis	Destructive upper respiratory tract lesions Acute alveolar and/or interstitial infiltrate
	Lupus-like reaction	*See* Procainamide

Table 1-1. (cont.)

Drug or Agent	Clinical-Pathologic Pattern	Roentgenographic Pattern
Pituitary snuff	Granulomatous reaction (Hypersensitivity pneu- monitis)	Diffuse micronodular or ground-glass infiltrate
	Asthma	
Procainamide	Lupus-like syndrome	Serositis with pleural and/ or pericardial effusions Pulmonary edema Infarction Atelectasis Interstitial pneumonitis
Propoxyphene	Pulmonary edema	*See* Heroin
Sulfonamides	Pulmonary infiltrates with eosinophilia (Vasculitis) (Lupus-like reaction)	*See* Penicillin

Entries in parentheses are the rare manifestations of reaction to the drug.

Table 1-2. Drugs Associated with Asthma

Allergenic extracts	Griseofulvin	Penicillin
Antisera	Indomethacin	Sodium dehydrocholate
Aspirin	Iodines	Streptomycin
β-Adrenergic antagonists	Iron dextran	Tartrazine
Bromsulphthalein	Local anesthetics	Tetracycline
Cephaloridine	Mercurials	Vaccines
Erythromycin	Neomycin	Vitamin K
Ethionamide	Parasympathomimetics	

Adapted from Davies (10)

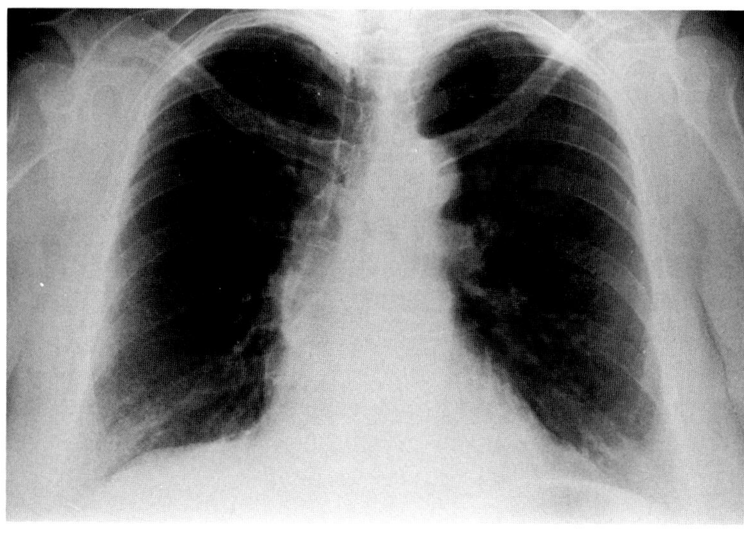

Fig. 1-1. Asthmatic reaction. The lungs are slightly overinflated. The basal interstitial markings are somewhat accentuated.

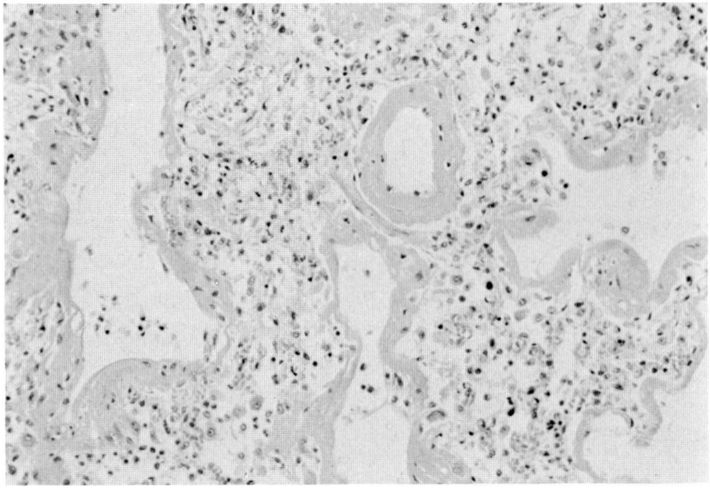

a

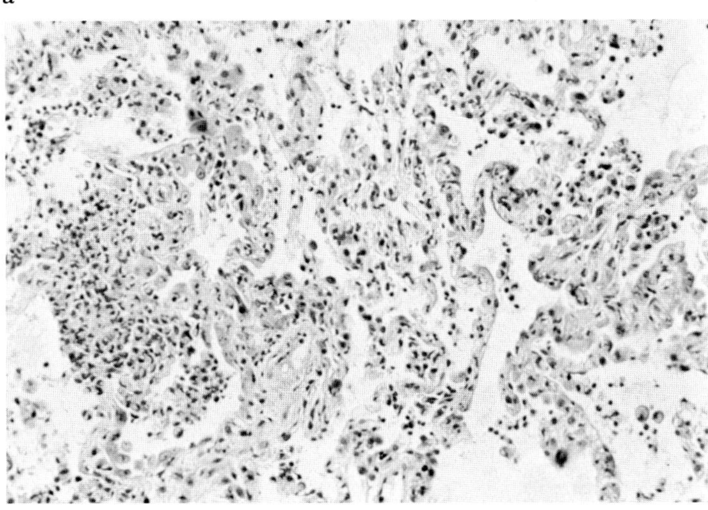

b

Fig. 1-2, a–d. The spectrum of diffuse parenchymal injury.

a Diffuse alveolar damage. Hyaline membranes line the alveolar septa. Type I pneumocytes have disappeared and focal intraalveolar hemorrhage is present. This pattern occurs acutely with oxygen toxicity and some chemotherapeutic agents.

b Interstitial pneumonitis. Chronic inflammatory cells are present in the interstitium and also within alveolar spaces, where they are accompanied by alveolar macrophages. Regenerating, large, atypical type II (granular) pneumocytes are prominent lining the alveolar septa. Cytotoxic drugs are most frequently responsible.

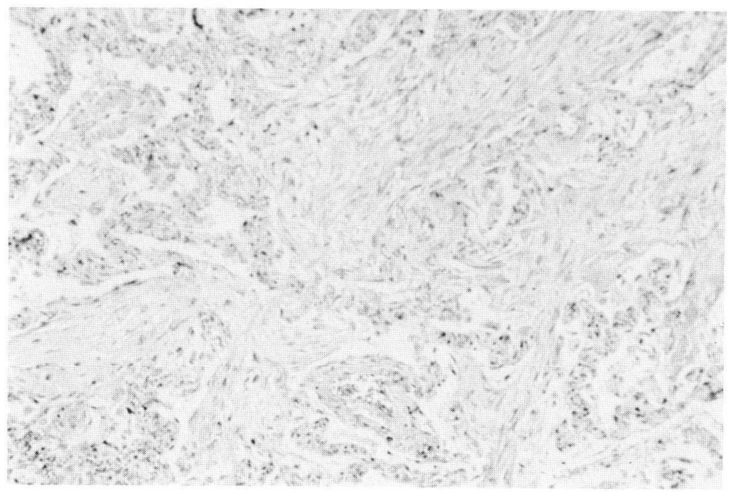

c

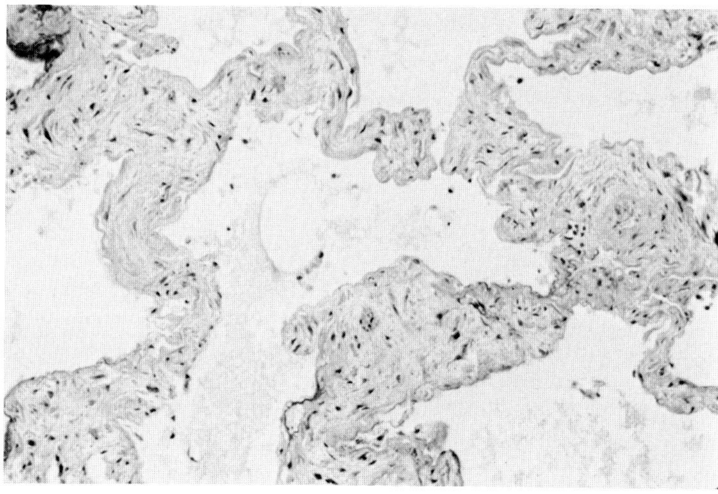

d

Fig. 1-2 (cont.)

   c Intraalveolar fibrosis. Loose cellular fibrous tissue fills the alveolar lumens; the septa are only slightly thickened. This pattern results from organization of intraalveolar fibrinous exudates, and may be seen with oxygen toxicity, busulfan, and ganglionic blocking agents.

   d Interstitial fibrosis. The pulmonary parenchyma has been remodeled with extensive septal connective tissue, obliteration of some alveoli, and dilatation of residual airspaces (honeycombing). This is an end-stage lesion that may be seen with any of the drugs that produce parenchymal injury (Masson's trichrome stain). All photomicrographs: H & E stain; original magnification ×50 unless indicated otherwise.

nent lining the alveolar septa (Fig. 1-2b). Cytotoxic drugs are most frequently responsible for this appearance.

Intraalveolar fibrosis is identified by loose cellular fibrous tissue in the alveolar lumens; the septa are only slightly thickened (Fig. 1-2c). This appearance results from organization of intraalveolar fibrinous exudates and may be seen with oxygen toxicity, busulfan, and ganglionic blocking agents.

In *interstitial fibrosis,* the pulmonary parenchyma has been remodeled with extensive septal connective tissue, obliteration of some alveoli and dilatation of airspaces (honeycombing) (Fig. 1-2d). This is an end-stage lesion that may be seen with many of the drug-induced reactions that produce parenchymal injury.

The patterns just described should be viewed as a continuum; both clinical and pathologic appearances often overlap. Because of this, we will discuss the individual drugs and therapeutic agents (Table 1-3) according to their therapeutic action rather than on the basis of the pathologic patterns.

Oxygen

Oxygen is probably the most commonly used therapeutic agent associated with adverse pulmonary reactions. Clinically, oxygen toxicity will manifest as progressive respiratory failure with decreased compliance, shunting, increased dead space, and decreased diffusing capacity. Both the onset and severity of symptoms are dependent on the inspired oxygen concentration. Because of the decreased arterial O_2 saturation, increased ventilatory pressure may be required, resulting in barotrauma (18,19).

Oxygen toxicity causes diffuse alveolar damage with intraalveolar fibrinous exudate, hyaline membranes, hemorrhage, congestion, and damage of the endothelial and type I epithelial cells (Fig. 1-2a). Proliferation of type II pneumocytes occurs early, followed by interstitial fibroblastic proliferation, organization of alveolar exudates, and pulmonary fibrosis. Earliest site of injury involves the capillary endothelial cells (20). Increased oxygen concentration within the airways predisposes to pulmonary infections by interfering with the mucociliary apparatus and by inhibiting phagocytosis.

The chest radiograph during the acute phase shows patchy and diffuse opacities or may have the appearance of an interstitial process. Extensive pulmonary fibrosis would indicate chronic injury.

Bronchopulmonary dysplasia (BPD) is a sequel of oxygen toxicity of infants with respiratory distress syndrome. Premature infants with birth weights under 2000 g are at greatest risk for development of BPD. Severe forms of the disease are usually fatal, while many milder cases may go undetected. While BPD is quite similar to oxygen toxicity seen in adults, the histologic injury in infants is more apparent in the distal airways, manifested by loss of cilia, epithelial necrosis, and bronchiolar squamous metaplasia. The natural history of this syndrome is complex because oxygen toxicity in infancy may interfere with lung growth and pulmonary vascular development, and the long-term prognosis for these children is uncertain (21,22).

Radiographically, early in the course only hyperexpansion and fine, diffuse, lacy opacities are seen. Larger fibrous streaks interspersed with lucent areas are only infrequently present (23). Complications of BPD may manifest as interstitial emphysema, atelectasis, pneumonic infections, and congestive heart failure. Pulmonary hypertension with right ventricular hypertrophy, an elevated cardiac apex, and enlarged central pulmonary arteries may also be seen.

Table 1-3. Drugs Associated with Diffuse Parenchymal Injury

Amphotericin B	6-Mercaptopurine
Azathioprine	Methotrexate
BCNU	Methysergide
Bleomycin	Mitomycin
Busulfan	Neocarzinostatin
Chlorambucil	Nitrofurantoin
Cyclophosphamide	Oxygen
Hexamethonium	Paraquat
Mecamylamine	Pentolinium
Melphalan	Procarbazine

Adapted from Davies (10)

Bleomycin

Concentrations of this drug on the skin and in the lung are six to ten times higher than in the blood. This may explain the abnormalities seen in bleomycin toxicity, such as stomatitis, alopecia, hyperkeratosis, and hyperpigmentation (which occurs in 50% of the cases). The clinical manifestations of pulmonary toxicity are varied. Pneumonialike symptoms have been reported in 5%–40% of patients receiving bleomycin. Only a small percentage, however (3.4%), will develop a pulmonary fibrosis that will become fatal in 1% to 2% of the cases. There is impairment reflected in the pulmonary function tests of about one-third of the patients who receive the drug for over 14 days (24–26). The pulmonary abnormalities are not entirely dose-related. However, pulmonary toxicity will sharply increase when the total dose exceeds 300–400 mg (27). Serious pulmonary reactions, however, have been noted at doses as low as 105 mg (28). Radiation therapy (directed to the thorax) (29) and systemic chemotherapy predispose to the development of pulmonary complications. Subsequent administration of oxygen will have similar effects (30). Pathologically, the acute reaction usually is associated with interstitial edema, hyaline membrane formation, and alveolar fibrinous edema. These changes may progress into a chronic phase marked by fibrosis and replacement of type I cells with type II cells (Fig. 1-2d). There will be a concomitant increase of the number of alveolar macrophages (31). The pathogenesis of the lung injury may be direct toxicity to the air-blood interface.

Chest x-ray usually reveals a symmetric, fine or moderately coarse, basal interstitial pattern. It may have a more reticular nodular appearance. The relatively high position of the domes of the diaphragm can be explained by loss of lung volume (32). Gallium-67 scanning (32) may accurately depict bleomycin-induced lung damage. Actually, the clinical symptoms and laboratory findings in one report (32) correlated better with gallium scans than with radiographic appearance.

Alkylating Agents (Busulfan, Cyclophosphamide, Chlorambucil, Melphalan)

While busulfan was one of the first drugs associated with pulmonary toxicity, all of these agents have been implicated in production of interstitial pneumonitis and fibrosis. Clinically, busulfan toxicity may present an Addisonianlike syndrome of hyperpigmentation, weakness, and weight loss, with dyspnea and chronic cough (33). Long-term busulfan administration (33) may result in pulmonary fibrosis. Subclinical busulfan injury predisposes to the development of radiation pneumonitis (34).

Acutely, "busulfan lung" will reveal accumulation of intraalveolar fibrinous edema. Subsequently, this edema becomes organized and may develop into striking intraalveolar fibrosis (Fig. 1-2c). Interstitial pneumonitis and fibrosis are the more common pathologic appearance seen with agents in this class (35–37). Radiologically, the early findings may resemble pulmonary edema, with patchy alveolar opacities or interstitial infiltrates. Apparently, if the drug is withdrawn early, the radiologic findings are completely reversible. Corticosteroids may have a useful role in treating early pulmonary toxicity. There have been reports (33) indicating progression of the interstitial infiltrates into a honeycomb appearance. Similar observations were made in a child treated with cyclophosphamide (38). In one report, disseminated pulmonary ossification was noted following busulfan treatment (39). In a large group of 195 patients receiving busulfan (average dose 464 mg) or cyclophosphamide, however, no radiologic abnormalities could be detected (40).

Methotrexate

The clinical syndrome associated with administration of this drug includes fever, cough, dyspnea, and blood eosinophilia (41). Pulmonary reactions are rare with doses that do not exceed 20 mg per week. Pulmonary toxicity may be present following intrathecal or oral administration (42). The reaction tends to be transient, and the patients improve following the discontinuation of the drug and glucocorticoid administration. Progressive fibrosis is rare. The histologic pattern indicates diffuse alveolar damage with hyaline membranes and proliferation of type II cells. The histologic pattern at times may resemble desquamative interstitial pneumonitis. It is assumed that the pathogenesis of methotrexate pneumonitis is either a hypersensitivity reaction or a direct toxic effect.

The radiologic presentation is a predominantly interstitial pattern; however, mixed airspace and interstitial opacities were also reported (43).

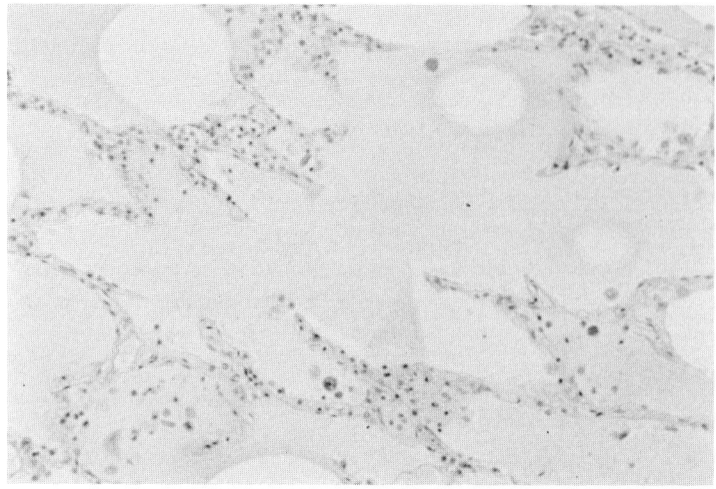

a

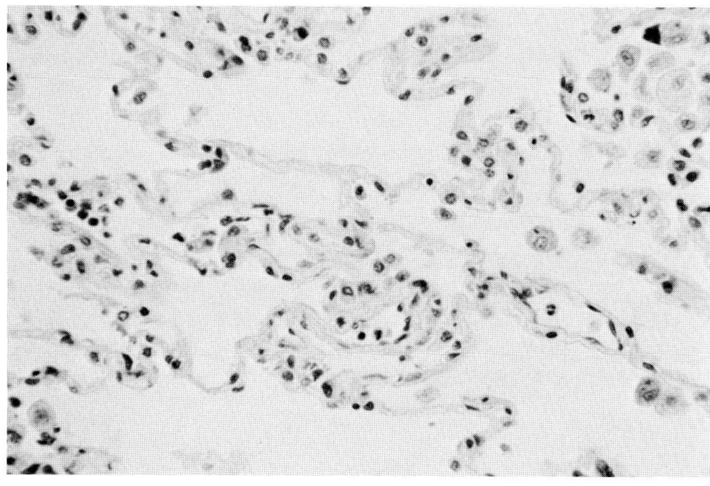

b

Fig. 1-3, a–d.

a Acute pulmonary edema. Fluid fills the alveolar spaces; the alveolar septa appear normal. This pattern occurs most frequently with narcotic overdose, transfusion reactions, or secondary to cardiac toxicity.

b Pulmonary infiltrates with eosinophilia. Pulmonary macrophages and eosinophils are present in the alveolar spaces; eosinophils and chronic inflammatory cells infiltrate the interstitium. This pattern occurs most frequently in response to sulfonamides and penicillins, para-aminosalicylic acid, and furadantoins (original magnification ×100).

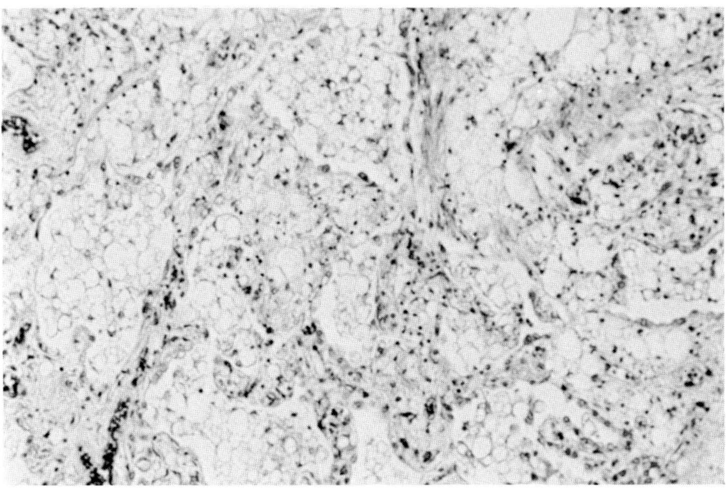

c

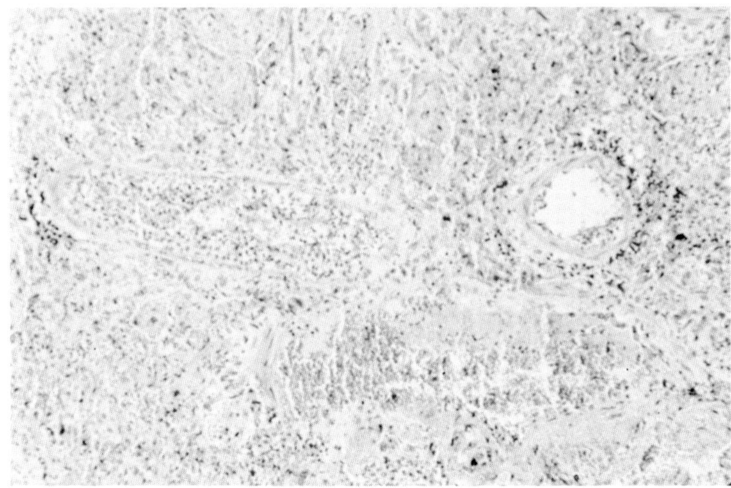

d

Fig. 1-3 (cont.)

   c Lipoid pneumonia. Numerous lipid-laden alveolar macrophages fill the alveoli. This reaction is a response to aspiration of exogenous lipid, usually from nose drops, cathartics, or contrast media (Masson's trichrome stain).

   d Pulmonary hypersensitivity vasculitis. Neutrophilic leukocytes infiltrate the wall and partially occlude the lumen of a pulmonary artery. Adjacent lung tissue shows recent and organizing hemorrhage. Pulmonary vasculitis may accompany a drug-induced systemic vasculitis affecting other organs. All photomicrographs: H & E stain, original magnification ×50, unless indicated otherwise.

Nitrosoureas (BCNU, CCNU, Methyl-CCNU)

Pulmonary toxicity from BCNU was first reported in 1976 and may occur in as many as 20% of patients receiving this agent (44,45). The onset of symptoms, usually progressive dyspnea and cough, occurs six months to three years after beginning therapy. Cumulative dosages associated with reactions range between 580mg/m² and 2100mg/m², and both total dose and dose per cycle may be important in predicting the likelihood of toxicity. Patients with preexisting lung disease develop symptoms at lower dosages and should be monitored with pulmonary function tests. In normal individuals, cumulative dosages up to 1400mg/m² are relatively safe. We have seen several cases of BCNU pulmonary toxicity of more rapid onset in patients who received single high doses of BCNU followed by transfusion of previously harvested, autologous bone marrow. Histologic changes are similar to those caused by other chemotherapeutic agents. Toxic synergism with other chemotherapeutic drugs and radiation therapy may also occur with BCNU. Pulmonary toxicity with methyl-CCNU has been reported only once. CCNU has not yet been implicated as a pulmonary toxin.

Procarbazine

This drug is commonly used in the MOPP combination chemotherapy regimen (with mechlorethamine, vincristine, and prednisone) for the treatment of Hodgkin's disease. Most likely it produces a reversible pneumonitis (Fig. 1-4); however, progression to interstitial fibrosis may occur, perhaps resulting from synergism with other chemotherapeutic agents (44). While the pathologic features are not well understood, in two cases the numbers of eosinophils and histiocytes were suggestive of a hypersensitivity reaction (46,47). Sarcoidlike granulomas were observed in one case (46).

Radiologically, procarbazine toxicity may appear as a nonspecific interstitial, alveolar or mixed pattern (47).

Mitomycin

This antibiotic produces interstitial pneumonitis and fibrosis which clinically, pathologically, and radiologically are indistinguishable from the effects of other anticancer drugs. Pulmonary toxicity may occur early with low doses. The outcome is unpredictable. Some patients will respond to steroids. Others progress to respiratory insufficiency.

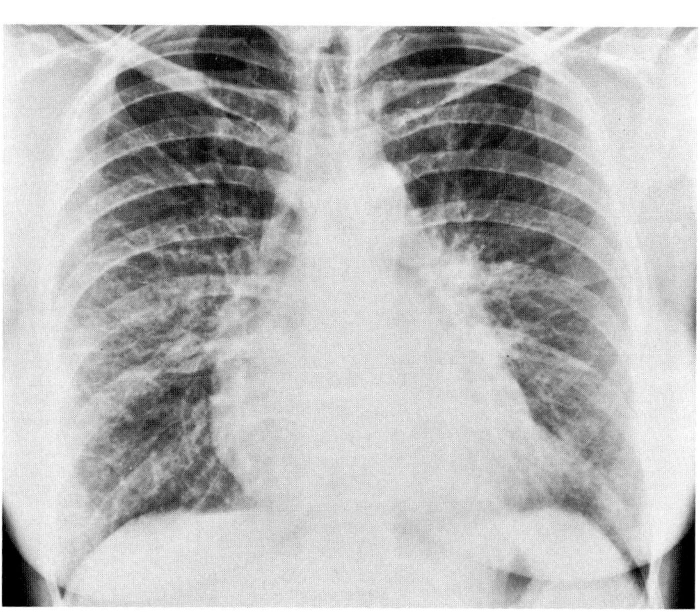

Fig. 1-4. Procarbazine-induced pneumonitis. Accentuated interstitial markings are seen.

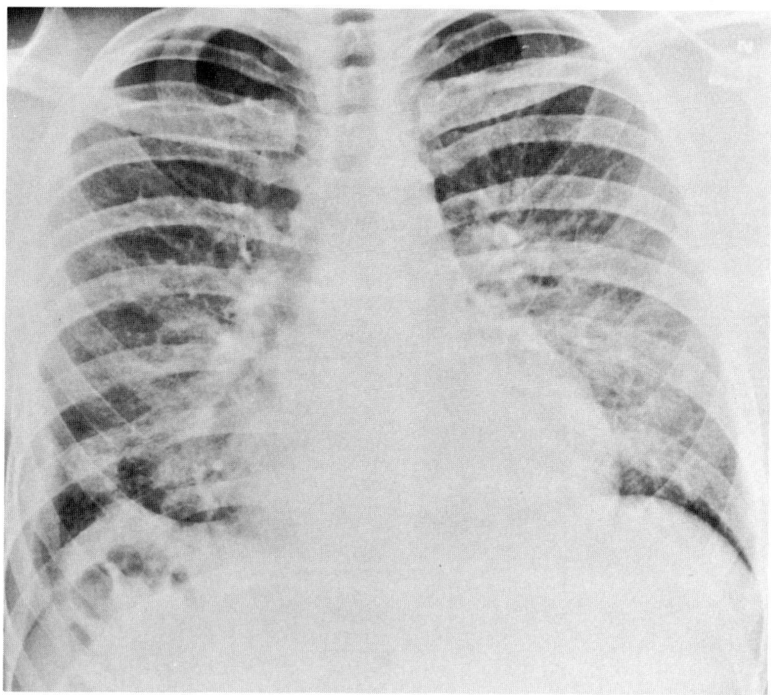

Fig. 1-5. Reaction to neocarzinostatin. Radiograph demonstrates findings of interstitial edema that developed secondary to drug therapy for hepatoma. Lung biopsy showed pulmonary vascular injury affecting venules, arterioles, and capillaries. The deformity of the right hemidiaphragm and right pleural thickening are due to previous surgery.

Zinostatin (Neocarzinostatin)

This drug may produce acute pulmonary endothelial damage affecting primarily the venules (with thrombus formation), arterioles, and capillaries (48) (Fig. 1-5).

Miscellaneous cytotoxic agents (49) have been implicated in the inducement of interstitial pneumonitis, such as 6-mercaptopurine and azathioprine.

Ganglionic Blocking Agents (Hexamethonium, Pentolinium, and Mecamylamine)

These drugs have been used in the treatment of malignant hypertension and may cause fibrinous intraalveolar edema, which eventually may lead to intraalveolar fibrosis (50–52) (Fig. 1-2c). The process resembles uremic pneumonitis and busulfan lung. Direct tissue injury is the most likely pathomechanism, considering the similarity of the chemical structure of hexamethonium and busulfan.

Radiologically, poorly defined lower lobe opacities or diffuse patchy infiltrates have been described.

Methysergide

This is used for migraine prophylaxis and it is well known to cause retroperitoneal fibrosis. Only 0.3% of the patients in one study complained of repeated episodes of chest pain, dyspnea, fever, pleural friction rubs, and effusions (53). Chest radiography shows pleural and disseminated pulmonary fibrosis appearing as a ground-glass pattern, in addition to localized areas of stranding. Both the clinical symptoms and the fibrosis may regress following discontinuation of the drug (54). Chronic pleural effusions, however, also may be present.

Acute Pulmonary Edema

The mechanism of development of pulmonary edema may be either direct injury of the alveolar-

Table 1-4. Drugs Associated with Pulmonary Edema

Amitriptyline	Iothalamate, sodium
Bleomycin	Methadone
Chlordiazepoxide	Methotrexate
Cyclophosphamide	Parathion
Cytosine arabinoside	Propoxyphene
Daunorubicin	Salicylates
Diatrizoate, meglumine	Transfusions
Doxorubicin	
Heroin	
Hydrochlorothiazide	

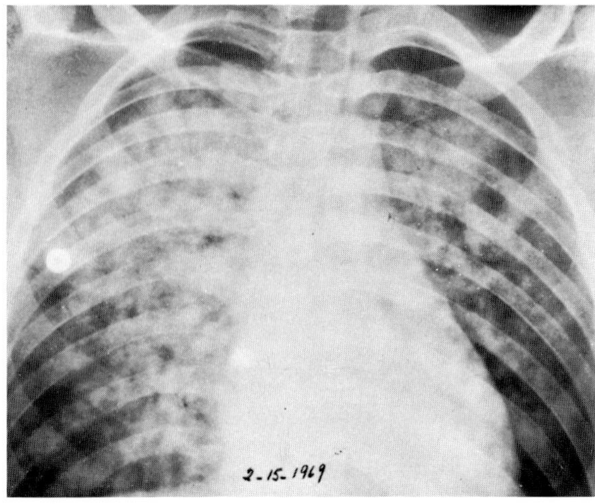

Fig. 1-6. **Methadone-induced pulmonary edema.** Bilateral alveolar densities are seen. (Courtesy of Dr. Yahya Berkmen, New York Medical College)

capillary membrane or cardiac toxicity, resulting in congestive heart failure (Table 1-4; Fig. 1-3a). The following classes of drugs have been implicated:

Heroin and Other Narcotics

In about 30%–40% of patients with acute intravenous heroin overdose, acute pulmonary edema develops (55,56). However, pulmonary edema also has been noted with intranasal heroin (57,58), oral and intravenous methadone (59,60) (Fig. 1-6), and propoxyphene (Darvon) (61,62). The onset following overdose is rapid, occurring within ten hours after drug administration. Occasionally, however, it may be delayed following the patient's recovery from coma.

The mechanism whereby pulmonary edema develops is still unknown. Many factors have been considered, particularly allergic or idiosyncratic reaction to the drug itself or to a contaminant. Other possibilities include a direct toxic effect on the lungs and myocardium and severe hypoxia.

Radiologically, heroin overdose should be considered in the appropriate clinical setting in the presence of central, bilateral, coalescent airspace or interstitial opacities. Usually the cardiac silhouette remains normal in size. Uncomplicated pulmonary edema secondary to heroin overdose will clear in 24 to 48 hours.

Other than pulmonary edema, heroin and similar substances may induce necrotizing angiitis and foreign body reactions due to talc, cotton fiber, or other drug impurities (63,64). This eventually may lead to pulmonary fibrosis in the so-called blue-velvet addicts (65,66). Other drugs that are associated with pulmonary edema are chlordiazepoxide (67), parathion (68–70), hydrochlorothia-

zide (69), salicylates (70), amitriptyline (71), iodinated contrast agents (72), methotrexate (73), cytosine arabinoside (74). We actually have encountered one case following administration of bleomycin.

Transfusion Reactions

Abrupt-onset pulmonary edema with fever, chills, tachycardia, dyspnea, and eosinophilia has been observed following transfusion (75). This may occur in patients with proper ABO matching, and antileukocyte antibodies are thought to be responsible.

The chest radiograph reveals nodular, perihilar opacities, somewhat favoring the lower lung zones, which persist for up to 48 hours. The cardiac silhouette usually is normal (Fig. 1-7).

The concomitant use of granulocyte transfusions and intravenous amphotericin B may cause an acute, potentially fatal, pulmonary reaction. Initial clinical manifestations are dyspnea, sudden onset or worsening of hypoxia, and the development of diffuse interstitial infiltrates on chest radiography. Wright et al. (76) reported that 14 of 22 patients (64%) who received both granulocyte transfusions and amphotericin B developed pulmonary complications. Only 5.7% of patients receiving leukocyte transfusions alone had pulmonary reactions, none of which were fatal. Respiratory difficulty in the 7 most severely affected patients, including all 5 deaths, began during or immediately after infusion

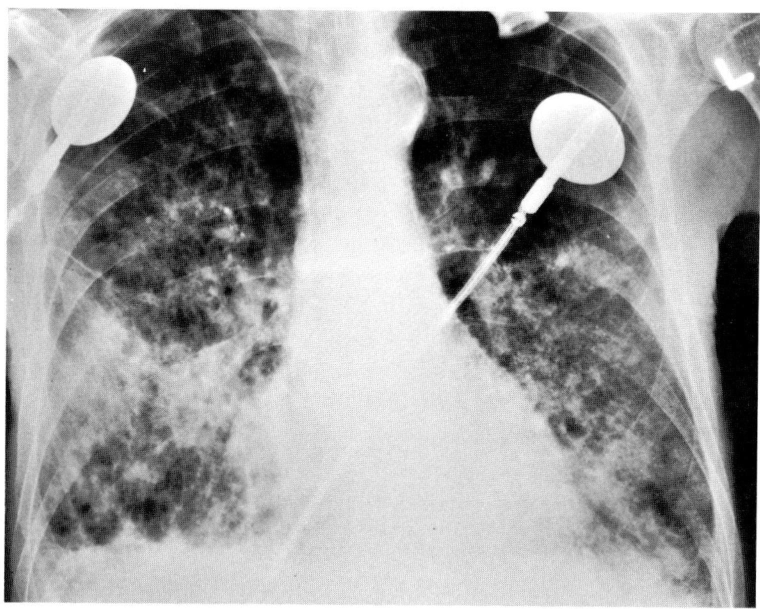

Fig. 1-7. Acute transfusion reaction. Bilateral alveolar and interstitial densities developed secondary to a reaction to a blood transfusion.

of amphotericin B. The pathologic findings were not specific, showing only diffuse intraalveolar edema and hemorrhage. This syndrome may result from intracapillary aggregation of the transfused leukocytes, followed by amphotericin B-mediated neutrophil cell membrane damage, which releases proteolytic enzymes and activates complement.

Cardiotoxins

Daunorubicin and doxorubicin, anthracycline antibiotics, may cause cardiac injury if the cumulative doses exceed 20 mg/kg and 550 mg/m², respectively. Patients with previous mediastinal irradiation are at a higher risk (77). Cyclophosphamide may produce acute cardiac toxicity at high doses (145 mg/kg or above) (78). Classical radiologic signs of congestive heart failure are present in these patients (79,80).

Pulmonary Infiltrates with Eosinophilia (PIE)

PIE syndrome has been observed following administration of numerous drugs (Table 1-5). Clinically, the syndrome is characterized by gradual onset of shortness of breath, cough, skin rash, and eosinophilia in the peripheral blood. The onset of this syndrome has been observed with the following classes of drugs:

Sulfonamides and Penicillins

The PIE syndrome may occur even following topical application (81) and has been observed following the first exposure to penicillin, which would make a hypersensitivity type of reaction unlikely (82). The symptoms rapidly improve following discontinuation of the drugs. The administration of glucocorticoids is beneficial. Following reexposure to the drugs, the symptoms may recur. Histologically, the alveolar spaces will be filled by macrophages, eosinophils, and fluids. Perivascular inflammatory infiltrates also will be present (Fig. 1-3b).

The chest radiograph demonstrates a fleeting, patchy, airspace process, more often noted on the periphery of the lung (Loeffler's syndrome). Pleural effusions are rare. The pulmonary infiltrates may persist for weeks following the withdrawal of the drug (83–86).

Table 1-5. Drugs Associated with Pulmonary Infiltrates with Eosinophilia

Chlorpropamide	Nitrofurantoin
Cromolyn sodium	Para-aminosalicylic acid
Furazolidone	Penicillin
Imipramine	Procarbazine
Mephenesin carbamate	Sulfonamides
Methotrexate	

Adapted from Davies (10)

Para-aminosalicylic Acid (PAS)

Drug reactions were reported in between 0.3% and 5.0% of patients. The manifestations include fever (98%), rash (72%), conjunctivitis, headache, joint pain, eosinophilia (30%), lymphadenopathy, and jaundice. The radiographic changes are similar to those of Loeffler's syndrome (87).

Nitrofurantoin

There have been at least 237 pulmonary reactions reported with use of this drug, including one fatality (88). The true incidence of pulmonary reactions is difficult to assess; however, it is known that over 44 million courses of nitrofurantoin have been prescribed. The acute reaction (89) mimics acute myocardial infarction (90), pumonary edema (91), pulmonary infarction (92), tracheobronchitis (93), or pneumonia (94). Several days following the drug ingestion, chills, fever, cough, and dyspnea may develop. Skin rash has been noted in 33% of the cases, and rales and wheezes are present in 12%. Mild blood eosinophilia occurs in 50% of the patients with pulmonary drug reaction.

The chest radiograph may be normal; however, patchy airspace opacities or an interstitial pattern at the lung bases has been noted (95–97). At times, there is an associated pleural effusion which may be unilateral. The chest x-ray findings may resemble chronic idiopathic eosinophilic pneumonia (98). In most instances, following discontinuation of the drug, the radiographic abnormalities will clear. There have been, however, cases reported where chronic nitrofurantoin therapy was associated with nonreversible pulmonary fibrosis (99). A pulmonary edema-like pattern has been occasionally noted (91). A similar acute reaction has also been seen following furazolidone (100).

The pathology and the radiologic findings in chronic nitrofurantoin reactions resembles the usual interstitial pneumonitis. Pathologically, in three cases a pattern resembling desquamative interstitial pneumonia was observed (101).

Granulomatous Reactions

Drug-induced granulomatous reactions in the lung occur as a foreign body reaction (lipoid pneumonia) or as an allergic reaction against organic antigens (extrinsic allergic alveolitis).

Lipoid pneumonia is the result of aspiration of oily nose drops or cathartics or may follow diagnostic examinations such as bronchography (Lipiodol (102), Visciodol (103))—and lymphangiography (Ethiodol) (104) (Fig.1-8). If these exogenous lipids enter through the airways, the abnormalities produced include acute and chronic pneumonitis, localized granulomas, and pulmonary fibrosis (105). Initially the patients are asymptomatic; however, repeated lipid exposure will lead to cough, dyspnea, and pulmonary fibrosis with impaired diffusing capacity. Radiologically, the aspirated lipids appear as oil-filled acinar shadows (rosettes). The aspirated oil tends to be localized in the lower lung zone (Fig. 1-9); however, oily nose drops may produce disseminated lesions. The intraalveolar lipids are phagocytized by alveolar macrophages (Fig. 1-3c), and the diagnosis may be made by identifying lipid-laden macrophages in the sputum. Chronic inflammation, fibrosis, and granulomas may follow. The areas of interstitial infiltrate or fibrosis may mimic a mass lesion which is difficult to distinguish from neoplasms.

Extrinsic allergic alveolitis (hypersensitivity pneumonitis) has been seen following usage of posterior pituitary snuff for the treatment of diabetes insipidus (106,107). Clinically, patients will develop increasing shortness of breath. The histologic pattern indicates chronic interstitial inflammation, poorly defined granulomas, and some interstitial fibrosis. A cell-mediated (type IV) immune reaction is most likely responsible. Since the introduction of synthetic antidiuretic hormone, new cases of "pituitary snuff-taker's lung" are unlikely. Radiology reveals a diffuse reticular nodular pattern or at times a ground-glass appearance.

Pulmonary Vascular Injury

Although many drugs may be associated with systemic vasculitis (108), involvement of the pulmonary vasculature is unusual (Table 1-6).

Sulfonamides and other drugs may induce hypersensitivity vasculitis (109,110). The involvement of the lungs, however, is less frequent than skin, kidney, and liver (110). Clinical and radiologic appearance sometimes resemble Wegener's granulomatosis or an allergic angiitis and granulomatosis (Churg and Strauss) (111). The systemic symptoms include arthralgias, edema, purpura, fever, weight loss, subcutaneous nodules, dermatitis, muscle tenderness, urticaria, neuritis, gastrointestinal bleeding, and renal failure. The typical pathologic feature is angiocentric inflammation and vascular necrosis, eventually leading to infarction or

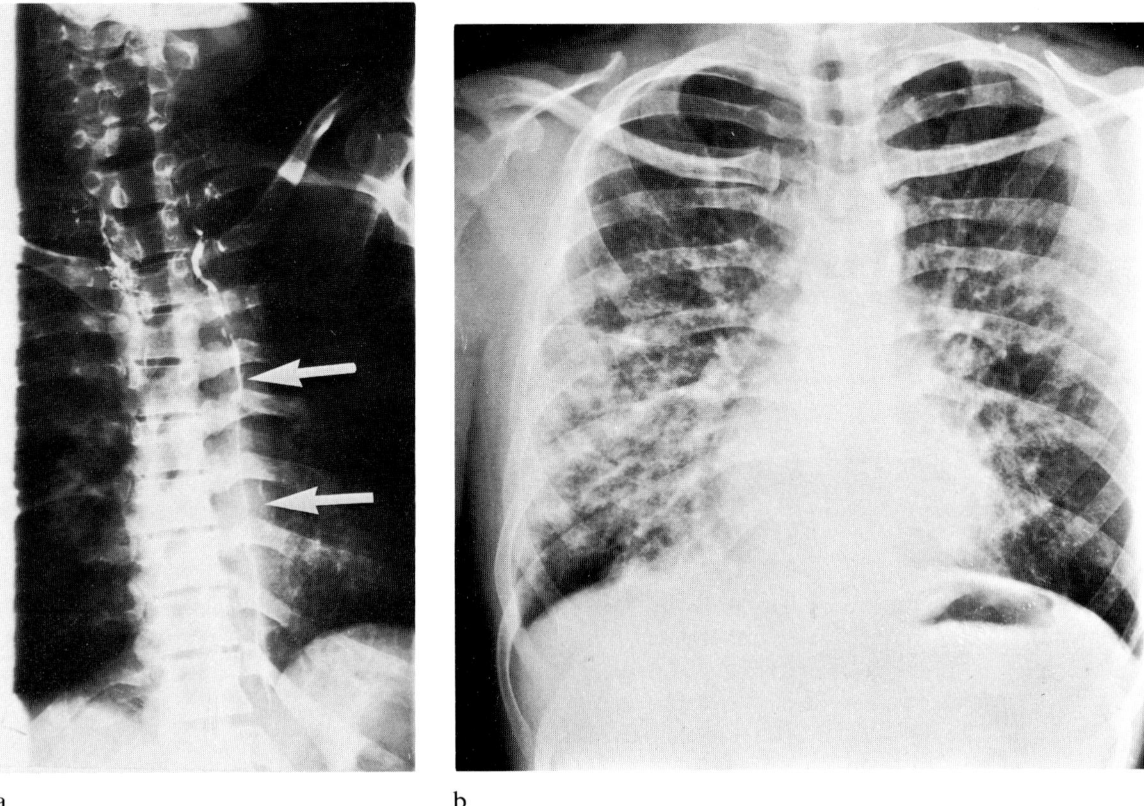

a   b

Fig. 1-8, a and **b. Ethiodol-induced pneumonitis. a** Film from a lymphangiogram shows opacification of the thoracic duct (*arrows*). **b** Chest radiographs became abnormal within 24 hours, and film 8 days after dye administration shows bilateral pneumonitis secondary to a reaction to the contrast agent.

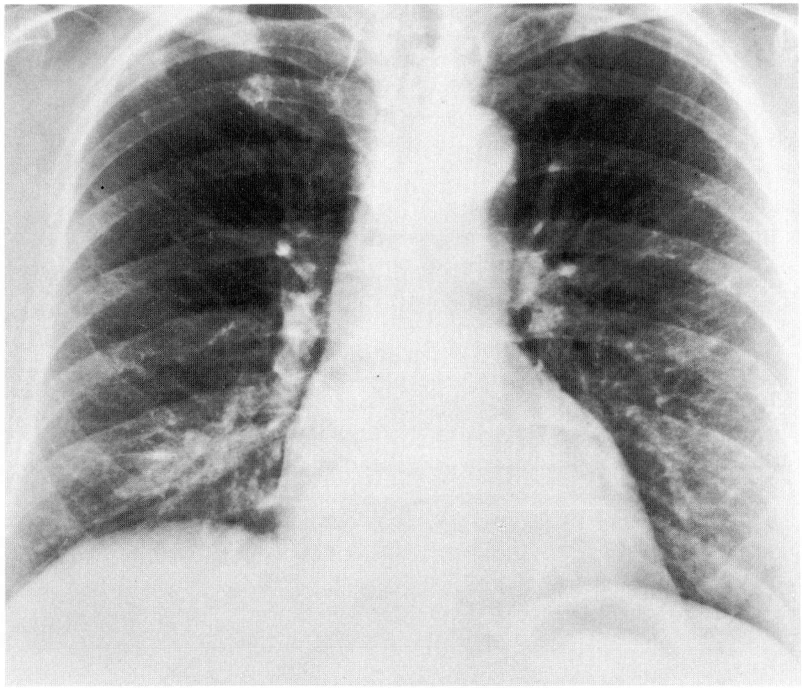

Fig. 1-9. Oil aspiration pneumonia. Development of irregular confluent opacity in right lower lobe after chronic use of mineral oil.

Table 1-6. Drugs Suspected of Causing Systemic Vasculitis That May Involve the
Lungs

Allopurinol	Diphenhydramine	Phenothiazines
Aminorex	Gold salts	Phenylbutazone/
Arsenicals	Griseofulvin	oxyphenbutazone
Busulfan	Hydantoins	Procainamide
Carbamazepine	Hydralazine	Quinidine
Casein	Indomethacin	Spironolactone
Chloramphenicol	Iodides/bromides/	Sulfonamides
Chlorothiazide	bismuth	Tetracycline/
Chlorpropamide	Isoniazid	chlortracycline
Chlorthalidone	Mercurials	Thiouracil
Colchicine	Methyldopa	Trimethadione
Cromolyn sodium	Penicillin/	
DDT	ampicillin	
Dextran		

Adapted from Davies (10)

hemorrhage in the adjacent lung parenchyma (Fig. 1-3d). Type III (immune complex) or type IV (cell-mediated) immune reactions may be responsible. Radiologically, it may present as an acute airspace or interstitial process.

Aminorex (2-amino-5-phenyloxazoline) has been linked to "primary" pulmonary hypertension in Europe, where it was widely used as an anorexic (112). Following administration of the drug, patients developed dyspnea and evidence of right heart failure. The pathomechanism is apparently vasoconstriction of the pulmonary vasculature. Most patients recovered following discontinuation of aminorex. The chest radiograph reveals right ventricular hypertrophy and large central pulmonary arteries. Chemically related substances such as monocrotaline can experimentally produce pulmonary hypertension in animals, and it is possible that cases of pulmonary hypertension considered to be idiopathic are actually produced by drugs or dietary substances.

Drug addicts can develop pulmonary vasculitis and pulmonary hypertension from embolization of the contaminants of street drugs or following intravenous administration of oral agents (64). Pathologically, different kinds of microcrystalline material including talc, starch, and cellulose may be seen. Septic pulmonary emboli may be present. Cor pulmonale will develop only rarely.

Lupus-like Syndrome

Numerous drugs have been associated with drug-induced systemic lupus erythematosus (SLE) (Table 1-7). Both clinically and pathologically it is similar to natural lupus (113,114). The mechanism whereby lupus is induced is uncertain but may be related to genetic abnormalities of drug metabolism (115). Radiologic findings are similar to natural lupus and include pleural and pericardial effusions, confluent pulmonary opacities which may represent a pneumonic process, and local edema. It often will respond to glucocorticoid treatment.

Table 1-7. Drugs That May Induce Systemic Lupus
Erythematosus

Carbamazepine	Penicillamine
Digitalis	Penicillin
Ethosuximide	Phenylbutazone
Gold	Phenytoin
Griseofulvin	Procainamide
Guanoxan	Streptomycin
Hydralazine	Sulfonamide
Isoniazid	Tetracycline
Methyldopa	Thiazides
Oral contraceptives	Thiouracil
Para-aminosalicylic acid	Trimethadione

Adapted from Davies (10)

Lung Injury Secondary to Drug-induced Disease in other Organs

Lungs may be involved secondarily by hemorrhage, embolization, infarction, and depression of respiration.

Diffuse Pulmonary Bleeding

Anticoagulants or similar drugs which interfere with the normal clotting mechanism or damage the microvasculature may induce pulmonary hemorrhage. Radiologically, a disseminated airspace process is seen. After several days, if there is no recurrent hemorrhage, the blood in the airspaces will be phagocytized by macrophages and cleared into the interstitium, resulting in a linear, reticular interstitial pattern. The lungs will clear in 10–14 days; however, interstitial fibrosis may develop after repeated bleeding episodes.

Pulmonary Embolism and Infarction

This complication may be associated with the use of estrogens or oral contraceptives. Emboli usually originate from the lower extremities or pelvis (116). Thromboembolic complications may occur from intravascular catheters. Contaminants of illicit drugs can also embolize. Following lymphography, stippling of the lung space is commonly seen, due to the deposition of oil droplets in the pulmonary vascular bed.

Respiratory Depression

Patients taking sedatives, hypnotics, narcotics, analgesics, and various other drugs will have both respiratory depression and loss of reflexes that help protect the airways. These patients are at risk to develop aspiration pneumonia.

Intrathoracic Extrapulmonary Abnormalities

Lymph Node Enlargement

Commonly prescribed anticonvulsant drugs such as hydantoins, especially diphenylhydantoin (Dilantin), can produce various hypersensitivity reactions (117). The clinical symptoms include fever, fatigue, rash, gingival hypertrophy, conjunctivitis, hepatosplenomegaly, lymphadenopathy, and eosinophilia. The generalized lymphadenopathy is usually manifest within weeks after the start of the therapy and regresses following discontinuation of the drug. Histologically, there is diffuse effacement of the nodal architecture with proliferation of immunoblasts, small lymphocytes, plasma cells, and eosinophils. At times the histology may be confused with Hodgkin's disease (118). There are case reports indicating malignant lymphoma developing in patients treated with diphenylhydantoin (119). Mediastinal lymphadenopathy following diphenylhydantoin administration also has been reported (120). In addition to lymph node enlargement, diphenylhydantoin may also produce acute pulmonary toxicity (121). In one case, the chest radiograph revealed diffuse reticulonodular opacities throughout both lung fields, which cleared following discontinuation of the therapy.

The long-term effects of diphenylhydantoin administration are not well documented (122). One report indicates reduced diffusing capacity and abnormal blood gas values in 45% of the subjects. Radiologically, accentuated bronchovascular markings and diffuse pulmonary fibrosis were reported in 27 of the 31 patients who have received the drug more than two years (123). A different report, however, found no evidence of radiographic abnormalities in a larger group of patients treated over two years (124). In a third report (125), accentuated lung markings were found only rarely.

Mediastinal Fat Accumulation

Long-term administration of corticosteroids can lead to fat deposition in the mediastinum (126–128). The chest radiograph shows mediastinal widening. Computed tomography, however, will reveal that the widened mediastinum is due to low-attenuation substance (fat) and therefore is diagnostic (Fig. 1-10).

Polyserositis

Dantrolene was reported to be associated with chronic pleural effusion, pericarditis, and eosinophilia without any primary lung involvement (129). We have observed a case of isoniazid-induced pericarditis (Fig. 1-11).

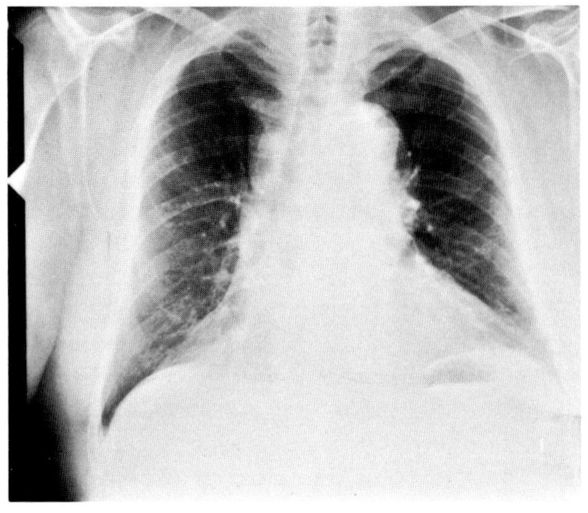

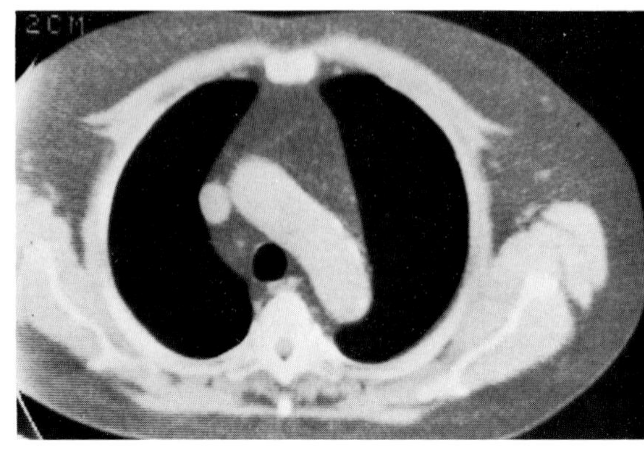

a   b

Fig. 1-10, a and **b. Steroid-induced mediastinal lipomatosis. a** Frontal chest radiograph demonstrating diffuse mediastinal widening. **b** CT scan demonstrating that the mediastinal widening is due to fat infiltration. (Courtesy of Dr. Robert Pugatch, Boston VA Medical Center, Tufts University School of Medicine)

Radiologic Patterns

It is apparent from this review that numerous drugs are associated with iatrogenic thoracic complications, which in turn may lead to an abnormal chest radiograph. Chest x-ray abnormalities in any patient who is receiving drugs may represent a drug reaction. Such abnormalities should be viewed with increased suspicion in the presence of clinical clues such as anaphylactic reaction, asthma, skin rash, or eosinophilia.

Since pulmonary drug reactions reflect various etiologies, pathomechanisms, and histopathologic manifestations, the radiologic findings are nonspecific. Even among commonly prescribed drugs, the x-ray findings of drug-induced reactions are incompletely documented and often based on limited experience. There have been efforts to classify the radiologic characteristics of pulmonary drug reactions into several categories (9,130) including Table 1-8.

1. *Acute, diffuse alveolar pattern.* Among the commonly prescribed drugs, cancer chemotherapeutic agents, anticoagulants and respiratory depressants may be responsible. The pathologic changes associated with this pattern are diffuse alveolar damage, PIE, pulmonary edema, vasculitis, hemorrhage, pneumonitis, and infarction.

2. *Acute, diffuse interstitial pattern.* This is seen with narcotics, antibiotics, certain cancer chemotherapeutic agents, and sulfa drugs. The pathologic findings represent pulmonary edema, interstitial pneumonitis, vasculitis, and similar interstitial processes.

3. *Chronic interstitial opacities.* These represent interstitial pneumonitis or fibrosis and are seen following oxygen toxicity, the use of antibiotics, cancer chemotherapeutic agents, and mineral oil.

4. *Pleuropulmonary pattern.* Drug-induced lupus and pulmonary drug reactions associated with fleeting airspace processes and pleural effusions fall into this pattern.

5. *Lymph node enlargement.* Enlarged lymph nodes may be produced by anticonvulsants.

The radiologist plays a central role in the recognition of pulmonary complications by drugs.

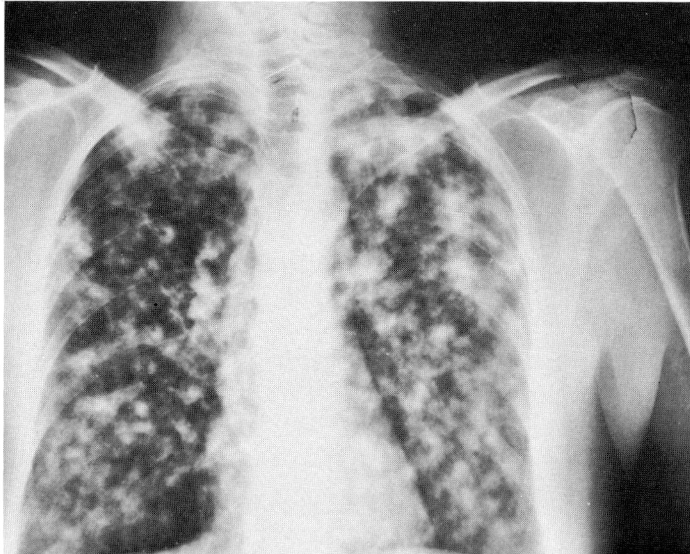

a

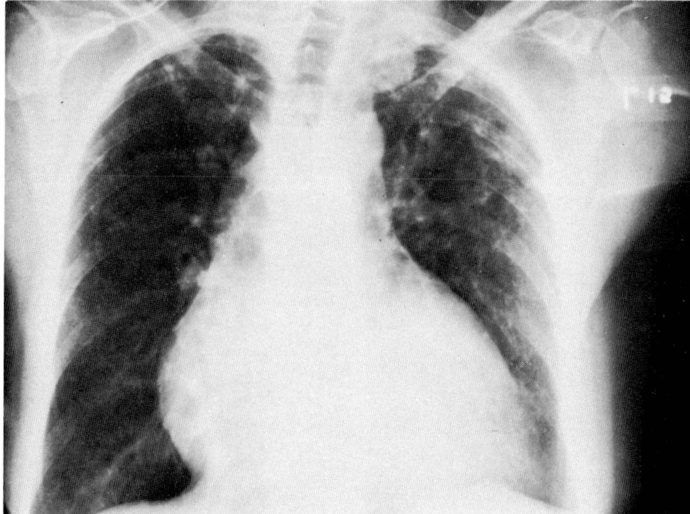

b

Fig. 1-11, a and **b. Isoniazid pericarditis. a** Chest radiograph shows patchy parenchymal densities secondary to disseminated tuberculosis. **b** Eight months later, the lungs have cleared, but a pericardial effusion has developed. (Courtesy of Dr. John Forrest, University of California, San Diego)

Table 1-8. Summary of Roentgenographic Manifestations of Drug Reactions in the Lungs

Acute Reactions

A. Confluent Opacities

Anticoagulants
Chemotherapy group[1]
Ganglionic blockers
Heroin group[2]
Mineral oil
Nitrofurantoin (acute)
Oral contraceptives
Oxygen
Para-aminosalicylic acid
Penicillin
Respiratory depressants
Sulfonamides

Other drugs in this group include those that cause

1. Pulmonary edema (*see* Table 1-4)
2. Diffuse parenchymal injury (*see* Table 1-3)
3. Pulmonary infiltrates with eosinophilia (*see* Table 1-5)
4. Vasculitis (*see* Table 6)
5. Lupus erythematosus (*see* Table 1-7)

B. Linear Opacities

Chemotherapy group[1]
Ganglionic blockers
Heroin group[2]
Methotrexate
Nitrofurantoin (acute)
Oxygen
Penicillin
Pituitary snuff
Sulfonamides

Other drugs in this group include those that cause

1. Diffuse parenchymal injury
2. Vasculitis (*see* Table 1-6)

C. Pleural Effusion

Dantrolene
Methotrexate
Methysergide
Nitrofurantoin
Penicillin
Sulfonamides

Other drugs in this group include those that cause

1. Lupus erythematosus (*see* Table 1-7)

D. Pulmonary Edema

Drugs in this group include those that cause
1. Acute Pulmonary Edema (see Table 1-4)

Chronic Reactions

A. Linear and Nodular Opacities

Chemotherapy group[1] (late)
Ganglionic blockers
Methysergide
Mineral oil
Nitrofurantoin (chronic)

Other drugs in this group include those that cause:

1. Diffuse parenchymal injury (*see* Table 1-3)
2. Granulomatous reactions (*see* Table 1-1)
3. Pulmonary vascular injury (*see* Table 1-6)

Table 1-8. (cont.)

B. Lymph Node Enlargement

  Diphenylhydantoin

C. Mediastinal Enlargement

  Steroids

[1] Chemotherapy group includes alkylating agents, bleomycin, methotrexate, nitrosoureas, procarbazine, and other cytotoxic agents.

[2] Heroin group includes heroin, methadone, propoxyphene.

Acknowledgments

We are grateful to Ms. Nancy Harrison for her help in preparation of the manuscript and Stephen Schroeder for the illustrations.

References

1. Editorial: Disease drugs cause. N Engl J Med 279:1286–1287, 1968.
2. De Swarte RD: Drug alergy. *In* Patterson R (ed): Allergic Diseases, Diagnosis and Management. Philadelphia: JB Lippincott, 1972, pp 393–493.
3. Rosenow EC: The spectrum of drug-induced pulmonary disease. Ann Intern Med 77:977–991, 1972.
4. Parker CW: Drug allergy. N Engl J Med 292:511–514, 732–736, 957–960, 1975.
5. Lakin JD: Hypersensitivity reactions. *In* Patterson R (ed): Allergic Diseases, Diagnosis and Management. Philadelphia: JB Lippincott, 1972, pp 1–30.
6. Ochsner SF, Hatch HB, Leonard GL: Hypersensitivity and the lung. AJR 107:390–399, 1969.
7. Ansell G: Radiological manifestations of drug-induced disease. Clin Radiol 20:133–148, 1969.
8. Brettner A, Heitzman ER, Woodin WG: Pulmonary complications of drug therapy. Radiology 96:31–38, 1970.
9. Heitzman ER: The Lung: Radiologic-Pathologic Correlation. St Louis: CV Mosby, 1973, pp 219–231.
10. Davies PDB: Drug induced lung disease. Br J Dis Chest 63:57–70, 1969.
11. De Weck AL: Drug reactions. *In* Samter M (ed): Immunological Diseases. Boston: Little Brown, 1971, pp 415–430.
12. Simon G: Type I immunologic reactions in the lung. Semin Roentgenol 10:21–31, 1975.
13. Freedman PJ: Idiopathic and auto-immune type III-like reactions: interstitial fibrosis, vasculitis and granulomatosis. Semin Roentgenol 10:43–52, 1975.
14. Samter M, Beers RF: Intolerance to aspirin: clinical studies and consideration of its pathogenesis. Ann Intern Med 68:975–983, 1968.
15. Shand DG: Propranolol, N Engl J Med 283:280, 1975.
16. Koelle GB: Anticholinesterase agents and parasympathomimetic agents. *In* Goodman LS, Gilman A (eds): The Pharmacological Basic of Therapeutics. New York: Macmillan, 1975, pp 454–470.
17. Szczekli A, Gryglewski RJ: Prostaglandins and aspirin-sensitive asthma. Am Rev Respir Dis 118:799–800, 1978.
18. Nash G, Blennerhassett JB, Pontoppidan H, et al: Pulmonary lesions associated with oxygen therapy and artificial ventilation. N Engl J Med 276:368–374, 1967.
19. Senior RM, Wessler S, Avioli LV: Pulmonary oxygen toxicity. JAMA 217:1373–1377, 1971.
20. Crapo JD, Peters-Golden M, Marsh-Salin J, Shelburne JS: Pathologic changes in the lungs of oxygen-adapted rats—a morphometric analysis. Lab Invest 39:640, 1978.
21. Stahlman MT: Clinical description of bronchopulmonary dysplasia. J Pediatr 95:829, 1979.
22. Reid L: Bronchopulmonary dysplasia-pathology. J Pediatr 95:823, 1979.
23. Edwards DK: Radiographic aspects of bronchopulmonary dysplasia. J Pediatr 95:829, 1979.
24. Kaufman SK, Nash G: Case records of the Massachusetts General Hospital. N Engl J Med 290:390–396, 1974.
25. Pascual RS, Mosher MB, Sikand RS, et al: Effects of bleomycin on pulmonary function in man. Am Rev Respir Dis 108:211–217, 1973.
26. Yagoda A, Mukherji B, Young C, et al: Bleomycin, an anti-tumor antibiotic. Ann Intern Med 77:861–870, 1972.
27. Rudders RA: Bleomysin: pulmonary toxicity. Ann Intern Med 78:618, 1973.
28. Iacovino JR, Leitner J, Abbas AK, et al: Fatal pulmonary reaction from low doses of bleomycin. JAMA 235:1253–1255, 1976.
29. Samuels ML, Johnson DE, Holoye PY, et al: Large dose bleomycin therapy and pulmonary toxicity. JAMA 235:1117–1120, 1976.
30. Goldiner PL, Carlon GC, Cvitkovic E, et al: Factors influencing postoperative morbidity and mortality in patients treated with bleomycin. Br Med J 1:1664, 1978.
31. De Lena M, Guzzon A, Monfardini S, et al: Clinical radiologic and histopathologic studies on pulmonary toxicity induced by treatment with bleomycin. Cancer Treat Rep (Part 1) 56:343–355, 1972.
32. Richman SD, Levenson SM, Bunn PA, et al: [67]Ga accumulation in pulmonary lesions associated with

bleomycin toxicity. Cancer 36:1966–1972, 1975.

33. Podoll LN, Winkler SS: Busulfan lung. AJR 120:151–156, 1974.

34. Soble AR, Perry H: Fatal radiation pneumonia following subclinical busulfan injury. AJR 128:15–18, 1977.

35. Patel AR, Shah PC, Rhee HL, Sasson H, Rao KP: Cyclophosphamide therapy and interstitial pulmonary fibrosis. Cancer 38:1542, 1976.

36. Cole SR, Myers TJ, Klatsky AV: Pulmonary disease with chlorambucil therapy. Cancer 41:455, 1978.

37. Taetle R, Dickman PS, Feldman PS: Pulmonary histopathologic changes associated with melphelan therapy. Cancer 42:1239, 1978.

38. Rodin AE, Haggard ME, Travis LB: Lung changes and chemotherapeutic agents in childhood. Am J Dis Child 120:337–340, 1970.

39. Kuplic JB, Higley CS, Niewoehner DE: Pulmonary ossification associated with long term busulfan therapy in chronic myeloid leukemia. Case report. Am Rev Respir Dis 106:759–769, 1972.

40. Stott H, Stephens R, Fox W, Vimon G, Roy DC: An investigation of the chest radiographs in a controlled trial of busulfan, cyclophosphamide, and a placebo after resection for carcinoma of the lung. Thorax 31:265–270, 1976.

41. Sostman HD, Matthay RA, Putman CE, Smith CJW: Methotrexate induced pneumonitis. Medicine (Baltimore) 55:371, 1976.

42. Gutin PH, Green MR, Bleyer WA, Bauer VL, Wiernik PH, Walker MD: Methotrexate pneumonitis induced by intrathecal methotrexate therapy. Cancer 38:1529, 1976.

43. Everts CS, Westcott JL, Bragg DG: Methotrexate therapy and pulmonary disease. Radiology 107:539–543, 1973.

44. Weiss RB, Muggia FM: Cytotoxic drug-induced pulmonary disease: update 1980. Am J Med 68:259, 1980.

45. Aronin PA, Mahaley MS Jr, Rudnick SA, Dudka L, Donohue JF, Selker RG, Moore P: Prediction of BCNU pulmonary toxicity in patients with malignant gliomas. N Engl J Med 303:183–188, 1980.

46. Farney RJ, Morris AH, Armstrong JD Jr, Hammer S: Diffuse pulmonary disease after therapy with nitrogen mustard, vincristine, procarbazine, and prednisone. Am Rev Respir Dis 115:135, 1977.

47. Ecker MD, Jay B, Keohane MF: Procarbazine lung. AJR 131:527–528, 1978.

48. Seltzer SE, Griffin T, D'Orsi C, Tryka F, Herman PG: Pulmonary reaction associated with neocarzinostatin (NCS) therapy. Cancer Treat Rep 62:1270–1271, 1978.

49. Willson JKV: Pulmonary toxicity of antineoplastic drugs. Cancer Treat Rep 62:2003–2008, 1978.

50. Rokseth R, Storstein O: Pulmonary complications during mecamylamine therapy. Acta Med Scand 167:23, 1960.

51. Heard BE: Fibrous healing of old iatrogenic pulmonary edema (hexamethonium lung). J Pathol 83:159, 1962.

52. Perry HM Jr, O'Neal RM, Thomas WA: Pulmonary disease following chronic chemical ganglionic blockade. Am J Med 22:37, 1957.

53. Graham JR, Suby HI, LeCompte PR, et al: Fibrotic disorders associated with methysergide therapy for headache. N Engl J Med 274:259–268, 1966.

54. Hinde W, Posner E, Sweetnam MT, et al: Pleural effusion and fibrosis during treatment with methysergide. Br Med J 1:605–606, 1970.

55. Morrison WJ, Wetherill S, Zyroff J: The acute pulmonary edema of heroin intoxication. Radiology 97:347–351, 1970.

56. Saba GP, James AE, Johnson BA, et al: Pulmonary complications of narcotic abuse. AJR 122:740–743, 1974.

57. Steinberg AD, Karliner JS: The clinical spectrum of heroin pulmonary edema. Arch Intern Med 122:122–127, 1968.

58. Duberstein JC, Kaufman DM: A clinical study of an epidemic of heroin intoxication and heroin induced pulmonary edema. Am J Med 51:704–714, 1971.

59. Zyroff J, Slovis TL, Nagler J: Pulmonary edema induced by oral methadone. Radiology 112:567–568, 1974.

60. Wilen SB, Ulreich S, Rabinowitz JG: Roentgenographic manifestations of methadone induced pulmonary edema. Radiology 114:51–55, 1975.

61. Bogartz J, Miller WC: Pulmonary edema associated with propoxyphene intoxication. JAMA 215:259–262, 1971.

62. Yound DJ: Propoxyphene suicides: report of nine cases. Arch Intern Med 129:62–66, 1972.

63. Halpern M, Citron BP: Necrotizing angitis associated with drug abuse. AJR 111:663–671, 1971.

64. Tomoshefski JF, Hirsch CS: The pulmonary vascular lesions of intravenous drug abuse. Hum Pathol 11:133, 1980.

65. Szwed JJ: Pulmonary angiothrombosis caused by "blue velvet" addiction. Ann Intern Med 73:771–774, 1970.

66. Douglas FG, Kafilmont KJ, Patt NL: Foreign particle embolism in drug addicts: respiratory pathophysiology. Ann Intern Med 75:865–872, 1971.

67. Richman S, Harris RD: Acute pulmonary edema associated with Librium abuse. Radiology 103:57–58, 1972.

68. Bledsoe FH, Seymour EQ: Acute pulmonary edema associated with parathion poisoning. Radiology 103:53–56, 1972.

69. Steinberg AD: Pulmonary edema following ingestion of hydrochlorothiazide. JAMA 204:825–827, 1968.

70. Broderick TW, Reinke RT, Goldman E: Salicylate-induced pulmonary edema. AJR 127:865–866, 1976.

71. Marshall A, Moore K: Pulmonary disease after amitriptyline overdosage. Br Med J 1:716–717, 1973.

72. Greganti MA, Flowers WM: Acute pulmonary edema after intravenous administration of contrast media. Radiology 132:583–585, 1979.

73. Lascari AD, Strano AJ, Johnson WW, Collins

JGP: Methotrexate induced sudden fatal pulmonary reaction. Cancer 40:1393, 1977.

74. Haupt JM, Hutchins GM, Moore GW: ARA-C lung: alveolar-capillary leak complicating cytosine arabinoside therapy of leukemia. Lab Invest 42:26, 1980.

75. Ward HN: Pulmonary infiltrates associated with leukoagglutinin transfusion reactions. Ann Intern Med 73:689–694, 1970.

76. Wright DG, Robichard KJ, Pizzo PA, Deisseroth AB: Lethal pulmonary reactions associated with the combined use of amphotericin B and leukocyte transfusions. N Engl J Med 304:1185–1189, 1981.

77. Eltringham JR, Fajardo LF, Stewart R: Adriamycin cardiomyopathy: enhanced cardiac damage in rabbits with combined drug and cardiac irradiation. Radiology 115:471–472, 1975.

78. Mills BA, Roberts RW: Cyclophosphamide-induced cardiomyopathy: a report of two cases and review of the English literature. Cancer 43:2223, 1979.

79. Raskin MM, Rajurkar MG, Altman DH: Daunomycin cardiac toxicity. AJR 118:68–71, 1973.

80. Calabresi P, Parks RE: Alkylating agents, antimetabolites, hormones, and other antiproliferative agents. *In* Goodman LS, Gilman A (eds): The Pharmacological Basis of Therapeutics. New York: Macmillan, 1975, p 1291.

81. Donlan CJ, Scutero JV: Transient eosinophilic pneumonia secondary to use of a vaginal cream. Chest 67:232, 1975.

82. Kilburn KH: Pulmonary disease induced by drugs. *In* Fishman AP (ed): Pulmonary Diseases and Disorders. New York: McGraw-Hill, 1979, p 717.

83. Ellis RV, McKenzie CA: Allergic pneumonia. J Lab Clin Med 26:1427–1432, 1941.

84. Fiegenberg HW, Weiss H, Kushman H: Migratory pneumonia with eosinophilia associated with sulphonamide administration. Arch Intern Med 120:85–92, 1967.

85. Klinghoffer JF: Loeffler's syndrome following use of vaginal cream. Ann Intern Med 40:343–350, 1954.

86. Riechlin S, Loveless MH, Kane EG: Loeffler's syndrome following penicillin therapy. Ann Intern Med 38:113–120, 1953.

87. Simpson DG, Walker JA: Hypersensitivity to paraaminosalicylic acid. Am J Med 29:297–306, 1960.

88. Hailey FJ, Glascock HW, Hewitt WF: Pleuropneumonic reactions to nitrofurantoin. N Engl J Med 281:1087–1090, 1969.

89. Ngan BH, Millard RJ, Lant AE, et al: Nitrofurantoin lung. Br J Radiol 44:21–23, 1971.

90. Risk AA: Brief recording: anaphylactoid reaction to nitrofurantoin. N Engl J Med 245:1054, 1957.

91. Murray MH, Kronenberg P: Pulmonary reaction simulating cardiac pulmonary edema caused by nitrofurantoin. N Engl J Med 273:1185–1187, 1965.

92. Israel HL, Diamont P: Recurrent pulmonary infiltration and pleural effusion due to nitrofurantoin sensitivity. N Engl J Med 266:1024–1026, 1962.

93. Bayer WL, Dawson RB, Kotin E: Allergic tracheobronchitis due to nitrofurantoin sensitivity. Dis Chest 48:429–430, 1965.

94. Wilson ES, McCarty RJ: Nitrofurantoin pneumonia. AJR 103:540–542, 1968.

95. Glueck MA, Janower ML: Nitrofurantoin lung disease. AJR 107:818–822, 1969.

96. Allen RW, Holt AH, Brown MG: Acute pulmonary sensitivity to nitrofurantoin. AJR 104:784–785, 1968.

97. Krush ED, Mostyn EM, Persky L: Nitrofurantoin pulmonary complications. J Urol 113:392–395, 1975.

98. Carrington CB, Addington WW, Goff AM, Madoff IM, Marks A, Schwaber JR, Gaensler EA: Chronic eosinophilic pneumonia. N Engl J Med 280:787, 1969.

99. Rosenow EC, De Remee RA, Dinen DW: Chronic nitrofurantoin pulmonary reaction. N Engl J Med 279:1258–1262, 1968.

100. Cortez LM, Pankey GA: Acute pulmonary sensitivity to furazolidone. Am Rev Respir Dis 105:823–826, 1972.

101. Bone RC, Wolfe J, Sobonya RE, Kerby GR, Strechschulte D, Ruth WE, Welch M: Desquamative interstitial pneumonitis following chronic nitrofurantoin therapy. Chest 69:296–297, 1976.

102. Felton WL II: The reaction of pulmonary tissue to Lipiodol. J Thorac Surg 25:530, 1953.

103. Smith TR, Frater R, Spataro J: Delayed granuloma following bronchography. Chest 64:122, 1973.

104. Fraimow W, Wallace S, Lewis P, Greening RR, Cathcart RT: Changes in pulmonary function due to lymphangiography. Radiology 85:231, 1965.

105. Weill H, Ferrans VJ, Gay RM, et al: Early lipoid pneumonia: roentgenologic, anatomic, and physiologic characteristics. Am J Med 36:370–376, 1964.

106. Pepys J, Jenkins PA, Lackman PJ, et al: An iatrogenic auto antibody immunological response to pituitary snuff in patients with diabetes insipidus. Clin Exp Immunol 1:377–389, 1966.

107. Harper LO, Burrell RG, Lapp NL, et al: Allergic alveolitis due to pituitary snuff. Ann Intern Med 73:581–584, 1970.

108. McCoombs RP, Patterson JF, MacMahon HE: Syndromes associated with allergic vasculitis. N Engl J Med 255:251–261, 1956.

109. Symmers WS: The occurrence of angiitis and of other generalized diseases of connective tissues as consequence of administration of drugs. Proc R Soc Med 55:20–28, 1962.

110. Mullick FG, McAllister HA Jr, Wagner BM, Fenoglio JJ: Drug related vasculitis, clinicopathologic correlations in 30 patients. Hum Pathol 10:313–325, 1979.

111. Churg J, Strauss L: Allergic granulomatosis, allergic angiitis and periarteritis nodosa. Am J Pathol 27:277, 1951.

112. Gurtner HP: Pulmonary hypertension produced by the ingestion of substances. Bull Physio-Pathol Resp 5:435, 1969.

113. Auerbach RC, Snyder NE, Bragg DG: The chest

roentgenographic manifestations of pronestyl-induced lupus erythematosus. Radiology 109:287–290, 1973.

114. Alarcon-Segovia D: Drug-induced lupus syndrome. Mayo Clin Proc 44:664–681, 1969.

115. Woosley RL, Drayer DE, Reidenberg MM, Nies AS, Carr K, Oates JA: Effect of acetylator phenotype on the rate at which procainamide induces antinuclear antibodies and the lupus syndrome. N Engl J Med 298:1157, 1978.

116. Brodelius A, Lorinc P, Nylander G: Localization of acute deep venous thrombosis in women taking oral contraceptives. Radiology 101:297–300, 1971.

117. Sparberg M: Diagnostically confusing complications of diphenylhydantoin therapy. Ann Intern Med 59:914–930, 1963.

118. Saltzstein SL, Ackerman LV: Lymphadenopathy induced by anticonvulsant drugs and mimicking clinically and pathologically the malignant lymphomas. Cancer 12:164–182, 1959.

119. Dorfman RF, Warnke R: Lymphadenopathy stimulating the malignant lymphomas. Hum Pathol 5:519, 1974.

120. Heitzman ER: Lymphadenopathy related to anticonvulsant therapy. Radiology 89:311–312, 1967.

121. Bayer AS, Targan SR, Pitchon HE, et al: Dilantin toxicity: miliary pulmonary infiltrates and hypoxemia. Ann Intern Med 85:475–476, 1976.

122. Hazlett DR, Ward GW, Madison DS: Pulmonary function loss in diphenylhydantoin therapy. Chest 66:660–664, 1974.

123. Moore MT: Pulmonary changes in hydantoin therapy. JAMA 171:1328–1333, 1959.

124. Low NL, Yahr MD: The lack of pulmonary fibrosis in patients receiving diphenylhydantoin. JAMA 174:1201–1202, 1960.

125. Livingston S, Whitehouse D, Panci LL: Study of the effects of diphenylhydantoin sodium on the lungs. N Engl J Med 264:648–651, 1961.

126. Teates CD: Steroid-induced mediastinal lipomatosis. Radiology 96:501–502, 1970.

127. Koerner HJ, Sun DI: Mediastinal lipomatosis secondary to steroid therapy. AJR 98:461–464, 1966.

128. Bodman SF, Condemi JJ: Mediastinal widening in iatrogenic Cushing's syndrome. Ann Intern Med 67:399–403, 1967.

129. Petusevsky ML, Faling LF, Rocklin RG, et al: Pleuropericardial reaction to treatment with Dantrolene. JAMA 242:2772–2774, 1979.

130. Morrison DA, Goldman AL: Radiographic patterns of drug-induced lung disease. Radiology 131:299–304, 1979.

131. Seltzer SE, Herman PG: Drug-induced pulmonary reactions associated with abnormal chest radiograph. J Contin Educ Radiol 1:25–42, 1979.

2 Nosocomial and Iatrogenic Infections of the Thorax

Cyrus C. Hopkins

Hospital-acquired infections of the lower respiratory tract are a major cause of mortality and morbidity. Many of these infections result from invasive techniques, especially respiratory assistance and to lesser degrees surgery and diagnostic procedures. All forms of invasive diagnostic or therapeutic intervention carry with them at least some risk of infection. The patterns of clinical presentation are not diagnostic, although some organisms and some modes of spread may cause distinctive manifestations. Though the potential range of pathogenic microorganisms is large, certain organisms are more common in specific settings. The clinical and especially the radiologic manifestations are affected by both the setting and the organism. Accordingly, one must consider the ecology, the pathogenesis, and the clinical manifestations of specific bacterial etiologies.

Incidence and Significance

Lower respiratory tract infections are the third most frequent among all nosocomial (hospital-acquired) infections, representing nationwide an overall estimated risk of about 5/1000 patients, as reported by the National Nosocomial Infection Study (1). However, this grossly underestimates the significance of such infections, and seems inappropriately low for many hospitals; the risk is variable and increases (as does the overall nosocomial infection rate) in referral hospitals.

General medical and surgical services provide the populations at highest risk. The risk is particularly prominent in intensive care units, where rates from 9% to 32% have been described following prolonged stays (2,3). This risk is not simply one of intensive care, geography, or crowding, but may be related to the nature of the underlying illness and the concomitant use, in these areas, of respiratory assistance or other invasive techniques (discussed later).

Furthermore, the medical, social, and economic importance of nosocomial pneumonia is far greater than the reported incidence would suggest; the rate of secondary bacteremia can be as high as 20% (2), and mortality is high. This ominous disease is observed in both university and community hospitals. In one study, more than half the deaths of hospitalized patients in both kinds of institution were felt to have been contributed to or caused by nosocomial infection (4), 60% of which were in the lower respiratory tract.

Source

Most hospital-acquired infections result from aspiration of pharyngeal contents. At least one-third will occur *without* the use of intubation or any respiratory assistance (5). However, if any tube is used to transgress the local defenses of the upper respiratory tract, the risk of acquiring infection increases. Such tubes provide two routes by which potentially pathogenic bacteria can reach the ordinarily sterile lower respiratory tract: via pharyngeal (or wound) secretions carried downward around the tube, and via contaminated fluids (usually in humidified air) infused through the lumen of the tube. Furthermore, some invasive techniques, such as bronchoscopy, can introduce upper airway flora into the lower respiratory tract and can also impair deeper bronchopulmonary host defenses, providing a site of decreased resistance to infection. Inadequately sterilized equipment may also introduce exogenous flora into the bronchi, and pathogenic bacteria can be directly implanted in the thorax at operation. Finally, organisms can be disseminated to the lung via a hematogenous route.

Etiology

The majority, perhaps two-thirds, of bacterial pneumonias acquired in the usual endemic hospital setting are caused by aerobic gram-negative bacilli (1) (Table 2-1). Generalizations regarding such numbers are not meaningful, as there is a wide range in reported studies, depending on the definitions used and the specific population at risk (6). In general, the greatest number, of those identified, are gram-negative bacilli of the Enterobacteriaceae. Staphylococci represent only 15% of the total, while *Streptococcus pneumoniae,* the most frequent cause of outpatient bacterial pneumonia, constitutes only 5%. In epidemics, on the other hand, marked changes in these proportions can occur. Deviations from the baseline data obtained

in any single unit or hospital can sometimes serve as important indicators of an epidemic problem, as may unexpectedly high endemic or procedure-associated rates (7).

The organisms isolated from a single case may also provide important clues as to which route might have been involved in the acquisition of the illness. Further consideration of individual routes is therefore appropriate.

Routes and Radiology

Aspiration

Frequency

Aside from invasive procedures or intubation, the most common pathway for lower respiratory infections is aspiration. The clinical problems associated with aspiration of food (8) or of gastric contents (9) are familiar ones and generally beyond the scope of this discussion. In neither case is infection a certain result. When it does occur, it is a result of concomitant aspiration of pharyngeal flora, with the site of infection made more susceptible by the damaging effects of gastric acid or the occlusive effects of particulate matter in food (10). Gross aspiration with coughing, choking, or respiratory distress (with or without a documented "positive" dye test) is not necessary for pharyngeal

Table 2-1. Incidence of Pathogens in Nosocomial Lower Respiratory Tract Infections

Organisms	Percent of Total Infections	Percent of Identified Organisms
Staph. aureus	10.8	15.2
Strep. pneumoniae	3.7	5.2
Klebsiella spp.	10.5	14.8
Pseudomonas aeruginosa	7.2	10.1
E. coli	7.1	10.0
Proteus-Providencia	6.1	8.6
Enterobacter spp.	5.5	7.7
Serratia spp.	2.7	3.8
Pseudomonas, nonaeruginosa	2.0	2.8
Candida spp.	3.5	4.9
(Other identified pathogens)	11.9	16.9
Unidentified pathogens	29.0	
Total	100%	100%

Results of a Nationwide Surveillance (NNIS 1977) (1)

flora to invade the lower respiratory tract. In fact, aspiration has been shown, by a number of techniques, to occur in normal adults during sleep or periods of diminished consciousness (11). Generally these small inocula are well tolerated, and the organisms neither reach the alveoli nor invade the mucosa of the normal tracheobronchial tree; they are swept upward, out of the trachea, by mucociliary defenses. In the presence of factors that decrease the efficacy of these protective mechanisms, such as alcohol or anesthesia, or in the presence of structural disease of the lung, the hazard of these aspirational events becomes much greater. In addition, diminished levels of consciousness may decrease the gag reflex. Aspiration has been documented in 70% of patients in stupor or coma (11). With the decreased respiratory effort of these patients, decreasing the effectiveness of coughing, the hazard of pneumonia is evident.

Following invasive procedures, the risk of aspiration is certainly increased. The use of nasotracheal or orotracheal tubes is not significantly associated with increased risk of frank aspiration, though the risk of infection is higher in these patients than in nonintubated hospitalized patients (5), which may be in part the function of other variables, including nature of illness and the use of anesthesia or other respiratory devices. Tracheostomy markedly increases the incidence of lower respiratory infection. Aspiration of contaminated secretions can come either from the pharynx or from the wound site, and infection of the stoma is quite common, 36% in one study (12). Frequencies of colonization or pneumonia as high as 87% have been reported with long-term care (13,14).

Flora

In the nonhospitalized patient, aspiration of pharyngeal flora will generally result in infection with gram-positive cocci such as *Streptococcus pneumoniae* or other streptococcal species. Pharyngeal flora and secondary infection will often include a large proportion of anaerobic organisms, including *Bacteroides melaninogenicus, Fusobacterium nucleatum,* and mixed gram-positive cocci. In perhaps half these patients, anaerobes may be the only organisms isolated (15).

However, the bacteriologic patterns associated with aspiration in the hospitalized patient include a much greater risk of infection with gram-negative bacilli, espeicaly Enterobacteriaceae. These also arise from the pharyngeal flora. Although found as part of the normal pharyngeal flora in significant numbers in only perhaps 2% of all patients before admission to the hospital, some patients may already be colonized (16) and still more, perhaps up to 20%–35%, promptly become colonized with these organisms, especially with *E. coli* and *Klebsiella* species (17). Some patients may be more susceptible to the acquisition of these organisms for various reasons, including age, debility, and severity and nature of the underlying illnesses (18,19). The association with prior use of broad-spectrum antimicrobial therapy is not clear, though these agents play a role in some cases (20,21). Once found colonizing the respiratory tract, these organisms are correlated with those producing subsequent pneumonias, probably following aspiration (17). Both in hospital and outside, uncommon organisms may occasionally appear in a primary pneumonia, either as a result of aspiration of pharyngeal flora or, especially for some organisms such as *Mycobacterium tuberculosis,* by means of the airborne route.

Clinical Patterns

The radiologic picture of aspirational events varies a great deal, depending on the material aspirated, the timing and source of illness, and the timing of radiographic studies. It should be emphasized, however, that virtually no radiologic or clinical picture is *diagnostic* either of the bacteriology involved or of the route of acquisition. Therefore, diagnostic conservatism and thorough bacteriologic evaluation are required to determine the cause of any pneumonia.

Nonhospital-acquired acute bacterial pneumonias, most commonly associated with pneumococci or streptococci, will produce a classic consolidation of a full lobe or bronchopulmonary segment. Effusion and empyema are now infrequently seen, though they have been reported in up to 15% of patients with pneumococcal pneumonia, and are perhaps more common in streptococcal infection. At some times, such as following influenza epidemics, other organisms, including staphylococci or *Hemophilus* species, may more frequently invade the lung, and will produce a clinical picture consistent with these organisms.

Following aspiration, the clinical picture is heterogeneous (10). Immediately following acute, large-volume aspiration, particularly involving gastric acid, a severely hypoxic, dyspneic clinical state may be associated with widespread areas of apparent infiltrate and with scattered areas of atelectasis in lower lobes or, in the supine patient, in posterior (dependent) portions of the lung. If infection does develop, both the clinical picture and the radiologic patterns will depend largely on the organisms involved, except that there remains a predisposition to the dependent bronchopulmonary segments.

In the most characteristic case of mixed or exclusively anaerobic infection, the development of infection is often insidious or subacute. Patients may not present with consolidation, but with a focal necrotizing process which may either be a lung abscess or empyema, depending on the time and extent of necrosis and probably on the location of the initial nidus.

Gram-negative bacilli cause generally more acute illnesses and provide different radiologic patterns (22,23). Though none of these are diagnostic, there are some weak correlations between radiologic observations and the bacteriologic isolates, such as the relative tendency of *Klebsiella* or *Proteus* pneumonias to produce lobar consolidation more commonly in the upper lobes. *Klebsiella* pneumonia may produce either a swollen lobe with a "bulging fissure" or a loss in volume. Still later, cavitation and abscess formation may occur. With sufficient time and severity, however, many gram-negative infections can progress to abscess and empyema formation. Such focal progression should be distinguished from the tendency of gram-negative bacillary infections associated with other pathogenic routes, such as respiratory apparatus, to provide a more diffuse pattern of necrotizing bronchopneumonia. These must, in turn, be distinguished from widely scattered, often peripheral, necrotizing lesions associated with the hematogenous acquisition of disease.

Staphylococcal infection is more likely to occur either following influenza or in the hospitalized patient particularly in the presence of a tracheostomy. In both cases the more characteristic pattern is a focal necrotizing bronchopneumonia, scattered in dependent segments of the lung. Necrosis may progress to abscess formation or empyema. If necrosis begins to develop within widespread areas of consolidation, small lucent areas surrounded by areas of infiltrate may appear, producing pneumatoceles, which are especially common in children.

Contaminated Fluid

Flora

Contaminated respiratory equipment, fluids, reservoirs, and circuits can also serve as a means of introducing bacteria in large numbers deep into the respiratory tract. Before the significance of this route was appreciated, and before adequate procedural means of dealing with and preventing these infections were developed, some centers were subject to high rates of a highly fatal necrotizing bronchopneumonia, often caused by *Pseudomonas aeruginosa* (24).

Source

The native ecosystem of these organisms is generally *not* the pharynx, and this is not the usual source of acquisition, at least in the setting of the immunocompetent host. Pseudomonads and certain other water-loving organisms have been found predominantly growing on the moist surfaces of the ventilatory circuit, particularly in the reservoir of water used to humidfy the air (24). *Pseudomonas aeruginosa* grows to high concentrations in such fluid systems and, particularly with nebulization of fluids, warmed fluid, or even cold mist vaporizers, can produce aerosols heavily contaminated with bacteria, actinomycetes, or yeast (25). Nebulizers used within the hospital setting can also become contaminated with hydrophilic gram-negative bacilli from the ambient air (26), and can serve as a source of subsequent dissemination of infectious organisms.

Clinical Pattern

The clinical pattern of these infections is that of a widespread, diffuse, rapidly necrotizing bronchopneumonia, progressing quickly to both large and small abscesses. Pneumatocele and pneumothorax may occur, and a wide variety of radiologic patterns can be observed (27).

Hematogenous

Predicted Patterns

The appearance of multiple peripheral pulmonary infiltrates can also result from hematogenous dissemination of an offending organism. These are uncommon in the hospitalized patient, and generally have been described as originating from sources releasing large numbers of organisms, with or without other embolic materials such as talc or thrombus, into the venous (or pulmonary arterial) circuit. The majority of these will appear in outpatients as a result of intravenous drug abuse, right-sided endocarditis (often together), or multiple septic pulmonary emboli, generally from retroperitoneal or pelvic sepsis.

Predisposing Hazards

While most of these settings are not iatrogenic, it should be recognized that bacteremia, especially with staphylococci, may occur as the result of a contaminated intravenous cannula. Some of these cases will result in septic phlebitis or seeding of the right side of the heart, and provide the potential for establishing the cycle of sepsis and pulmonary infiltrates (28). Preliminary data regarding colonization of both venous and pulmonary arterial catheters increase the concern about this hazard, which can occur with any such catheter.

Direct Introduction

The occurrence of thoracic infections following an operation will vary depending upon the type of surgery; but in clean thoracic wounds, the wound infection rate is reported as less than 5%, depending on case definitions and how carefully such complications are sought for and documented (29).

The patterns found clinically represent a large variety of conditions, depending upon the anatomic site of infection, and most often present as superficial wound infection with abscess or cellulitis. Deeper infections, such as empyema in the pleural operative site or mediastinitis in a sternum-splitting procedure, occur in less than 1% of cases, and are generally beyond the scope of this discussion. These have been reviewed elsewhere (29). Briefly, however, it should be recognized that the sources of the bacteria again correlate with the organisms found, while the clinical picture reflects the site of inoculation. Most of such intraoperative infections originate in the operative incision and field with *Staphylococcus aureus* and enteric gram-negative rods providing the predominant flora. Contaminated procedures become infected with the adjacent flora. Therefore, many organisms may gain access to the pleural space from the tracheobronchial tree, particularly following an incision across colonized tracheal or bronchial mucosa.

The wide variety of postoperative pulmonary changes following thoracic surgery, including atelectasis and fluid accumulation, have been recently reviewed elsewhere (30).

Complications of Specific Procedures

Relative Risks

Three serious methodologic flaws limit the ability of a reviewer to compare the relative risks of various procedures, and direct comparison of usually cited rates is inappropriate. First, several risks are time-related, increasing with duration of exposure, and these risks (intubation, tracheostomy, ventilatory assistance) cannot be compared with rates following single events, such as biopsy or bronchoscopy. Second, the risk factors are interrelated, with two or more often appearing in a single individual, either together or consecutively, e.g., tracheostomy following prolonged intubation. Finally, a major discrepancy exists, in those procedures studied, between prospective data and large retrospective or questionnaire surveys, which will produce lower recalled rates.

Assisted Ventilation

Assisted ventilation alone has been associated with the development of nosocomial tracheobronchitis or pneumonia, in both endemic and epidemic fashion. The risk of infection would be expected to vary with the disease process requiring intubation, but this has not always been observed. The risk is significantly increased with increasing time on a ventilator and with attempted self-extubation (5, 31). The association with the ventilator alone is most convincingly demonstrated in outbreaks involving contaminated fluid or tubing (32). Even in the endemic situation, however, the relative risk of the use of assisted ventilation has been carefully documented, with 12% of patients requiring intubation for at least 24 hours developing nosocomial pneumonia (5). The addition of a respirator either to a tracheostomy or to endotracheal intubation nearly tripled the overall risk of each of these procedures. Even without intubation, 10% of patients using IPPB or nasal mask oxygen alone develop nosocomial pneumonia. This seems to support the potential risk of ventilation alone, but it seems equally likely that the nature of the underlying disease requiring this therapy may be more significant.

Endotracheal Intubation and Tracheostomy

The introduction of endotracheal tubes or tracheostomy significantly increases the risk of altering pharyngeal flora (33) and subsequently of acquiring pneumonia. There is a significant risk in the use of an endotracheal tube alone, and this risk increases with time. The risk associated with tracheostomy is still higher (5), though this may also be a function of time and confounded by other factors, especially since tracheostomy often follows a period of increased hazard in the form of prolonged intubation (12). Indeed, with prolonged intubation by either route, the rate of pharyngeal colonization and pneumonia increases with time, reaching 60%–70% after 10 days, or perhaps virtually all patients with prolonged intubation (13).

Bronchoscopy and Biopsy

Relative Risk

The risk of infectious complications following bronchoscopy, even when combined with invasive procedures such as bronchopulmonary lavage or biopsy, appears to be very low, though the few cases reported demonstrate that there is a potentially significant problem when infection does occur. The risk now is certainly much less than that with the use of the rigid bronchoscope, when Berman noted that 50% of his patients, prospectively followed, had fever following the procedure, and one-third of these had transient bacteremia (34). The current baseline figure cannot be clearly delineated, since the largest series documenting complications of bronchoscopy are retrospective and often obtained by questionnaire. In such surveys, the occurrence of pneumonia or infection is often

not mentioned (even after 48,000 cases surveyed) (35) or, when mentioned, would seem to be as low as 2 cases of pneumonia in 24,521 cases reviewed (36).

In similar series documenting the results of bronchoscopy with biopsy, infection is often simply not mentioned as a complication, in spite of 6000 cases being so summarized (37–39). Prospective series appear in small numbers, but show transient fever following the procedure in as many as 16% (40). Only 6% of the total had subsequent pulmonary infiltrates, and most of these were mild and transient. One patient in this series did develop rapidly progressive pneumonia leading to death. A subsequent prospective collaborative study of larger magnitude showed a much smaller risk, estimated at less than 1%, though this may be an underestimate since cases were followed for only 24 hours (41). It is of note that four of the five patients who developed pneumonia in this series may have been immunodepressed, suggesting that there may be a subpopulation at especially high risk.

Clinical Patterns

Single case descriptions of complications of bronchoscopy do appear, however, and show two predictable patterns. In one, bacteremia may ensue, especially following bronchial biopsy (42–45). In such cases, the organism was often found in the bronchial secretions at the time of the procedure, but the bacteremia is not necessarily preventable by the use of prophylactic antibiotics (45). The incidence of bacteremia alone is so low as to make further studies probably impractical, except for high-risk patients (46).

The other pattern represents local extension of disease into the lung or into the bronchopulmonary segment intubated. Excluding those outbreaks associated with contaminated bronchoscopes (47), this complication also appears to be very uncommon. The largest prospective series, cited earlier, found 5 patients with pneumonia in 908 cases followed (41). Individual cases, however, are noted in which it is suggested that pneumonia appeared secondary to the procedure (48), and this may occur with bacteremia as well (43).

Quite a different potential problem occurs with bronchoscopy to establish drainage of an abscess, which occasionally will result in massive dissemination of infected pus throughout the tracheobronchial tree, giving a characteristic radiologic picture of widespread scattered alveolar infiltrates concomitant with the disappearance of the previously observed air-fluid level (49).

Percutaneous Biopsies

Percutaneous biopsies, which do not transgress the contaminated oropharynx, are much less often associated with infection, as determined by questionnaire (50); and the small series thus far reporting complications have discussed the risks of pneumothorax and hemorrhage, but not of infection (51–53). Even percutaneous biopsies performed on patients with documented infections seem relatively safe (52,53), though these have not yet been studied as thoroughly or prospectively as has bronchoscopy, nor has the incidence of bacteremia been determined.

Vascular Catheterization

With increasing concern about the cause and significance of nosocomial bacteremias, studies similar to those documenting the incidence of contamination of venous catheters (54) have been extended to arterial catheters, which show an 18% incidence of local infection and 4% of bacteremia (55). Recent studies on pulmonary artery catheters reflect similar rates of catheter colonization or contamination (56). Though such studies establish that the risk of contamination of the catheter is significant, and there is always a potential risk of septicemia, the magnitude of this risk is not yet clear.

References

1. Center for Disease Control: National Nosocomial Infections Study Report, 1977 (6-month summaries), issued November 1979.
2. Caplan ES, Hoyt N, Cowley RA: Changing patterns of nosocomial infections in traumatized patients. Am Surg 45:204–210, 1979.
3. Thorp JM, Richards WC, Telfer ABM: A survey of infection in an intensive care unit; "forewarned is forearmed." Anesthesia 34:643–650, 1979.
4. Gross PA, New HC, Aswapokee P, Van Antwerpen C, Aswapokee N: Deaths from nosocomial infections: experience in a university hospital and a community hospital. Am J Med 68:219–223, 1980.
5. Cross AS, Roup B: Role of respiratory assistance devices in endemic nosocomial pneumonia. Am J Med 70:681–685, 1981.
6. Sanford JP, Pierce AK: Lower respiratory infections. *In* Bennett JV, Brachman PS (eds): Hospital Infections. Boston: Little, Brown & Co., 1979.
7. Dixon RE: Investigation of endemic and epidemic infections. *In* Bennett JV, Brachman PS (eds): Hospital Infections. Boston: Little, Brown & Co, 1979.
8. Irwin RS, Ashba JK, Braman SS, Lee H, Corrao W: Food asphyxiation in hospitalized patients. JAMA 237:2744–2745, 1977.
9. Wynne JW, Modell JH: Respiratory aspiration of stomach contents. Ann Intern Med 87:466–474, 1977.
10. Bartlett JG, Gorbach SL: The triple threat of aspiration pneumonia. Chest 68:560–566, 1975.
11. Huxley EJ, Viroslav J, Gray WR, Pierce AK: Pharyngeal aspiration in normal adults and patients with depressed consciousness. Am J Med 64:564–568, 1978.
12. Stauffer JL, Olson DE, Petty TL: Complications and consequences of endotracheal intubation and tracheotomy; a prospective study of 150 critically ill adult patients. Am J Med 70:65–76, 1981.
13. Brook I: Bacterial colonization, tracheobronchitis, and pneumonia following tracheostomy and long term intubation in pediatric patients. Chest 76:420–424, 1979.
14. Schwartz SN, Dowling JN, Benkovic C, Dequittner-Buchanan M, Prostko T, Yee RB: Sources of gram-negative bacilli colonizing the tracheae of intubated patients. J Infect Dis 138:227–231, 1978.
15. Bartlett JG, Gorbach SL, Finegold SM: The bacteriology of aspiration pneumonia. Am J Med 56:202–207, 1974.
16. Rosenthal S, Tager IB: Prevalence of gram-negative rods in the normal pharyngeal flora. Ann Intern Med 83:355, 1975.
17. Johanson WG, Pierce AK, Sanford JP: Changing pharyngeal bacterial flora of hospitalized patients: emergence of gram-negative bacilli. N Engl J Med 281:1137–1140, 1969.
18. MacKowiak PA, Martin RM, Jones SR, Smith JW: Pharyngeal colonization by gram-negative bacilli in aspiration-prone persons. Arch Intern Med 138:1224–1227.
19. Valenti WM, Trudell RG, Bentley DW: Factors predisposing to oropharyngeal colonization with gram-negative bacilli in the aged. N Engl J Med 298:1108–1111, 1978.
20. Tillotson JR, Finland M: Bacterial colonization and clinical superinfection of the respiratory tract complicating antibiotic treatment of pneumonia. J Infect Dis 119:597–624, 1969.
21. Schlenker JD: Gram-negative pneumonias in surgical patients: complication of antibiotic treatment. Arch Surg 106:267–272, 1973.
22. Tillotson JR, Lerner AM: Pneumonias caused by gram-negative bacilli. Medicine 45:65–76, 1966.
23. Valdivieso M, Gil-Extremera B, Zornoza J, Rodriguez V, Bodey, GP: Gram-negative bacillary pneumonia in the compromised host. Medicine 56:241–254, 1977.

24. Reinarz JA, Pierce AK, Mays BB, Sanford JP: The potential role of inhalation therapy equipment in nosocomial pulmonary infection. J Clin Invest 44:831–829, 1965.

25. Solomon WR: Fungus aerosols arising from cold-mist vaporizers. J Allergy Clin Immunol 54:222–228, 1974.

26. Kelsen SG, McGuckin M, Kelsen DP, Cherniack NS: Airborne contamination of fine-particle nebulizers. JAMA 237:2311–2314, 1977.

27. Renner RR, Coccaro AP, Heitzman ER, Dailey ET, Markarian B: *Pseudomonas* pneumonia: prototype of hospital-based infection. Radiology 105:555–562, 1972.

28. Nolan CM, Beaty HN: *Staphylococcus aureus* bacteremia: current clinical patterns. Am J Med 60:495–500, 1976.

29. Kirsh MM, Rotman H, Behrendt DM, Orringer MB, Sloan H: Complications of pulmonary resection. Ann Thorac Surg 20:215–236, 1975.

30. Goodman LR: Postoperative chest radiograph II: Alterations after major intrathoracic surgery. Am J Radiol 134:803–812, 1980.

31. Zwillich CW, Pierson DJ, Creagh CE, Sutton FD, Schatz E, Petty TL: Complications of assisted ventilation: a prospective study of 354 consecutive episodes. Am J Med 57:161–170, 1974.

32. Mertz JJ, Scharer L, McClement JH: A hospital outbreak of *Klebsiella* pneumonia from inhalation therapy with contaminated aerosol solutions. Am Rev Respir Dis 94:454–460, 1966.

33. Harris H, Wirtschafter D, Cassady G: Endotracheal intubation and its relationship to bacterial colonization and systemic infection of newborn infants. Pediatrics 58:810–823, 1976.

34. Burman SO: Bronchoscopy and bacteremia. J Thorac Cardiovasc Surg 40:635–639, 1960.

35. Suratt PM, Smiddy JF, Gruber B: Deaths and complications associated with fiberoptic bronchoscopy. Chest 69:747–751, 1976.

36. Credle WF Jr, Smiddy JF, Elliott RC: Complications of fiberoptic bronchoscopy. Am Rev Respir Dis 109:67–72, 1974.

37. Herf SM, Suratt PM, Arora NS: Deaths and complications associated with transbronchial lung biopsy. Am Rev Respir Dis 115:708–711, 1977.

38. Zavala DC: Diagnostic fiberoptic bronchoscopy: techniques and results of biopsy in 600 patients. Chest 68:12–19, 1975.

39. Ellis JH Jr: Transbronchial lung biopsy via the fiberoptic bronchoscope: experience with 107 consecutive cases and comparison with bronchial brushing. Chest 68:524–532, 1975.

40. Pereira W, Kovnat DM, Khan MA, Lacovino, JR, Spivack ML, Snider GL: Fever and pneumonia after flexible fiberoptic bronchoscopy. Am Rev Resp Dis 112:59–64, 1965.

41. Pereira W Jr, Kovnat DM, Snider GL: A prospective cooperative study of complications following flexible fiberoptic bronchoscopy. Chest 73:813–816, 1978.

42. Alexander WJ, Baker GL, Hunter FD: Bacteremia and meningitis following fiberoptic bronchoscopy. Arch Intern Med 139:580–582, 1979.

43. Beyt BE Jr, King DK, Glew RH: Fatal pneumonitis and septicemia after fiberoptic bronchoscopy. Chest 72:105–107, 1977.

44. Timms RM, Harrell JH: Bacteremia related to fiberoptic bronchoscopy: a case report. Am Rev Respir Dis 111:555–557, 1975.

45. Robbins H, Goldman AL: Failure of a "prophylactic" antimicrobial drug to prevent sepsis after fiberoptic bronchoscopy. Am Rev Respir Dis 116:325–326, 1977.

46. Kane RC, Cohen MH, Fossieck BE Jr, Tvardzik AV: Absence of bacteremia after fiberoptic bronchoscopy. Am Rev Respir Dis 111:102–104, 1975.

47. Webb SF, Vall-Spinosa A: Outbreak of *Serratia marcescens* associated with the flexible fiberbronchoscope. Chest 68:703–708, 1975.

48. Muers M, Lane D: Acute pneumonia and pneumothorax as a complication of transbronchial biopsy. Endoscopy 12:183–187, 1980.

49. Hammer DL, Aranda CP, Galati V, Adams FV: Massive intrabronchial aspiration of contents of pulmonary abscess after fiberoptic bronchoscopy. Chest 74:306–307, 1978.

50. Herman PG, Hessel SJ: The diagnostic accuracy and complications of closed lung biopsies. Radiology 125:11–14, 1977.

51. Zornoza J, Snow J Jr, Lukeman JM, Libshitz HI: Aspiration biopsy of discrete pulmonary lesions using a new thin needle. Results in the first 100 cases. Radiology 123:519–20, 1977.

52. Berguist TH, Bailey PB, Cortese DA, Miller WE: Transthoracic needle biopsy: accuracy and complications in relation to location and type of lesion. Mayo Clin Proc 55:475–481, 1980.

53. Zavala DC, Schoell JE: Ultrathin needle aspiration of the lung in infections and malignant disease. Am Rev Respir Dis 123:125–131, 1981.

54. Maki DG, Goldmann DA, Rhame FS: Infection control in intravenous therapy. Ann Intern Med 79:867–887, 1973.

55. Band JD, Maki DG: Infections caused by arterial catheters used for hemodynamic monitoring. Am J Med 67:735–741, 1979.

56. Michel L, Marsh HM, McMichan JC, Southorn PA, Brewer NS: Infection of pulmonary artery catheters in critically ill patients. JAMA 245:1032–1036, 1081.

Table 3-2. Most Frequent Opportunistic Pulmonary Infections in the Immunocompromised Host

Pathogen	Usual Underlying Condition	Usual Diagnostic Methods	Treatment	Mortality (Range Reported)
Bacteria				
Gram-negative bacilli (*Klebsiella, E coli, Pseudomonas*)	Hematologic; neoplasia with neutropenia	Blood culture, sputum culture, "response" to antibiotics	Cephalosporin or ticarcillin, plus aminoglycoside	40% to 80%
Staphylococcus	Hematologic neoplasia	Same	Semisynthetic penicillin or cephalosporin	10% to 20%
Legionnaires' disease	Transplant; steroids; lymphoma	IFA,* DFA,* charcoal yeast extract media	Erythromycin ± rifampin	25%
Nocardia	Transplant; lymphoma	Invasive procedure (rarely sputum)	Sulfa or trimethoprim-sulfamethoxazole	5 to 80%
Fungi				
Aspergillus and phycomycetes	Neutropenia	Lung aspirate or biopsy	Amphotericin B	80% to 90%
Cryptococcus	Transplant; lymphoma	Spinal fluid (indirect), serum latex agglutination, lung biopsy or aspirate	Amphotericin B	
Parasite				
Pneumocystis carinii	Steroids	Lung biopsy or aspirate	Trimethoprim-sulfamethoxazole	40% to 60%
Viruses				
Cytomegalovirus	Transplant; lymphoma	Lung biopsy, serology	None proven	Usually low, but up to 50% in bone marrow transplant
Herpes zoster	Hodgkin's	Associated skin lesions	Possibly adenine arabinoside or acyclovir (investigated)	Low

* IFA = indirect fluorescent antibody titer;
  DFA = direct fluorescent antibody preparation.

noninfectious diseases. Some of the noninfections processes require no specific therapy, and the correct management of the patient is to stop potentially toxic empirically chosen drugs.

Infections

Bacteria

Table 3-2 lists the most frequently encountered infectious agents in immunocompromised hosts, the usual method of diagnosis, and the treatment and prognosis. It should be noted that the most frequent of infectious causes appears to be typical bacteria (3–6). The clinical presentation of bacterial pneumonia in the neutropenic patient is distinctly different from that in nonmyelosuppressed populations (6,7). Cough occurs in less than half of cases and, when present, is usually nonproductive. Dyspnea may be the only indication of chest disease in a febrile, neutropenic host, and the radiographic appearance of an infiltrate may be discovered unexpectedly during the routine work-up of fever.

Even if sputum is unavailable, presumptive therapy with broad-spectrum antibiotics is generally instituted for new cases of pneumonia, since bacterial causes are so common. In fact, the most common method by which the diagnosis of bacterial pneumonia is made is actually an indirect method. A prompt clinical response to institution of broad-spectrum antibiotics is generally taken as a sign that bacterial infection was present. Thus, many cases of "bacterial pneumonia" are actually diagnosed by inference rather than microbiologically. Of course, this is perfectly acceptable practice, since it obviates the need for invasive procedures to secure a truly specific diagnosis.

Radiologically, the chest x-ray may be normal early, particularly in patients with neutropenia. In the gram-negative pneumonias, patchy multilobar alveolar-type infiltrates are most common. Purely lobar consolidation is rather infrequent. Pleural effusions and empyema are rare. In the *Legionella* infections a pseudonodular appearance has been also described.

The prognosis for bacterial infection in these patients appears to be improving. One report documented up to 60% survival among cancer patients with gram-negative pneumonia (7). However, certain pathogens, such as *Pseudomonas aeruginosa,* and certain high-risk settings, such as profound neutropenia, continue to be associated with mortalities exceeding 80% (13).

Our therapeutic approach has generally been to utilize two bactericidal agents for gram-negative pneumonia. For example, a cephalosporin plus aminoglycoside for *Klebsiella,* or ticarcillin plus aminoglycoside for *Pseudomonas.* In addition, some evidence exists that granulocyte transfusion therapy may be beneficial for refractory cases of bacterial pneumonia in neutropenic patients (14).

Recently, several atypical bacteria have been associated with pulmonary infections in patients receiving glucocorticosteroids. These organisms, known as *Legionella*-like organisms (LLO), include *Legionella pneumophila,* Pittsburgh bacillus, Tex-KL, and others (9–11, 15–17). They are all small, aerobic, gram-negative rods, which require special media for in vitro cultivation (e.g., charcoal yeast extract media). Serologic techniques, such as indirect fluorescent antibody titers or direct fluorescent antibody stains, are also available as diagnostic tools. Radiographically, Legionnaires' disease (LD) resembles usual bacterial pneumonias, often beginning with focal consolidation and spreading rapidly to invade one or more lobes. Cavitation and pleural effusions are not unusual. If these atypical bacterial agents are suspected or identified, erythromycin is the drug of choice. Intravenous erythromycin may be needed during early therapy, and rifampin has been useful as a second agent for difficult cases (16). A minimum of three weeks treatment is recommended. Mortality for LD in immunocompromised hosts not treated with erythromycin has been reported to be 80%, while erythromycin treatment results in a mortality of 24% (18).

Nocardia asteroides

Nocardia asteroides is a gram-positive higher bacterium, which grows aerobically, and has a predilection for the lungs of patients receiving glucocorticosteroids (19,20). Thus, pulmonary nocardiosis generally occurs among organ transplant recipients and patients with advanced lymphomas. Cardiac transplant recipients have been a particularly high-risk group for nocardiosis (20).

Nocardial infection of the lung generally is a subacute disease, presenting with intermittent fever. Cough and other respiratory symptoms may or may not be present. Although sputum cultures are occasionally helpful, mouth flora often overgrow the culture, obscuring the more slowly grow-

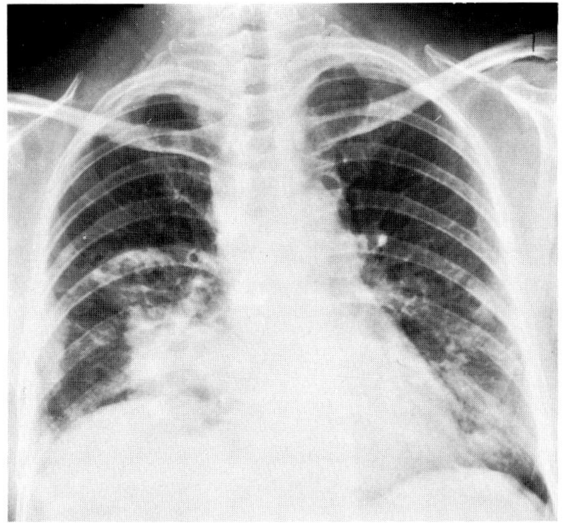

a

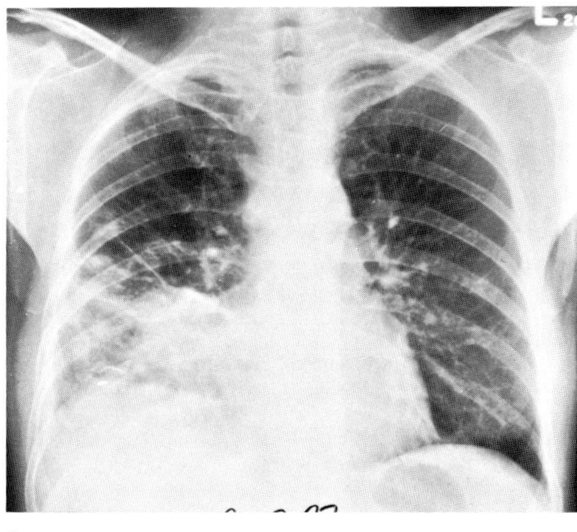

c

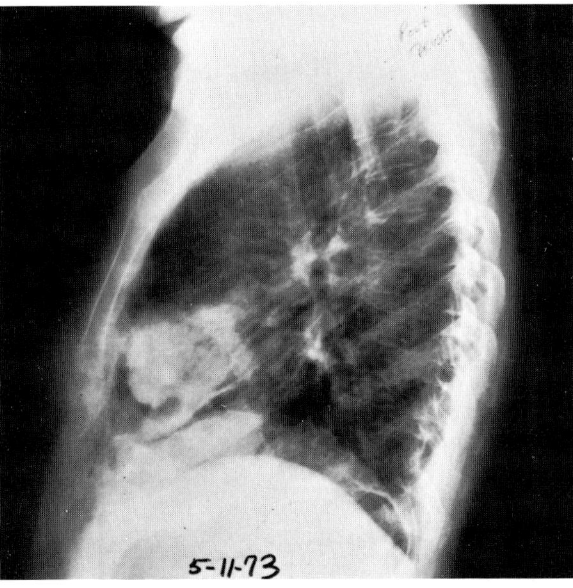

b

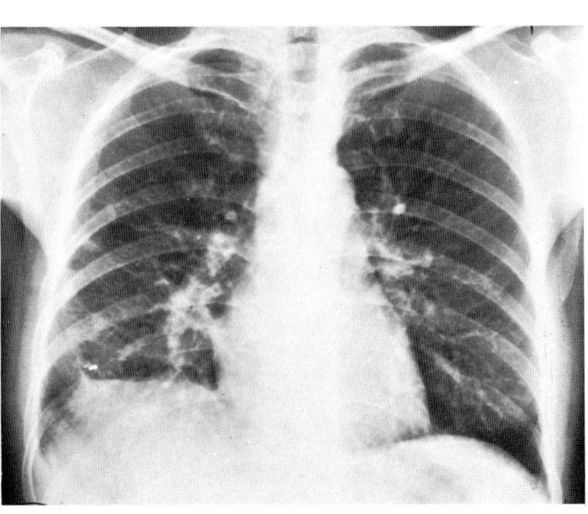

d

Fig. 3-1, a-d. Nocardiosis. A 45-year-old woman received 30 mg of prednisone over one year. **a,b** Nodular slowly progressing opacity in the right middle lobe. Diagnosis was made by transthoracic and open lung biopsies. **c** Four months following therapy there was persistent opacity on the chest x-ray, but the patient was asymptomatic. **d** Eight months later the pulmonary infiltrate had cleared.

ing *Nocardia.* The clinical progression is usually slow and some patients may be asymptomatic. Radiologically, a single or multiple nodules with or without cavitation may suggest a diagnosis; however, focal or more diffuse infiltrates are also seen (22) (Fig. 3-1). Thus, invasive diagnostic procedures are usually needed to confirm the diagnosis of nocardia.

This infection is particularly important to diagnose, since early therapy is associated with an excellent prognosis, whereas a delay in proper therapy has been associated with mortalities of up to 80%. The usual therapy for nocardiosis is high-dose sulfonamides, given for at least five months. (21) Longer courses of treatment are not unusual.

Fungi

The most common primary fungal pneumonia among immunocompromised patients is *Aspergillus* pneumonia (1,3,5,23). This pneumonia is only about one-tenth to one-twentieth as common as bacterial pneumonia, however. *Aspergillus* species are ubiquitous in nature; thus exposure to aerosols of *Aspergillus* spores is inevitable. Additionally, it appears that effluent air from certain air-conditioning systems, as well as the environment surrounding building and excavation projects, is particularly dense with *Aspergillus*. Such conditions have been associated with outbreaks of *Aspergillus* pneumonia, and it is occasionally encountered in immunosuppressed patients.

Aspergillus is rarely an invasive pathogen in normal hosts, occasionally occurring as a chronic, indolent infestation of old cavitary lung disease (aspergilloma, mycetoma). However, in immunosuppressed and, in particular, myelosuppressed patients, this organism can cause a rapidly progressive, invasive, and necrotizing lung infection (24). Dissemination is occasionally encountered, but a primary lung infection is generally the only clinical manifestation.

A typical presentation of *Aspergillus* pneumonia involves a neutropenic patient with underlying hematologic malignancy. Frequently the patient is on, or has recently been on, broad-spectrum antibiotics for fever of uncertain origin. Suddenly the patient develops dry cough and increased fever. Radiologically, areas of consolidation, sometimes with cavitation and crescent-shaped radiolucencies, are seen. This is caused by a fulminant necrotizing infection, usually with hemorrhagic pulmonary infarction. The most common radiologic manifestation, however, is the presence of patchy confluent opacities, which may rapidly cavitate. Infrequently a diffuse reticular pattern may be encountered on the chest x-ray (Figs. 3-2, 3-3).

The misdiagnosis of presumed bacterial pneumonia is frequently made. Lack of response to usual antibiotics in this setting should alert the clinician to the possibility of aspergillosis. While an invasive diagnostic procedure is needed to confirm the diagnosis, a strong suspicion of *Aspergillus* pneumonia should exist if either sputum or nasal swabs contain *Aspergillus*. Unfortunately, reliable *Aspergillus* serologic tests are not yet available for this type of patient, nor are blood cultures helpful.

Treatment for proven or suspected *Aspergillus* pneumonia is with amphotericin B. 5-Fluorocytosine may be synergistic but also may be myelosuppressive. The experience to date with miconazole or ketoconazole in this setting is too limited for comment. Likewise, no prospective study has doc-

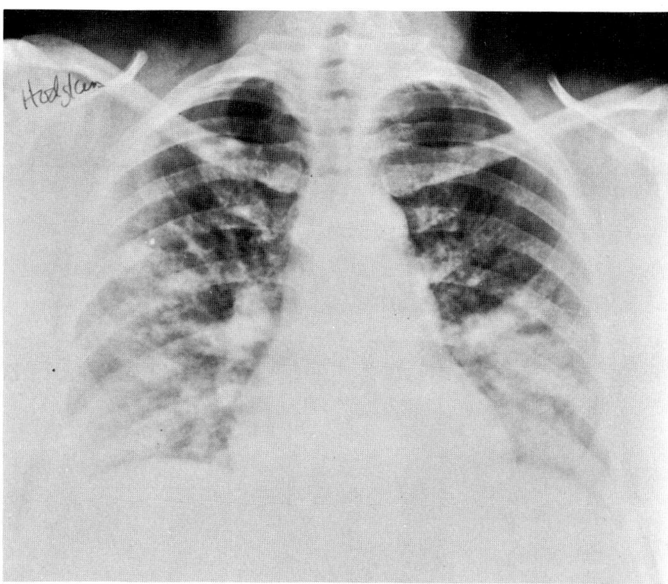

Fig. 3-2. Invasive aspergillosis. Multifocal confluent opacities in a patient receiving chemotherapy for acute myelocystic leukemia who was granulocytopenia. Diagnosis was confirmed at autopsy.

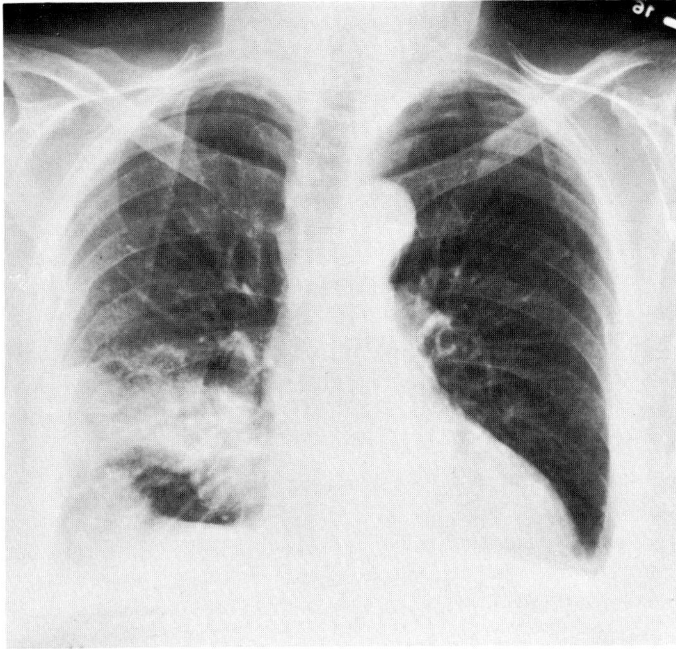

a

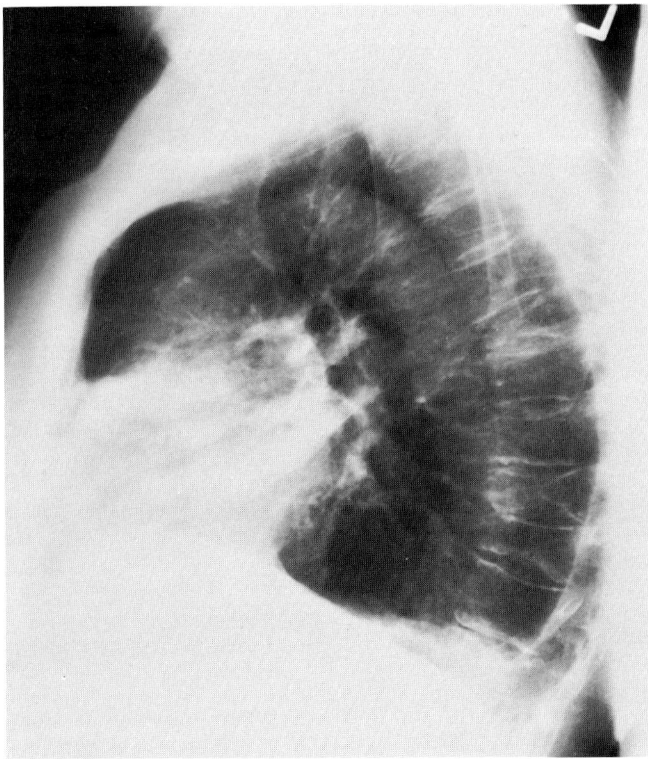

b

Fig. 3-3, a and **b. Invasive aspergillosis.** Rapidly progressing multifocal confluent opacity in the right middle lobe in a patient receiving chemotherapy for non-Hodgkin's lymphoma. Diagnosis was made by transthoracic needle biopsy and confirmed at autopsy. **a** Anteroposterior view. **b** Lateral view.

umented clinically important synergistic effects of rifampin or tetracycline when added to amphotericin B.

While mortality from *Aspergillus* pneumonia remains greater than 80% in this setting, earlier diagnosis and therapy have resulted in a number of clinical successes (25–29). Thus, every effort should be made to diagnose and treat this infection correctly. Calling this condition "hopeless," as was done in the past, is no longer tenable.

Other fungi occasionally encountered in the compromised host include *Mucor, Cryptococcus,* and rarely *Histoplasma* and *Coccidioides* (30–34). Most of the comments made for aspergillosis obtain for mucormycosis (Fig. 3-4). However, this organism is even more difficult to cultivate in culture, is almost always lethal when infecting the lung, and fortunately is much less common than *Aspergillus.*

Cryptococcus neoformans almost always present as meningitis in noncompromised patients, but can be a fulminant pneumonia in immunocompromised patients. Often, meningeal and pulmonary cryptococcal infection coexist, and the CNS infection may initially overshadow the pulmonary lesion. Diagnosis can occasionally be made by sputum culture but usually requires an invasive procedure. The serum latex agglutination test for cryptococcal antigen is helpful to evaluate pulmonary lesions for the possibility of *Cryptococcus* (e.g., "coin" lesion in renal transplant patient with fever) (35).

Clinical and autopsy experience has disclosed that primary candidiasis of lung tissues is rarely encountered in immunocompromised patients. This is surprising, since sputum cultures from these patients often contain *Candida.* Certainly positive sputum cultures for *Candida* by no means should prompt institution of amphotericin B. Occasionally, disseminated candidiasis from gastrointestinal sites will result in hematogenous spread to lungs. This is generally a late and terminal event, however.

Another yeast, *Torulopsis glabrata,* has been implicated in an occasional primary pneumonia of immunosuppressed patients. This also seems to be a rare event, however.

Finally, in endemic areas, *Histoplasma* and *Coccidioides* may cause particularly severe pneumonia when acquired in the compromised host. Again, these are infrequent causes compared with *Aspergillus.*

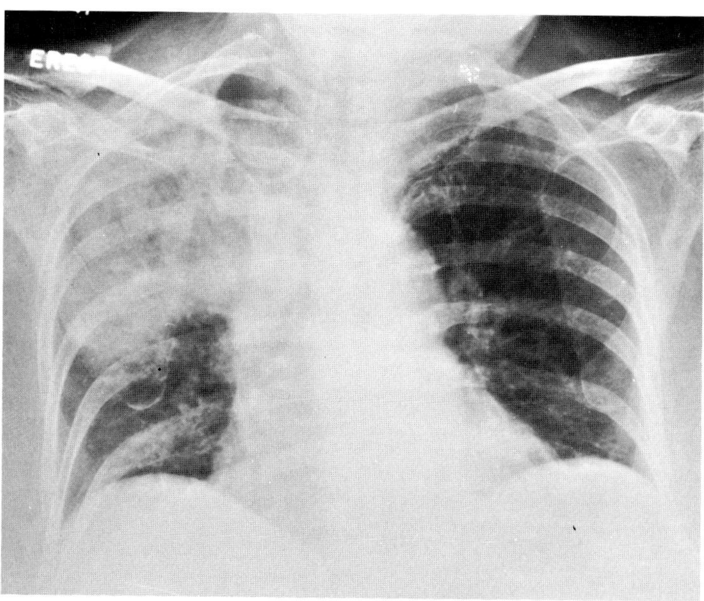

Fig. 3-4. Pulmonary mucormycosis. Lobar opacity in a patient receiving chemotherapy for chronic myelogenous leukemia. Diagnosis was made by transthoracic needle biopsy and confirmed at autopsy.

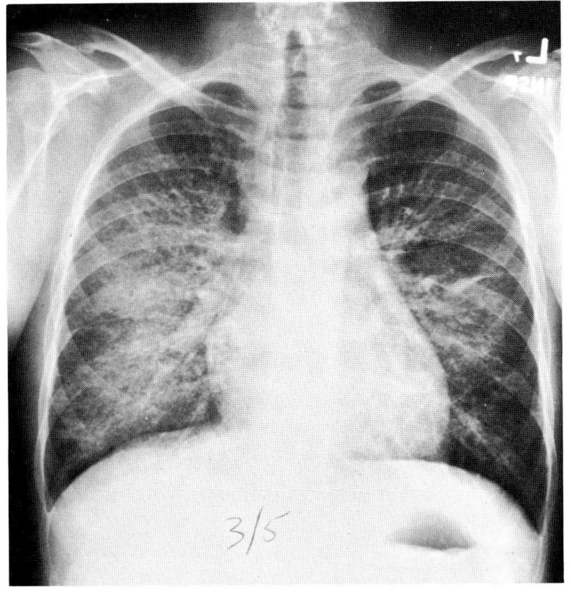

a

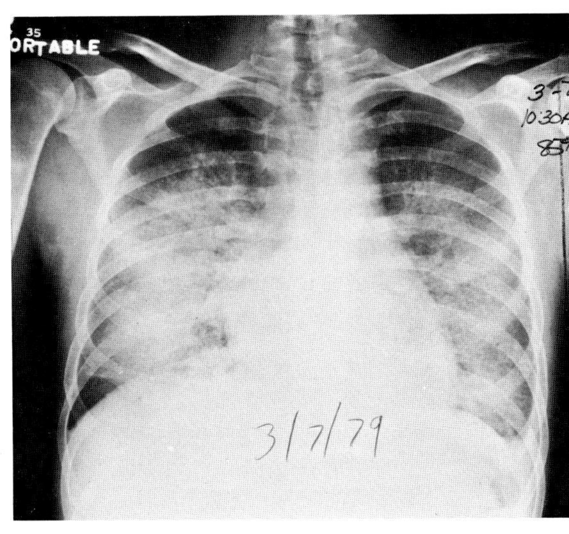

b

Fig. 3-5, a and b. Pneumocystosis pneumonia. a Disseminated interstitial process resembling pulmonary edema appeared in a middle-aged man treated for non-Hodgkin's lymphoma. **b** Two days later, significant progression is present. Appearance is suggestive of airspace edema. Diagnosis was made by open lung biopsy.

Pneumocystis carinii

Although *Strongyloides* and *Toxoplasma gondii* may rarely cause pneumonia in the compromised host, the only parasitic pneumonia that occurs with any frequency in this country is due to *Pneumocystic carinii* (36–38). The natural reservoir and life cycle of this protozoan are poorly understood. There is some evidence that dormant foci of *Pneumocystis* may exist in the lungs of many normal healthy humans and that immunosuppression, particularly glucocorticosteroids, may allow an active infection to become unmasked. In any event, *Pneumocystis* pneumonia generally presents in patients receiving, most typically tapering, high doses of glucocorticosteroid agents (39).

A typical presentation of this illness involves rapidly progressive dyspnea, falling arterial blood oxygen saturation, and abnormal chest roentgenogram. Radiologically, initially a bilateral reticular process is seen which in three to five days progresses to a more homogeneous consolidation. The initial radiographic involvement may be patchy or can present as a fine reticulogranular pattern. The infiltrates typically are perihilar and radiate into the lung fields (Fig. 3-5). Atypical radiographic presentations are not uncommon, such as unilateral predominance, lobar or segmental consolidation.

Many such patients are initially diagnosed as having pulmonary edema (Fig. 3-5b). However, lack of response to diuretics and a normal heart size should eliminate that possibility. Sputum is rarely available, and culture of blood or serologic tests are useless. The diagnosis can only be made with certainty using invasive diagnostic procedures and subjecting the specimens to special stains (such as methenamine silver nitrate).

Treatment in past years has consisted of pentamidine isethionate, a rather toxic drug. However, recent experience has shown that high doses of trimethoprim (20 mg/kg/day) plus sulfamethoxazole (TMP-SMX) result in equivalent or superior clinical results and offer less potential for serious side effects (40–42). Erratic gastrointestinal absorption of orally administered TMP-SMX has accounted for treatment failure in some patients; thus the parenteral form of this drug (currently investigational) should be employed when possible.

Despite less toxic therapy for pneumocystosis, mortality remains high. Although children with acute lymphocytic leukemia experience mortalities of 25%, other patient populations continue to exhibit mortality exceeding 40% to 50%.

Viruses

Viral pneumonias in the immunosuppressed patient are less common than bacterial or fungal, but occasionally can be fatal. The most common viral pneumonia is caused by cytomegalovirus (CMV). This is almost exclusively a disease of transplant and lymphoma patients, implying that cell-mediated immunity must be critical in containing this pathogen (43–48). In many ways, the presentation of CMV pneumonia resembles *Pneumocystis* pneumonia, with fever, dyspnea, and hypoxemia. Radiologically, a symmetric, bilateral interstitial process is seen, with a tendency to begin in the periphery of the lower lobes and extend centrally and superiorly. It may appear in a patchy, pseudonodular pattern. CMV pneumonia is rarely fatal in renal transplant patients but appears to predispose to more serious secondary pneumonias with bacteria, *Pneumocystis,* or fungi (49). In contrast, CMV alone may cause fatal pneumonia in bone marrow transplant recipients (45,47). Up to half of all cases of interstitial pneumonitis in marrow transplant recipients are caused by CMV, and the mortality in these patients is 50% (45). Unfortunately, no effective therapy has yet been devised for CMV pneumonia.

Other viral pneumonias encountered include herpes zoster in Hodgkin's disease patients, generally associated with disseminated zoster (Fig. 3-6), and rarely adenovirus pneumonia. There is little evidence that the common viral pneumonias of nonimmunosuppressed patients (e.g., influenza, parainfluenza) occur with increased frequency in the immunocompromised host.

Noninfectious

A partial list of noninfectious causes of fever and lung infiltrates in the immunosuppressed patient includes drug toxicity, pulmonary embolism and infarct, pulmonary leukoagglutinin reaction, pulmonary hemorrhage, tumor infiltrate, radiation pneumonitis, pulmonary edema, and nonspecific interstitial pneumonitis (NIP). The latter entity (NIP) is among the most frequent tissue diagnoses found at lung biopsy or autopsy, ranking second after infection at our institution (1). This is a rather frustrating fact, since it is clearly possible that after such extensive diagnostic efforts as open lung biopsy are made, there still will not be a specific microbiologic or histologic diagnosis. Our approach to management of patients with NIP has been to discontinue empirically chosen antibiotics. If the patient has deteriorating lung function, a short course of glucocorticosteroids may be tried. Mortality from NIP in our hands has been about 25% (Fig. 3-7).

Differential Diagnosis Based Upon Radiographic Patterns

In approaching the immunocompromised host with pneumonia, the two major clinical clues for diagnostic possibilities are, first, the underlying risk factor (Table 3-1) and, second, the radiographic pattern of the lung infiltrate(s) (Table 3-3). As mentioned previously, such a statistically oriented approach is often necessary, since traditional methods of diagnosis, such as sputum examination and culture, are generally unavailable.

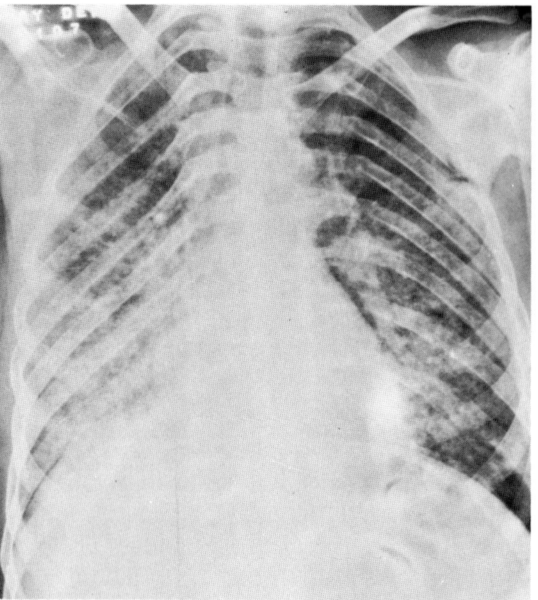

Fig. 3-6. Varicella-zoster pneumonia. Disseminated reticular nodular process in a young adult treated with chemotherapy for Hodgkin's disease. Diagnosis was confirmed at autopsy.

Table 3-3. Causes of Diffuse and Focal Infiltrates

Diffuse Infiltrate	Focal (or Cavitary) Infiltrate

Common:
  Nonspecific interstitial
    pneumonitis (NIP)
  Cytomegalovirus
  Pneumocystis carinii
  Drug reaction
	Common:
	  Gram-negative rods
	  Staphylococcus aureus
	  Aspergillus
	  Malignancy
	  Nonspecific interstitial
	    pneumonitis (NIP)

Uncommon:
  Bacteria
  Aspergillus
  Cryptococcus
  Malignancy
  Radiation pneumonitis
  Leukoagglutinin reac-
  tion
	Uncommon:
	  Cryptococcus
	  Nocardia
	  Mucor
	  Pneumocystis carinii
	  Tuberculosis
	  ? *Legionella pneumo-
	  phila*

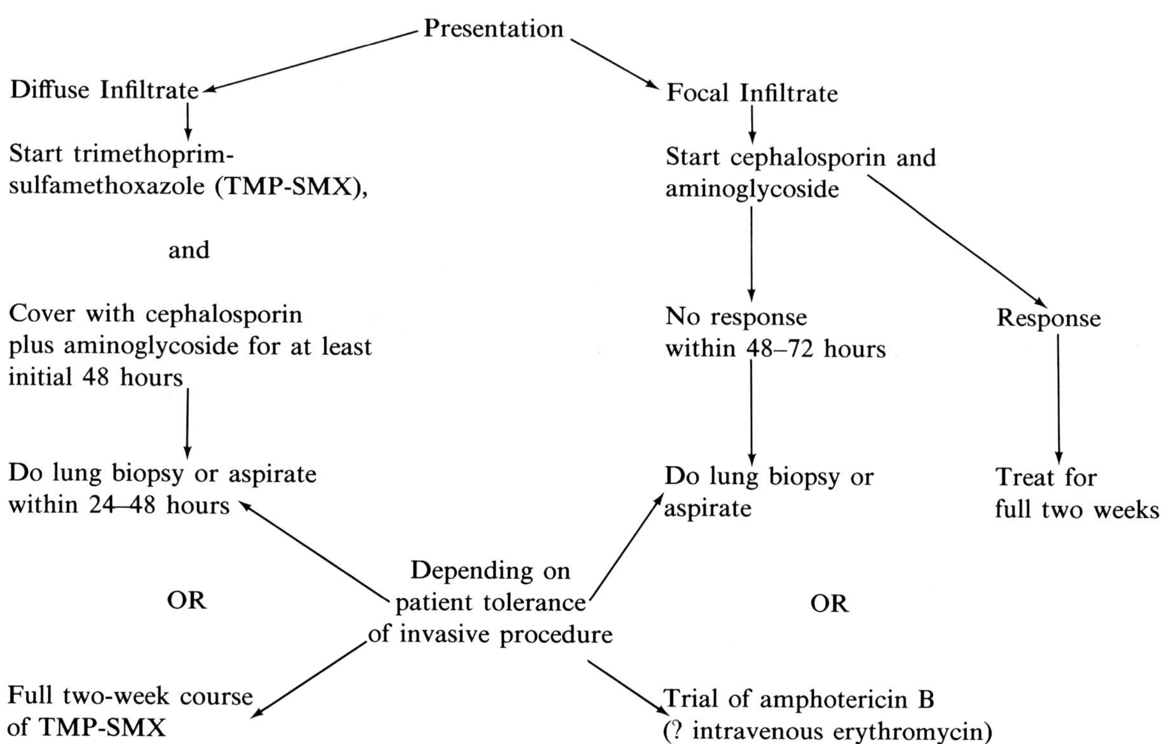

Fig. 3-7. Scheme for management of the immunocompromised host with fever and new lung infiltrates.

References

1. Fanta CH, Pennington JE: Fever and new lung infiltrates in the immunocompromised host. Clin Chest Med 2:19–39, 1981.
2. Pennington JE: Infection in the compromised host: recent advances and future directions. Semin Infect Dis 1:142–168, 1978.
3. Pennington JE, Feldman NT: Pulmonary infiltrates and fever in patients with hematologic malignancy: assessment of transbronchial biopsy. Am J Med 62:581–587, 1977.
4. Williams DM, Krick JA, Remington JS: Pulmonary infection in the compromised host. Am Rev Respir Dis 114:359–392, 593–627, 1976.
5. Levine AS, Schimpff SC, Graw RG Jr, et al: Hematologic malignancies and other marrow failure states: progress in the management of complicating infections. Semin Hematol 11:141–202, 1974.
6. Sickles EA, Young VM, Greene WH, et al: Pneumonia in acute leukemia. Ann Intern Med 79:528–534, 1973.
7. Valdivieso M, Gil-Extremera B, Zornoza J, et al: Gram-negative bacillary pneumonia in the compromised host. Medicine 56:241–254, 1977.
8. Bode FR, Paré JAP, Fraser RG: Pulmonary diseases in the compromised host: a review of clinical and roentgenographic manifestations in patients with impaired host defense mechanisms. Medicine 53:255–293, 1974.
9. Myerowitz RL, Pasculle AW, Dowling JN, et al: Opportunistic lung infection due to "Pittsburgh pneumonia agent." N Engl J Med 301:953–958, 1979.
10. Beaty HN, Miller AA, Broome CV, et al: Legionnaires' disease in Vermont, May to October 1977. JAMA 240:127–131, 1978.
11. Haley CE, Cohen ML, Halter J, et al: Nosocomial Legionnaires' disease: a continuing common-source epidemic at Wadsworth Medical Center. Ann Intern Med 90:583–586, 1979.
12. Singer C, Armstrong D, Rosen PP, et al: Diffuse pulmonary infiltrates in immunosuppressed patients: prospective study of 80 cases. Am J Med 66:110–120. 1979.
13. Pennington JE, Reynolds HY, Carbone PP: Pseudomonas pneumonia: a retrospective study of 36 cases. Am J Med 55:155–160, 1973.
14. Dale DC, Reynolds HY, Pennington JE, et al: Granulocyte transfusion therapy of experimental *Pseudomonas* pneumonia. J Clin Invest 54:664–671, 1974.
15. Rogers BH, Donowitz GR, Walker GK, et al: Opportunistic pneumonia: a clinicopathological study of five cases caused by an unidentified acid-fast bacterium. N Engl J Med 301:959–961, 1979.
16. Saravolatz LD, Burch KH, Fisher E, et al: The compromised host and Legionnaires' disease. Ann Intern Med 90:533–537, 1979.
17. Bock BV, Kirby BD, Edelstein PH, et al: Legionnaires' disease in renal-transplant recipients. Lancet 1:410–413, 1978.
18. Kirby BD, Snyder KM, Meyer RD, et al: Legionnaires' disease: report of sixty-five nosocomially acquired cases and review of the literature. Medicine 59:188–205, 1980.
19. Young LS, Armstrong D, Blevins A, et al: *Nocardia asteroides* infection complicating neoplastic disease. Am J Med 50:356–367, 1971.
20. Krick JA, Stinson EB, Remington JS: *Nocardia* infection in heart transplant patients. Ann Intern Med 82:18–26, 1975.
21. Geiseler PJ, Check F, Lamothe F, et al: Failure of trimethoprim/sulfamethoxazole in invasive *Nocardia asteroides* infection. Arch Intern Med 139:2271–2276, 1975.
22. Balikian JP, Herman PG, Kopit S: Pulmonary nocardiosis. Radiology 126:569–573, 1978.
23. Mirsky HS, Cuttner J: Fungal infection in acute leukemia. Cancer 30:348–352, 1972.
24. Pennington JE: Aspergillus lung disease. Med Clin North Am 64:475–490, 1980.
25. Aisner J, Schimpff SC, Wiernik PH: Treatment of invasive aspergillosis: relation of early diagnosis and treatment to response. Ann Intern Med 86:539–543, 1977.
26. Pennington JE: Successful treatment of aspergillus pneumonia in hematologic neoplasia. N Engl J Med 295:426–427, 1976.
27. Pennington JE: Aspergillus pneumonia in hematologic malignancy: improvements in diagnosis and therapy. Arch Intern Med 137:769–771, 1977.
28. Gercovich FG, Richman SP, Rodriguez V, et al: Successful control of systemic *Aspergillus niger* infections in two patients with acute leukemia. Cancer 36:2271–2276, 1975.
29. Sinclair AJ, Rossof AH, Coltman CA Jr: Recognition and successful management in pulmonary aspergillosis in leukemia. Cancer 42:2019–2024, 1978.
30. Meyer RD, Armstrong D: Mucormycosis-changing status. CRC Crit Rev Clin Lab Sci 4:421–451, 1973.
31. Kaplan MH, Rosen PP, Armstrong D: Cryptococcosis in a cancer hospital: clinical and pathological correlates in forty-six patients. Cancer 39:2265–2274, 1977.
32. Schröter GPJ, Temple DR, Husberg BS, et al: Cryptococcosis after renal transplantation: report of ten cases. Surgery 79:268–277, 1976.
33. Kauffman CA, Israel KS, Smith JW, et al: Histoplasmosis in immunosuppressed patients. Am J Med 64:923–932, 1978.
34. Deresinski SC, Stevens DA: Coccidioidomycosis in compromised hosts: experience at Stanford University Hospital. Medicine 54:377–395, 1974.
35. Fisher BD, Armstrong D: Cryptococcal interstitial pneumonia: value of antigen determination. N Engl J Med 297:1440–1441, 1977.
36. Hughes WT: *Pneumocystis carinii* pneumonia. N Engl J Med 297:1381–1383, 1977.
37. Goodell B, Jacobs JB, Powell RD, et al: *Pneumocystis carinii:* the spectrum of diffuse interstitial pneumonia in patients with neoplastic diseases. Ann Intern Med 72:337–340, 1970.
38. Rosen PP, Martini N, Armstrong D: *Pneumocystis carinii* pneumonia: diagnosis by lung biopsy. Am J Med 58:794–802, 1975.
39. Johnson HD, Johnson WW: *Pneumocystis carinii*

pneumonia in children with cancer. JAMA 214:1067–1072, 1970.

40. Winston DJ, Lau WK, Fale RP, et al: Trimethoprim-sulfamethoxazole for the treatment of *Pneumocystis carinii* pneumonia. Ann Intern Med 92:762–769, 1980.

41. Sattler FR, Remington JS: Intravenous trimethoprim-sulfamethoxazole therapy for *Pneumocystis carinii* pneumonia. Am J Med 70:1215–1222, 1981.

42. Hughes WT, Feldman S, Chaudhary SC, et al: Comparison of pentamidine isethionate and trimethoprim-sulfamethoxazole in the treatment of *Pneumocystis carinii* pneumonia. J Pediatr 92:285–291, 1978.

43. Andersen HK, Spencer ES: Cytomegalovirus infection among renal allograft recipients. Acta Med Scand 186:7–19, 1969.

44. Fiala M, Payne JE, Berne TV, et al: Epidemiology of cytomegalovirus infection after transplantation and immunosuppression. J Infect Dis 132:421–433, 1975.

45. Neiman PE, Reeves W, Ray G, et al: A prospective analysis of interstitial pneumonia and opportunistic viral infection among recipients of allogeneic bone marrow grafts. J Infect Dis 136:754–767, 1977.

46. Neiman PE, Thomas ED, Reeves WC, et al: Opportunistic infection and interstitial pneumonia following marrow transplantation for aplastic anemia and hematologic malignancy. Transplant Proc 8:663–667, 1976.

47. Winston DJ, Gale RP, Meyer DV, et al: Infectious complications of human bone marrow transplantation. Medicine 58:1–31, 1979.

48. Betts RF, Hanshaw JB: Cytomegalovirus (CMV) in the compromised host(s). Ann Rev Med 28:103–110, 1977.

49. Rand KH, Pollard RB, Merigan TC: Increased pulmonary superinfections in cardiac-transplant patients undergoing primary cytomegalovirus infection. N Engl J Med 298:951–953, 1978.

4 Traumatic Complications of Endotracheal Intubation and Cardiopulmonary Resuscitation

I. J. Isaacson and R. Fortunato

There is little question that the techniques of intubation of the trachea and prompt cardiopulmonary resuscitation (CPR) have saved countless lives. As with all invasive procedures in medicine, there are risks associated with both endotracheal intubation and CPR.

The purpose of this chapter is to review the complications associated with endotracheal intubation and CPR and to describe how such complications may be diagnosed both clinically and radiographically.

Endotracheal Intubation

Endotracheal intubation is performed for a variety of reasons. These include: a) to relieve upper airway obstruction (e.g., acute epiglottitis); b) to protect the airway from aspiration (e.g., the obtunded patient with a full stomach); c) to maintain adequate bronchial-pulmonary hygiene in an individual whose own ability to effectively clear secretions is impaired (e.g., a tetraplegic unable to cough); d) to provide positive pressure to the airway for mechanical ventilation or continuous positive-pressure breathing; e) for administration of oxygen to assure a precise inspired oxygen concentration; and f) intraoperatively, when the patient's position or procedure is such that the anesthesiologist would be unable to maintain an adequate airway with mask alone.

Intubation may be necessary in elective as well as emergent situations. Complications are seen under both poor and optimal conditions. Unfortunately it is often difficult to predict precisely who is at risk for complications.

Early Complications That Occur During Intubation

Diverse early complications, during the act of intubation, have been reported. Many of these complications can be documented radiographically. They include retropharyngeal dissection, development of subcutaneous and mediastinal emphysema, perforation of the esophagus or pharynx, and laceration of the trachea.

A tragic example of a retropharyngeal dissection occurred in an otherwise healthy patient who presented in the emergency ward with a multiple drug overdose. She was obtunded and exhibited shallow ventilatory efforts and was therefore intubated. The endotracheal intubation was surprisingly difficult and required several attempts, both orally and nasally. There were no apparent anatomic abnormalities to account for the difficulties. Finally, an 8-mm (internal diameter) endotracheal tube was placed with the aid of a stylet. The patient regained consciousness and was extubated 48 hours later. During the ensuing 24 hours the patient developed fever, chills, as well as a sore throat and sore neck. Soft-tissue x-rays of the neck revealed a large retropharyngeal abscess which required surgical drainage. The patient required a tracheostomy to alleviate airway compromise secondary to edema. The radiograph in Figure 4-1 demonstrates the typical findings with retropharyngeal inflammation. Al-

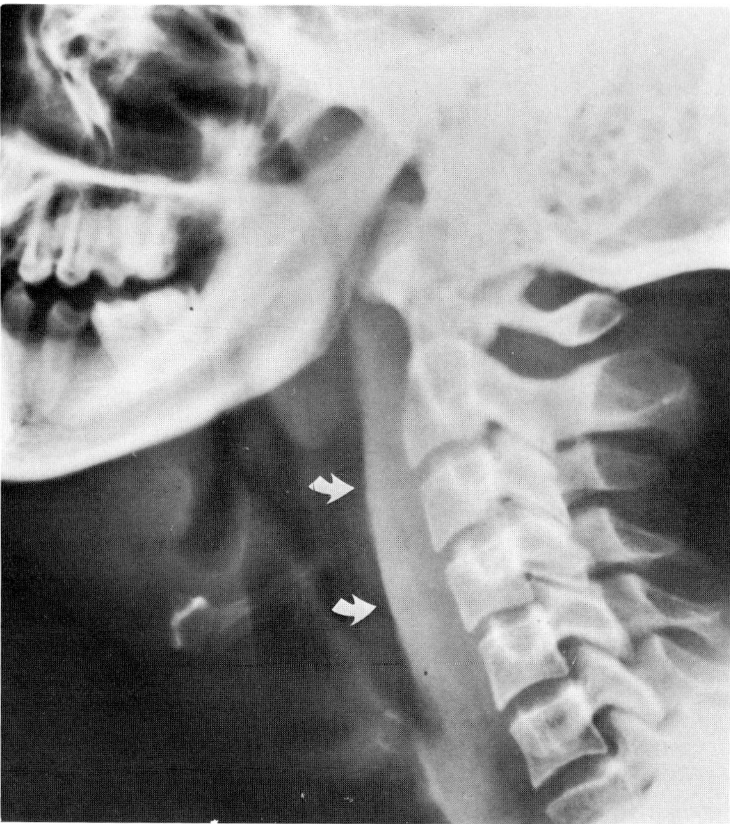

Fig. 4-1. Retropharyngeal inflammation. Lateral soft-tissue view of neck demonstrates diffuse swelling of the retropharyngeal prevertebral soft tissues (*arrows*). The soft-tissue stripe measured 11 mm in width, while the average is 3 mm with a usual range of 1 to 7 mm.

though such abscess formation is admittedly a rare complication of traumatic endotracheal intubation, it is one that necessitates prompt recognition and treatment (1).

The incidence of subcutaneous and mediastinal emphysema as a result of positive pressure applied to an airway traumatized during intubation is unknown. Inadvertent hypopharyngeal injury, accidental intubation of the pyriform sinus, and esophageal perforation can all be the source of the emphysema (2–4). An early universal hallmark of such a disaster is the development of crepitations in the cervical area. Frequently an immediate diagnosis can be made, even in the absence of symptoms, if there is a high index of suspicion for such trauma, with the development of subcutaneous emphysema shortly after the intubation attempt. When such perforation is suspected, radiologic examination will often confirm the presence and location of the perforation. Roentgenograms

of the neck and thorax in the frontal and lateral planes will demonstrate a) cervical or cervicomediastinal emphysema, b) widening of the upper mediastinum, and c) occasionally pleural extravasation or a pneumothorax. Figure 4-2 is an example of the cervicomediastinal emphysema associated with esophageal rupture which occurred during a traumatic intubation.

Tracheal laceration has occurred with repeated attempts at a difficult intubation, with overdistention or rupture of endotracheal tube cuffs, with tracheal abnormalities, as well as in uneventful intubations in otherwise normal people (5). Again, the diagnosis has to be suspected if subcutaneous emphysema and pneumothorax develop (usually tension pneumothorax). With a tracheal laceration it is imperative to define the source of the air leak. Bronchoscopy offers the best means of finding the exact location and extent of the lesion.

Lung disruption, when it occurs, usually results

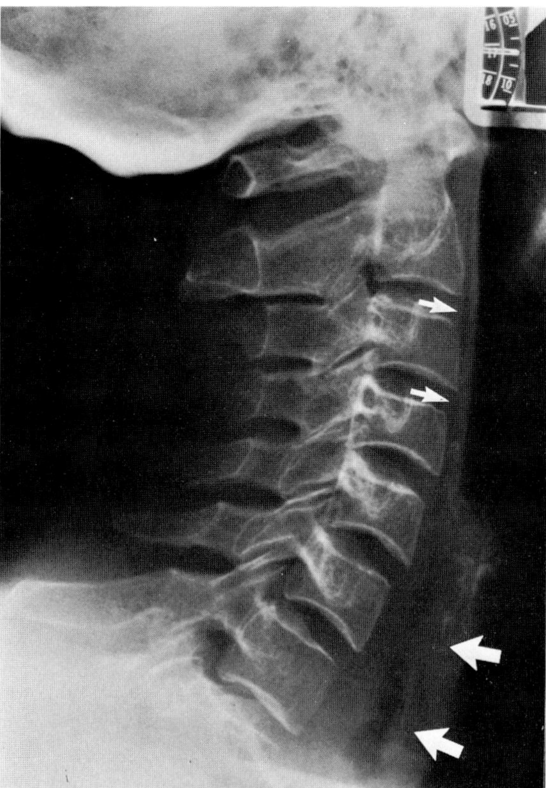

Fig. 4-2. Cervical emphysema. Air is seen tracking along the prevertebral soft tissues from the second to the seventh cervical vertebra (*arrows*). This followed esophageal rupture and results from air being forced into the soft tissues during swallowing. Eventually, air may track into the soft tissues of the thorax, the mediastinum, and even the pleural spaces, causing a pneumothorax.

from positive-pressure ventilation applied after the endotracheal tube is in place. Lung disruption from mechanical ventilation is the subject of another chapter of this book and will not be covered further here.

Aspiration is a common complication during endotracheal intubation. Stimulation of the larynx may promote vomiting and aspiration of stomach contents. Teeth that have been chipped or dislodged during laryngoscopy as well as foreign objects, such as a laryngoscope bulb, have all been seen on chest radiographs after intubation. Figure 4-3 shows an aspirated tooth fragment in the right mainstem bronchus. In a traumatic intubation the aspiration of blood may be seen on the chest radiograph relatively soon after placement of the endotracheal tube; however, the distinction radiographically between blood and stomach content

aspiration is not possible. Figure 4-4 shows a blood aspiration which occurred during intubation. There have been reports of endotracheal tubes being swallowed by infants when the tube was disconnected from its adapter during an attempted tracheal intubation. In one such case, a chest radiograph revealed the tube to be lodged beneath the cricopharyngeal sphincter, extending down the esophagus into the antrum of the stomach (6). Rigid esophagoscopy under general anesthesia was required to remove the swallowed tube. The endotracheal tube can be aspirated into the tracheobronchial tree if dislodged from its connector. This is a startling and potentially fatal complication. One such case required emergency tracheotomy for removal.

Pneumothorax without lung disruption may result from perforation of the trachea, larynx, pharynx, or esophagus. Air may dissect along the fascial planes of the neck and reach the chest, resulting in pneumothorax and lung collapse.

Inadvertent esophageal intubation should be detected at the bedside, before radiographic evidence is obtained. After the endotracheal tube is removed from the esophagus and inserted properly into the trachea, residual gaseous distention of the stomach may be obvious radiographically.

Bronchial intubation is one of the more common complications of endotracheal intubation. When the endotracheal tube is inserted too far into the trachea it will usually slip into the right mainstem bronchus, since the right bronchus comes off the trachea at a less acute angle than the left. Bronchial intubation can usually be recognized by asymmetry of chest wall movement and by absent or diminished breath sounds over half of the chest. It is remedied by withdrawing the tube from the bronchus, to a tracheal position. Endotracheal tubes should ideally be placed 2–3 cm above the carina, as measured radiographically. Figure 4-5a shows an endotracheal tube in the right mainstem bronchus, and Figure 4-5b shows the tube repositioned in the midtrachea 2–3 cm above the carina. The chest should be auscultated immediately after tube placement and periodically thereafter as well, especially whenever the patient's position is changed. After endotracheal intubation in a critically ill patient, a chest radiograph is obtained. This is done to confirm the midtracheal position of the tube and to exclude any of the previously discussed traumatic complications that may be radiographically apparent.

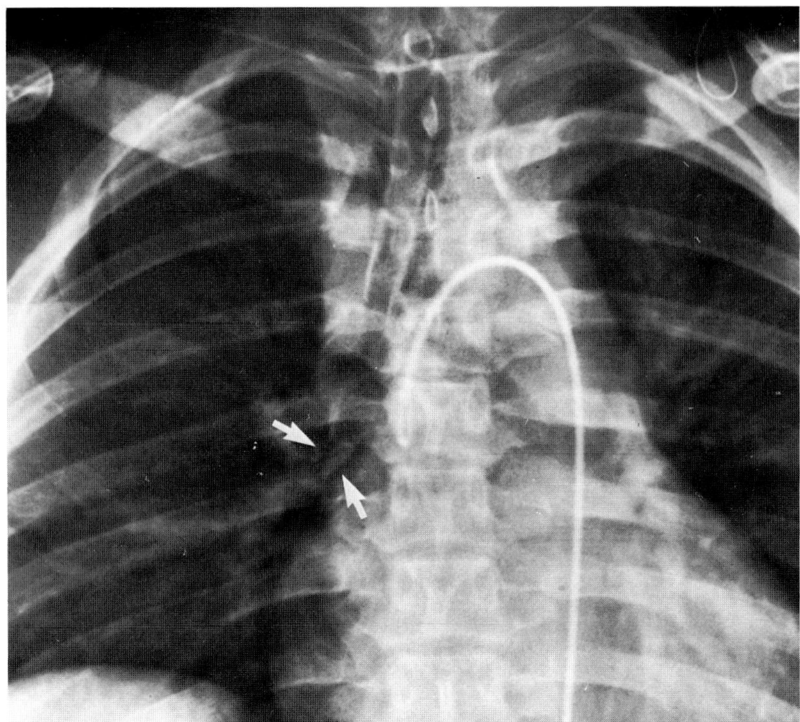

Fig. 4-3. Tooth fragment in right mainstem bronchus. Film from an arteriogram following a motor vehicle accident shows a radiodensity in the right mainstem bronchus just at the takeoff of the upper lobe bronchus (*arrows*). Intubation was difficult and it was not certain at what point the tooth was aspirated. Endotracheal tube is placed too low, ending at the origin of the right mainstem bronchus.

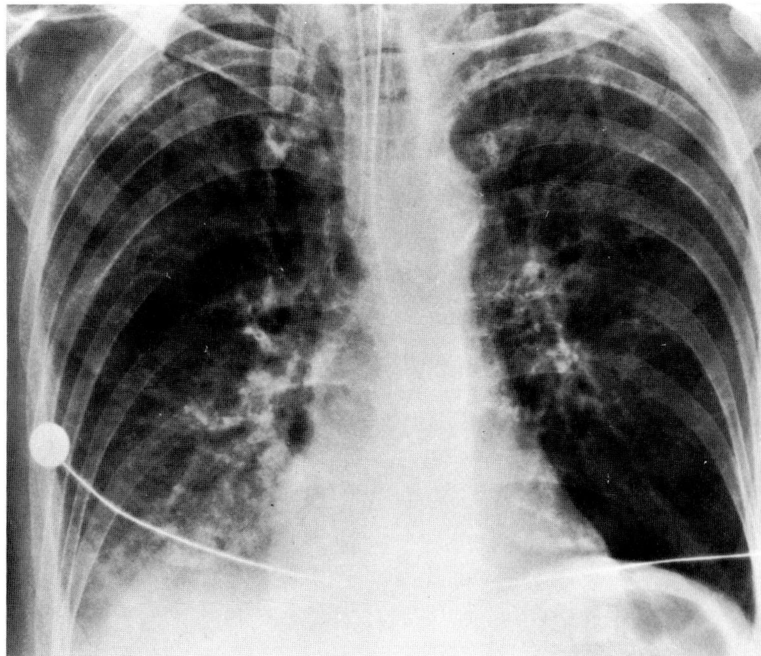

Fig. 4-4. Blood aspiration pneumonia. There is a patchy infiltrate involving the right lower lobe with obliteration of the right hemidiaphgram on this PA chest radiograph. The infiltrate developed as a result of blood aspiration following tracheal rupture due to tracheostomy cuff overdistention. The right side is more often involved in aspiration pneumonia, as the right mainstem bronchus forms a straighter angle with the trachea.

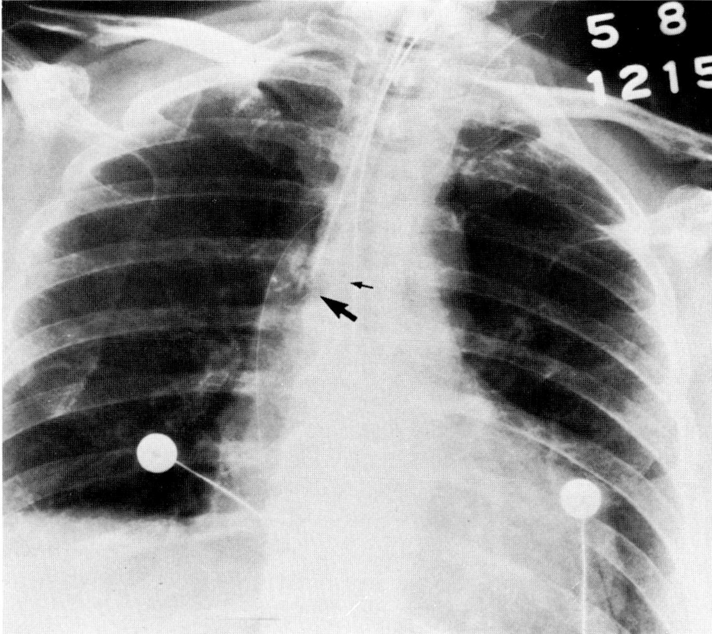

a

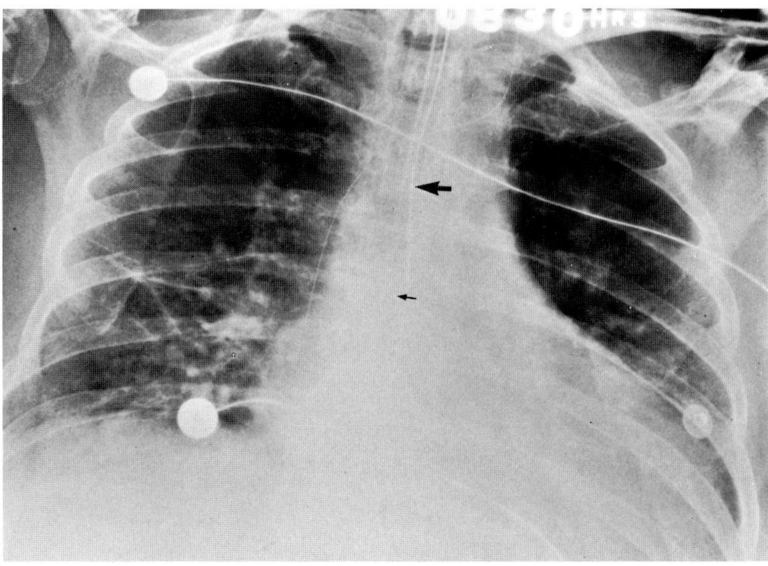

b

Fig. 4-5. a Right endobronchial intubation. This portable chest radiograph demonstrates right endobronchial intubation. Arrows mark the end of the endotracheal tube (*large arrow*) and the carina (*small arrow*).

b Proper endotracheal tube position. Large arrow denotes the end of the tube properly placed 2–3 cm above the carina (*small arrow*).

Early Complications That Occur with Tube in Place

After the endotracheal tube has been successfully placed and secured, the risk of complications persist. Many of the complications that can occur during this period are the same as those that occur during the act of intubation. These include rupture of the trachea or bronchus, the development of subcutaneous emphysema and/or pneumothorax, as well as a potential risk of aspiration pneumonia.

Tracheobronchial rupture is certainly one of the most serious complications of endotracheal intubation. This complication has been associated with predisposing pathologic changes in the major airways and traumatic intubation; however, albeit rarely, tracheobronchial rupture has occurred in the absence of trauma (7). The use of a double-lumen endotracheal tube for selective bronchial intubation may increase the risk of tracheobronchial rupture. Guernelli et al. (8) reported 5 such cases in a series of 2700 intubations with a double-lumen Carlen endotracheal tube. The most common site of rupture in their series was the distal portion of the trachea and the left main bronchus. The most common sign was an inexhaustible pneumothorax.

Finally, with the tube in place and the cuff inflated, it is important to keep in mind that aspiration can still occur (9). This may explain the sudden appearance of a new infiltrate in a dependent area of the lung even days after the placement of the endotracheal tube.

Late Complications of Tracheal Intubation

Various late complications of translaryngeal intubation can occur; however, we will limit our discussion to problems related to damage of tracheal structures.

After extubation, the most common complications are hoarseness and dysphagia, usually of short (less than 24 hours) duration. Pathologic changes, which include abrasions of the mucosa in the supraglottic, glottic, and subglottic regions, have been reported and can lead to serious complications. The least incidence of damage is in patients intubated for less than 48 hours (10). Frequently the mucosal damage is in the supraglottic region, manifested by edema and swelling. Granulation tissue may form in these regions, further complicating the course. Occasionally these changes may be detected on lateral films of the neck as well as by lateral xerograms of the cervical region.

Persistent tracheal dilatation can occur after intubation and may occur within 48 hours of intubation (11). This complication is less frequent now with the widespread use of low-pressure, high-compliance, soft-cuffed endotracheal tubes. Acute tracheal dilatation can be recognized radiographically. It is incumbent upon the radiologist to make this diagnosis. The need for increasing amounts of air inflation into the endotracheal tube cuff to maintain a seal is found concomitantly with the radiographic finding. The diagnosis is important because the lesion is asymptomatic but may predispose to aspiration, dysphagia, tracheal rupture, tracheomalacia, or tracheoesophageal fistula. If the trachealis muscle or cartilages are damaged, malacia is likely to persist and may be present for years after extubation.

The primary factor in the development of persistent tracheal dilatation is excessive pressure from the cuff against the tracheal wall. This pressure may be transmitted by a low-compliance cuff or overinflation of a high-compliance cuff. A minimal-leak technique should be used when inflating endotracheal tube cuffs: The cuff is inflated until no air or gas is heard escaping through the airway from around the tube on application of positive pressure. It is then slowly deflated until a barely audible air escape is heard; the cuff is then maintained in this volume.

The diameter of the endotracheal tube cuff and the diameter of the trachea can be measured on radiographs. It has been shown that the ratio of the endotracheal tube cuff diameter to the tracheal diameter may be valuable in the early prediction of severe tracheal damage (12). Marked tracheal damage was found only in those patients who had a cuff diameter to trachea diameter (C/T) ratio above 1.5. Figure 4-6 illustrates a radiograph with a C/T ratio greater than 1.5. It seems prudent to measure on the radiograph, and to record, the C/T ratio whenever chest radiographs are obtained on intubated critically ill patients. A C/T ratio of higher than 1.5 requires a) decreasing the cuff pressure, b) changing the tube, c) decreasing the cuff volume, d) early extubation or decannulation, and e) after extubation, follow-up with a suspicion of possible tracheal damage.

Tracheal stenosis is a complication that may occur with both translaryngeal intubation and tracheostomy and will be discussed under complications of tracheostomy.

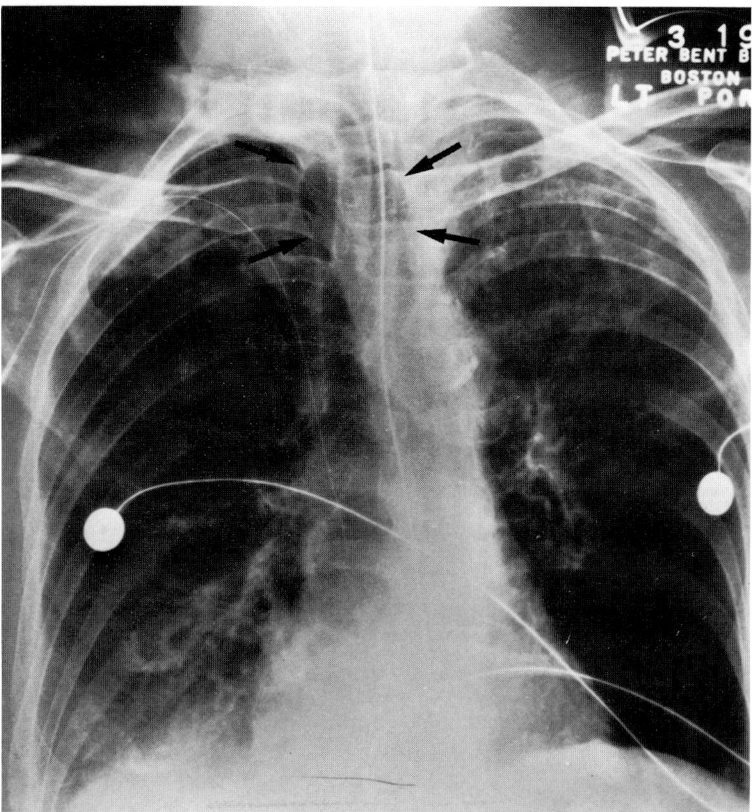

Fig. 4-6. Tracheostomy cuff overdistention. The cuff is markedly distended (*arrows*), with a cuff-to-trachea ratio in excess of 3.0. This patient went on to develop a traumatic tracheoesophageal fistula, one of the common sequelae of traumatic tracheal rupture.

Tracheotomy

The complications of tracheotomy can be divided into immediate and delayed complications.

Immediate Complications

The immediate complications of tracheotomy that are of import to the radiologist include an obstructed displaced tube, subcutaneous emphysema, pneumothorax and pneumomediastinum, aspiration, atelectasis, and tracheoesophageal fistula. The overall incidence of these and other complications varies from 6.7% to 48%. In adults the most frequent complications are hemorrhage (3.7%), tube obstruction (2.7%), and tube displacement

(1.5%). However, in children, pneumothorax (4.3%), tube displacement (2.0%), and subcutaneous emphysema are most frequent (13).

Subcutaneous emphysema localized in the neck is a common finding after tracheotomy. Usually the air remains in the neck, but it may spread to involve the face, neck, and abdominal wall, thus becoming quite apparent on routine chest or abdominal films. Subcutaneous emphysema is not a serious problem and usually requires no therapy. If present, however, it should raise the suspicion that air may also be present in the chest.

Pneumomediastinum after tracheotomy is caused by air that dissects through the fascial planes of the neck to enter the mediastinum. Vigorous ventilatory efforts, both spontaneous and with positive-pressure ventilation, may force air escaping around the tube into the tissue planes of the neck and into the mediastinum. Extensive dissection of pretracheal fascia during tracheotomy may also predispose to development of pneumomediastinum. As with subcutaneous emphysema, pneumomediastinum usually is not a serious complication, but if excessive it may rupture the pleura, leading to pneumothorax with its complications.

Another mechanism, producing pneumothorax during tracheotomy, is more common in infants and children. In these young patients, the domes of the pleura reach the base of the neck, making them vulnerable to inadvertent trauma during tracheotomy. Routine chest radiography shortly after tracheotomy will detect this complication. It is recommended for all patients.

Aspiration and atelectasis may occur both during tracheotomy and anytime after the procedure. The aspirate may be gastric contents, blood, or crusts that may develop in the trachea or in the tracheostomy tube. As with translaryngeal endotracheal tubes, an inflated cuff helps to reduce the incidence of aspiration, but is not a guarantee against it.

A tracheoesophageal fistula can develop if at the time of tracheotomy the posterior tracheal wall is penetrated and the esophagus entered. The risk of this complication is lessened if tracheotomy is done with a translaryngeal endotracheal tube previously placed. Tracheoesophageal fistula is a very serious, albeit rare, early complication of tracheotomy.

Delayed Complications

Delayed complications of tracheotomy include hemorrhage, obstruction, aspiration pneumonia, and tracheoesophageal fistula. Figure 4-7 is a barium swallow radiograph showing a tracheoesophageal fistula as a late complication of tracheotomy.

Tracheal stenosis is a delayed complication of tracheotomy or translaryngeal endotracheal intubation. Obstructive granulomas may develop at the level of the tracheostomy stoma. The stenosis is most frequently at the level of the inflatable cuff used to seal the trachea. Between the levels of the stoma and cuff, varying degrees of inflammatory changes can develop, sometimes with irregular narrowing seen on a radiograph. A lesion distal to the position of the cuff can be seen at the site where the tip of the tracheostomy tube has eroded the wall of the trachea. This frequently occurs in children, in whom a cuffless endotracheal tube is often used. Major reconstructive surgery is nec-

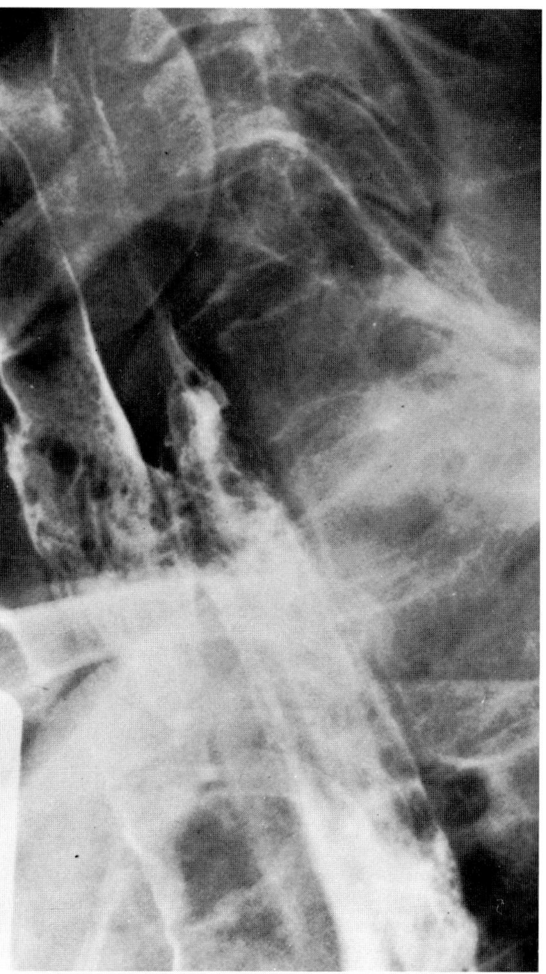

Fig. 4-7. Tracheoesophageal fistula. In this view from a barium swallow, barium is seen in both the trachea and the esophagus, with demonstration of the fistulous tract. The fistula developed as a complication of the overdistention of the tracheostomy tube cuff in Figure 4-6.

essary to repair the resulting stenosis (14). Figure 4-8 shows the common site of tracheal narrowing.

Cardiopulmonary Resuscitation

Multiple complications of cardiopulmonary resuscitation are seen by the radiologist. We shall specifically look at the complications of external cardiac

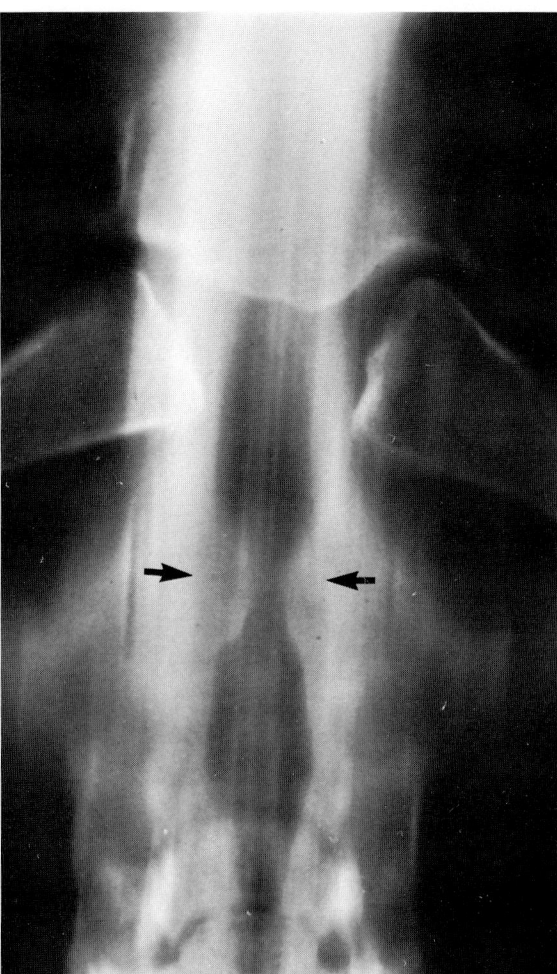

Fig. 4-8. Common site of tracheal stenosis. There is marked narrowing of the tracheal air column (*arrows*) seen on this frontal tomogram of the neck, with a diagnosis of tracheal stenosis. (Courtesy of Massachusetts Eye and Ear Infirmary)

compression. Chest trauma can occur not only with excessive and misplaced compression but also with proper technique. Fractures of the ribs, sternum or spine, flail chest, fat embolization, pulmonary infarction, laceration of lungs, liver, spleen, as well as pneumothorax, hemothorax, and hemopericardium are among the many complications that can occur.

Bony Injuries with Closed-Chest Massage

Among 209 cases that came to autopsy after resuscitative treatment had been started outside the hospital, the overall complication rate was 40%. Bone fractures were present in *36%* of the group. Among 25 patients who sustained a cardiopulmonary arrest while in the hospital and could not be resuscitated, rib fractures were seen in 6, with sternal fractures occurring in one (15). There is little doubt that rib fractures are frequent sequelae of CPR; they should be looked for on postresuscitation radiographs. However, fractures of ribs and sternum can easily be missed on the radiograph. Myocardial imaging using ^{99m}Tc pyrophosphate has been reported to detect, as a side benefit, skeletal trauma after CPR (16).

Flail chest after CPR is not as rare an occurrence as once thought. An incidence of 5.6 per 100 survivors has been reported. There was no difference in age, frequency, and duration of resuscitation between the patients who did have a flail chest after CPR and those who did not have this complication. The occurrence of the flail chest, however, did not seem to contribute to mortality (17).

Barotrauma

Lung disruption or barotrauma is another frequent complication of CPR. Clearly seen on the chest radiograph is the development of pneumothorax. It is caused more often by attempted intracardiac puncture for injection of drugs than by rib fractures. Once recognized, either clinically or radiographically, it is treated by insertion of a chest tube.

Pneumomediastinum may also develop, with or without the presence of a pneumothorax, and is usually benign.

Pneumoperitoneum is a rare complication which may create sufficient intraabdominal pressure to severely compromise ventilation. Recognition of the complication is usually first made by the radiologist. Air may enter the peritoneal cavity by several mechanisms. Rupture of a hollow viscus such as the stomach may occur during the resuscitation attempt. Air penetrating from the pulmonary parenchyma to the mediastinum may dissect within the esophageal wall to the stomach or intestine and enter the peritoneal cavity via the serosal surface of the viscus. Furthermore, pneumomediastinum may lead to retropneumoperitoneum, which can then lead to perforation of the parietal peritoneum, with subsequent pneumoperitoneum.

Pericardial Tamponade

Pericardial tamponade has been reported on several occasions during and after CPR. Most frequently this is associated with intracardiac drug injection. The treatment involves pericardial aspiration. A large cardiac silhouette may be seen on the chest radiograph suggesting a pericardial collection of fluid.

Organ Injury

Injuries to the heart, lung, liver, spleen, and stomach during CPR have all been reported; fortunately they are rare. A rupture of the spleen was recognized 13 days postresuscitation and required emergency splenectomy. When looking at abdominal films in a patient who has undergone resuscitation, an enlarged splenic shadow or a downward displacement of the splenic flexure may be the only initial sign that splenic rupture has occurred (18). Additionally, abdominal ultrasound provides a rapid, efficient means for evaluation of organ rupture, and can be performed at the bedside.

Conclusion

The types of complication that can occur with either endotracheal intubation or cardiopulmonary resuscitation are protean. Many of the unfortunate complications are first discovered by the radiologist when the routine postintubation or post-CPR radiograph is seen. For those wishing further information, the references listed will serve as thorough reviews of the subject.

General References

Applebaum EL, Bruce DL: Tracheal Intubation. Philadelphia: WB Saunders Co, 1976.

Blanc VF, Tremblay NA: The complication of tracheal intubation: a new classification with a review of the literature. Anesth Analg (Cleve) 53:202–213, 1974.

McIntyre KM, et al: Pathophysiologic syndromes of cardiopulmonary resuscitation. Arch Intern Med 138:1130–1133, 1978.

Cited References

1. Heath LK, Peirce TH: Retropharyngeal abscess following endotracheal intubation. Chest 72:776–777, 1977.
2. Hirsch M, et al: Hypopharyngeal injury as a result of attempted endotracheal intubation. Radiology 128:37–39, 1978.
3. Dubost C, et al: Esophageal perforation during attempted endotracheal intubation. J Thorac Cardiovasc Surg 78:44–51, 1979.
4. O'Neill D, Syman DN: Pneumopericarcium and pneumomediastinum complicating endotracheal intubation. Postgrad Med J 55:273–275, 1979.
5. Kumar SM, et al: Tracheal laceration associated with endotracheal anesthesia. Anesthesiology 47:298–299, 1977.
6. Mitchell SA, et al: Deglutition of an endotracheal tube: case report. Anesth Analg (Cleve) 57:590–591, 1978.
7. Patel KD, et al: Mainstem bronchial rupture during general anesthesia. Anesth Analg (Cleve) 58:59–61, 1979.
8. Guernelli N, et al: Tracheobronchial ruptures due to cuffed Carlen's tubes. Ann Thorac Surg 28:66–67, 1979.
9. Menta S: The risk of aspiration in presence of cuffed endotracheal tubes. Br J Anaesth 44:601–605, 1972.
10. Burns HP, et al: Laryngotracheal trauma: observations on its pathogenesis and its prevention following prolonged orotracheal intubation in the adult. Laryngoscope 89:1316–1325, 1979.
11. Honig EG, Francis PB: Persistent tracheal dilatation: onset after brief mechanical ventilation with a "soft-cuff" endotracheal tube. South Med J 72:487–490, 1979.
12. Khan F, Reddy NC: Enlarging intratracheal tube cuff diameter: a quantitative roentgenographic study of the value in the early prediction of serious tracheal damage. Ann Thorac Surg 24:49–53, 1977.
13. Tucker JA, Silberman HD: Tracheostomy in pediatrics. Ann Otol 81:818–824, 1972.
14. Grillo HC: Surgical treatment of post-intubation lesions of the trachea. Acta Chir Belg 76:361–369, 1977.
15. Poulsen H, et al: Discussion on complications of cardiopulmonary resuscitation. Acta Anaesthesiol Scand 29:319–322, 1968.
16. Lockett FC, et al: Detection of bone trauma after cardiopulmonary resuscitation. Md State Med J 26:78–79, 1977.
17. Enarson DA, et al: Flail chest as a complication of cardiopulmonary resuscitation. Heart Lung 6:1020–1022, 1977.
18. Berlinerblau R, et al: Delayed rupture of the spleen after cardiac massage. JAMA 243:364–365, 1980.

5 Thoracic Complications of Respiratory Intensive Care

Gale S. Pasternack and
Charles F. O'Cain

Intensive care units (ICUs) came into being after World War II and were modeled after postoperative recovery rooms. The polio epidemic of the 1950s spurred the growth of ICUs when anesthesiologists in Copenhagen reduced the death rate from 87% to 40% by applying to victims of respiratory paralysis principles learned in the recovery room (30). Today the increased use of mechanical ventilation reflects two trends. First, more poor-risk patients have surgery and require postoperative ventilatory support. Second, with better survival rates of patients treated for acute respiratory failure (ARF), prevention of ARF and early treatment of pulmonary vascular congestion have become frequent indications for artificial ventilation (49).

Although there is little doubt that more patients survive catastrophic illness since the advent of the intensive care unit, complications such as improper placement of catheters and tubes contribute to morbidity and mortality (1,13).

Technical Considerations of Portable Radiography

Physical examination is frequently difficult in the ICU. The radiograph may be the first indicator of malposition or malfunction of diagnostic and therapeutic devices. Unfortunately, bedside radiographs are almost always technically inferior to those obtained in the radiology department. Stationary equipment generates higher kilovoltage and milliamperage, allowing decreased exposure time and less motion degradation. In addition, stationary equipment allows more precise patient positioning, the use of grids as needed, and produces less geometric distortion. The ICU patient is either supine or semierect and usually unable to suspend respiration. The focus-film distance at the bedside is necessarily short. A portable chest film delivers to the patient two to four times the dose of a comparable stationary film (24,25), and the scattered radiation affects physicians, nurses, and other patients. Portable x-ray machines should obtain a well-penetrated chest film with the shortest possible exposure time and with good penetration of the ribs and mediastinum.

Because of the inherently poor quality of bedside radiographs, consistency in technique and positioning must be maintained for better assessment of the patient over a series of examinations. Therefore, it may be desirable to take a baseline or preoperative portable chest x-ray with exposure timed at full inspiration.

Other necessary or desirable ICU imaging equipment includes a portable C-arm fluoroscopy unit for insertion and localization of intravenous pacemakers and pulmonary artery catheters, a gamma camera and portable pulmonary angiographic equipment for the detection of pulmonary embolism at the bedside, and a portable ultrasound unit for evaluation of pleural and pericardial effusions.

Interpretation of films in the ICU calls for modification of the criteria employed for standard erect posteroanterior films. In supine films, artifacts such as apparent widening of the mediastinum, pulmonary venous hypertension, and elevation of the diaphragm are no cause for alarm. Postoperative changes, including subcutaneous emphysema and minimal pleural effusion following thoracotomy, are usual. There must be close correlation of clinical and radiologic findings. A viewing area in the ICU for displaying films on an alternator in temporal sequence provides easy access for both the radiologist and the ICU clinical staff. Daily working conferences will help to maximize diagnostic and therapeutic efficacy.

The interpretation of ICU chest films should answer the following questions: 1) Is the film technically adequate regarding degree of inspiration, rotation, exposure factors, and effective vertical x-ray beam? 2) Are there rib fractures, flail chest? 3) Are the lines and tubes correctly positioned, e.g., is the central venous pressure (CVP) catheter in the superior vena cava or right atrium; is the endotracheal tube at least 2 cm above the carina? 4) Is there pulmonary parenchymal disease, with or without air bronchograms? 5) Is there pulmonary collapse, including retrocardiac density? 6) Is there pleural fluid or elevation of a hemidiaphragm? 7) Is there a pneumothorax (note that the supine position is most unfavorable for detection)? The clinician not only should compare the current radiograph with the immediately previous one but, whenever possible, should review the patient's entire course to avoid missing slowly developing pathology (2).

The utility of routine daily chest x-rays in intubated ICU patients is not well established. In one study, 200 routine ICU chest x-rays were evaluated (26). Seventy-four (37%) were suboptimal or were available too late for rounds. Of the remaining 126 films, 54 (43%) showed worsening of known pathology, development of a new cardiopulmonary abnormality, or unexpected misplacement of an invasive device. Therefore, routine daily chest x-rays were judged valuable in identifying abnormalities in critically ill patients.

Mechanical Ventilation

The treatment of respiratory failure, very generally, consists of establishing an airway, administering O_2, and maintaining adequate alveolar ventilation. Positive-pressure mechanical ventilators, usually volume-cycled, provide assistance until treatment of the underlying cause allows a return to spontaneous breathing. Many thoracic compli-

cations of intensive care result directly from this form of life support.

Intubation

Longer-term mechanical ventilation requires the placement of a cuffed endotracheal tube (ET tube, ETT) of appropriate size to ensure an adequate airway. Nasotracheal tubes are usually more comfortable and more stable in position than are orotracheal tubes, but nasotracheal tubes require greater skill for insertion, whether done "blindly" or under direct laryngoscopic vision with the aid of McGill forceps. In emergencies, orotracheal intubation is faster. When patients have markedly abnormal clotting studies, nasotracheal intubation may cause brisk bleeding from nasopharyngeal trauma.

Upper Airway Trauma

Major injuries of the upper airway during intubation are uncommon but may occur with difficult intubations by unskilled operators under emergency circumstances. Lacerations or perforations of the oropharynx or hypopharynx, which occur especially with the use of a rigid stylet to stiffen the tube, may cause cervical and mediastinal emphysema, hematoma, and occasionally abscess formation. The lateral soft-tissue radiograph of the neck will demonstrate subcutaneous emphysema or a mass separating the trachea from the cervical spine. Laryngeal fracture or unilateral or bilateral cord paralysis may be recognized only following extubation. Foreign bodies, including teeth chipped or broken during the laryngoscopic blade insertion, may lodge in the esophagus or trachea, occasionally requiring endoscopic removal. Facial pain, nasal stuffiness, purulent secretions, or fever following nasotracheal intubation should alert the physician to the possibility of maxillary sinusitis resulting from nasal mucosal edema impeding sinus drainage. Bedside radiographs with horizontal beam may demonstrate air-fluid levels in the paranasal sinuses.

Endotracheal Tube Position

The normal adult trachea is 10–13 cm in length from cricoid cartilage to carina (64). The ideal endotracheal tube position is in the midtrachea, 5–7 cm from the carina with the head in neutral position, which allows a safe margin for tube tip movements. The endotracheal tube moves approximately 2 cm downward with flexion of the neck and 2 cm upward during extension. There is an approximately 1 cm of motion during head rotation (12). When the carina is not visible, examine prior films or approximate its position from the vertebral bodies. On 95% of portable radiographs, the carina projects over T5, T6, or T7 (23). The tip of the ET tube should therefore project at the T2 or T3 level. The position of the chin relative to the vertebrae provides a clue to neck position. The chin is usually projected over T1 or T2 with flexion, at C5 to C6 in the neutral position, and above C4 with neck extension.

Frequent follow-up radiographs will ensure that the tube position has not changed, because of either head and neck motion, patient's coughing, or loss of anchoring at the nose or mouth. The width of the endotracheal tube as seen on the radiograph should be one-half to two-thirds the width of the trachea (48). The inflated cuff should not bulge at the lateral tracheal wall, compress the ETT wall inward, nor deflect the tube bevel toward the lateral tracheal wall.

As many as 10%–15% of intubations result in poor initial position (68). Higher than ideal positioning of the tube risks cuff injury to the larynx or accidental dislodgement of the tube into the oropharynx, with consequential disruption of ventilation, gastric dilatation, and possible aspiration of gastric contents. Lower placement may traumatize the carina or allow migration of the tube into a mainstem bronchus (usually the right, because of the narrower angle of origin and larger size of the right mainstem bronchus). As many as 10% of intubations may be accidental right mainstem intubations (68). Although endobronchial intubation may be diagnosed clinically, the radiograph is often the first indicator of malposition. The early film may show normal aeration. Following the absorption of air in the nonventilated left side, the left lung increases in density, the right lung becomes hyperlucent, and the mediastinum may shift to the left, with right tension pneumothorax or pneumomediastinum (Fig. 5-1). Fifteen percent of patients with right mainstem bronchus intubation develop pneumothorax (68). Occasionally, the right upper lobe will collapse if the tube tip passes the origin of the right upper lobe bronchus (Fig. 5-2). Esophageal intubation with laceration will present radiographically as gastric dilatation, subcutaneous emphysema, and pneumomediastinum. Delayed manifestations include mediastinitis or mediastinal or cervical abscess, with air-fluid levels demonstrable on erect or horizontal-beam radiographs.

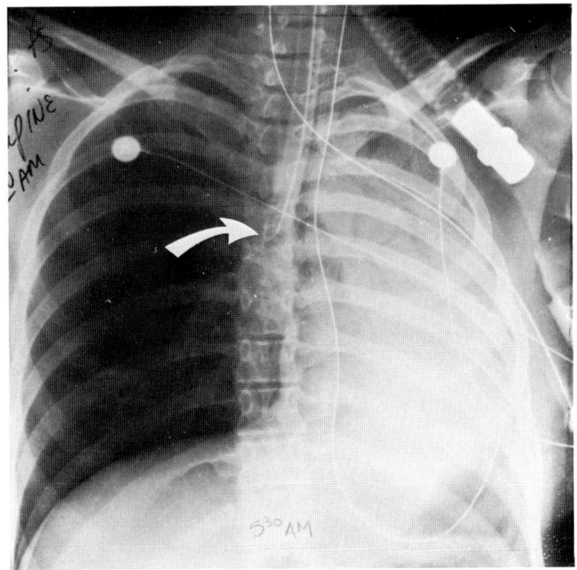

a

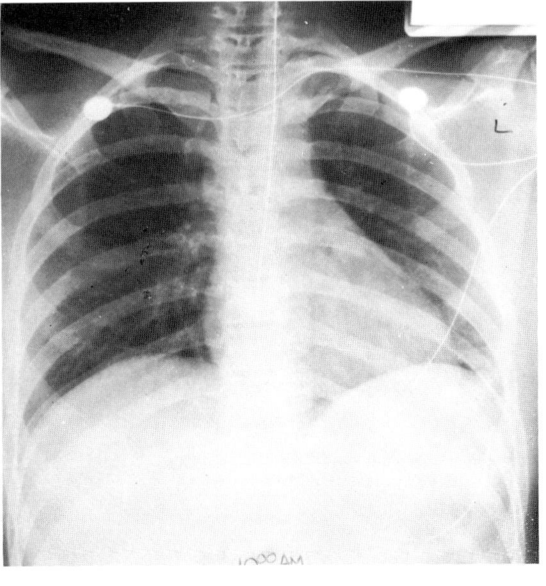

b

Fig. 5-1, a and b. Atelectasis. a Endotracheal tube terminates in the right mainstem bronchus (*arrow*), resulting in complete atelectasis of the left lung. **b** Same patient six hours following extubation with complete reaeration of the left lung. (Courtesy Dr. Paul Spirn, Massachusetts General Hospital)

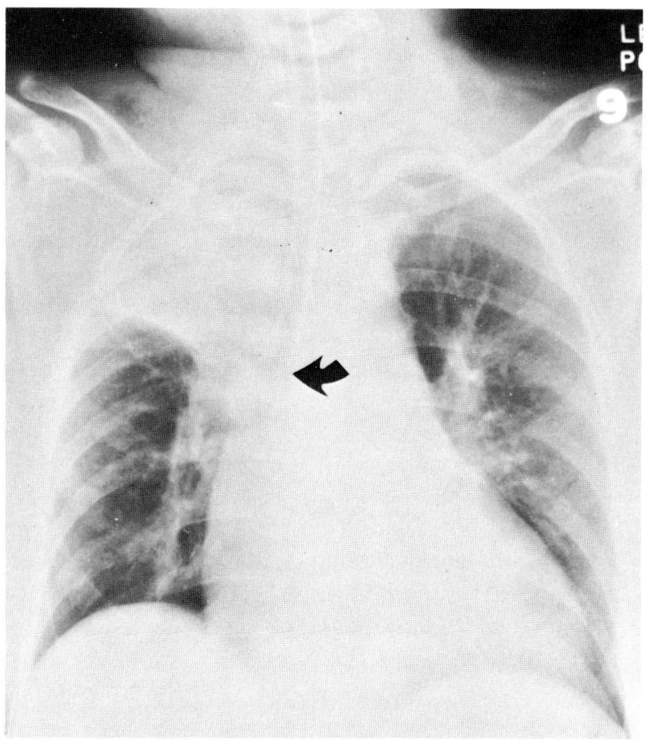

Fig. 5-2. Atelectasis. Endotracheal tube beyond the right upper lobe bronchus (*arrow*), resulting in right upper lobe atelectasis.

Tracheostomy

Most tracheostomies in the intensive care setting are performed following prolonged nasal or oral intubation when continuing ventilator support is required or when ineffectual cough necessitates access for tracheal suctioning.

Position

The tip of the tracheostomy tube should be located one-half to two-thirds the distance between the tracheal stoma and the carina, at about the level of T3. Neck flexion and extension will not affect tube position. The lumen of the tracheostomy tube should be about two-thirds the tracheal diameter and the cuff should hug but not distend the tracheal wall.

The short-term complication rate of tracheostomy has been estimated at 30%–40% and the long-term complication rate as high as 60%; the procedure is thought to cause or contribute to death in 5%–10% of patients with tracheostomies (24). Table 5-1 lists some frequently reported complications.

Immediately following tracheostomy, the radiograph should be checked for tube position and for pneumothorax, pneumomediastinum, and sub-

cutaneous emphysema. A small amount of gas in the neck is not uncommon, but large amounts may signify direct injury to the lung apex or air leakage into subcutaneous tissue during mechanical ventilation when the stoma is too tight. Should the tube be misplaced in the pretracheal soft tissues, subcutaneous and mediastinal air may dissect into

Table 5-1. Tracheostomy Complications

Complication	Manifestation
Operative	
Recurrent laryngeal nerve injury	Unilateral or bilateral vocal cord paralysis
Lung apex injury	Pneumothorax (frequently tension)
Fascial plane disruption	Pneumomediastinum and pneumothorax (frequently tension)
Postoperative	
Infection	Fever, cervical abscess
Tracheoinnominate-artery fistula	Hemoptysis
Tracheoesophageal fistula	Aspiration and gastric distention
Late	
Stricture and granulomas	Dyspnea and stridor

the pleural space, causing bilateral tension pneumothorax. Mediastinal widening in the immediate posttracheostomy setting may portend mediastinal hemorrhage.

Daily radiographs should be obtained early in the course following tracheostomy, then as clinically indicated. Tracheoinnominate-artery fistula is a potentially lethal complication of tracheostomy. If the tube veers to the right and anteriorly, it may erode the innominate artery, resulting in massive fatal hemoptysis in two-thirds of patients. This complication is estimated to occur in approximately 0.7% of all tracheostomy patients. Posterior erosion, resulting in tracheoesophageal, tracheopleural, or tracheomediastinal fistula, can occur in 0.5% of patients with tracheostomies, usually in the second to fourth week following intubation (24).

Late Complications of Intubation

The development of endotracheal tubes made of polyvinyl chloride rather than rubber with high-compliance, low-pressure cuffs has reduced laryngeal and tracheal injuries from 17% to 1% in patients requiring long-term intubation (64). Today, late complications are on the rise because of longer-term mechanical ventilation (10). Injury to the glottis and trachea during intubation produces granuloma formation, tracheal stenosis, tracheomalacia, and rarely perforation (39). After extubation, approximately 5%–15% of patients develop clinically significant tracheal obstruction occurring at the level of the stoma, the level of the inflatable cuff, or rarely where the tip of the tracheostomy tube impinges on the mucosa (25). Necrosis of the tracheal wall develops when lateral wall pressure on the trachea at the cuff site exceeds capillary perfusion pressure (Fig. 5-3). Histologic inflammatory changes are seen at 24–48 hours, and mucosal ulceration can occur within one week (64). With continued insult there may be fragmentation and loss of cartilage, granulation tissue with granuloma formation (Figs. 5-4, 5-5), or fibrosis with stricture. Narrowing may be fixed, as by circumferential scarring, or dynamic, when the supporting cartilage is destroyed. Symptoms of upper airway obstruction may occur within the first few months after extubation or may arrive years later.

While the high-compliance, low-pressure endotracheal tube cuffs have diminished the incidence of tracheal stenosis and tracheoesophageal fistulas, the possibility of introducing a nasogastric tube into the tracheobronchial tree has emerged as a new hazard (58). Futhermore, the high-volume, low-pressure tracheal cuffs, properly inflated, may not prevent aspiration of orotracheal contents if the net hydrostatic gradient is appropriate for lungward migration of fluid.

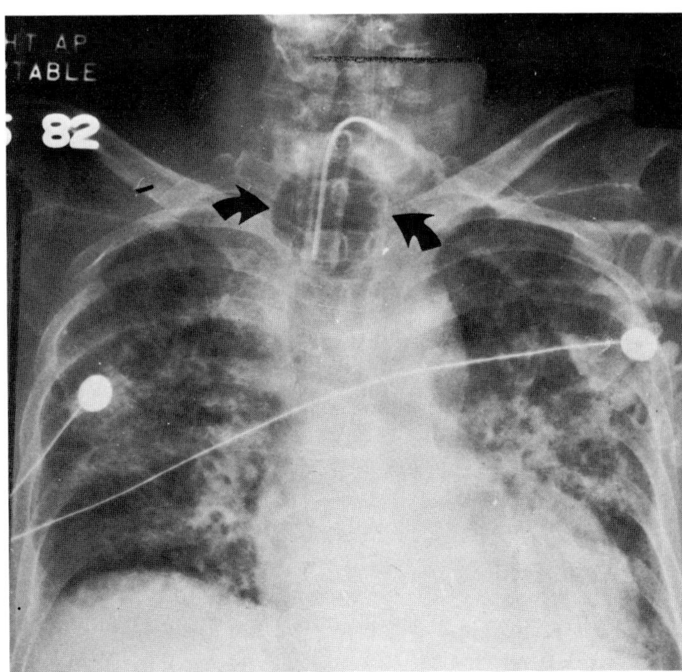

Fig. 5-3. Tracheal wall necrosis. Following long-term tracheostomy, there is necrosis of the tracheal wall. Note that the balloon (*arrows*) is three times wider than the native trachea.

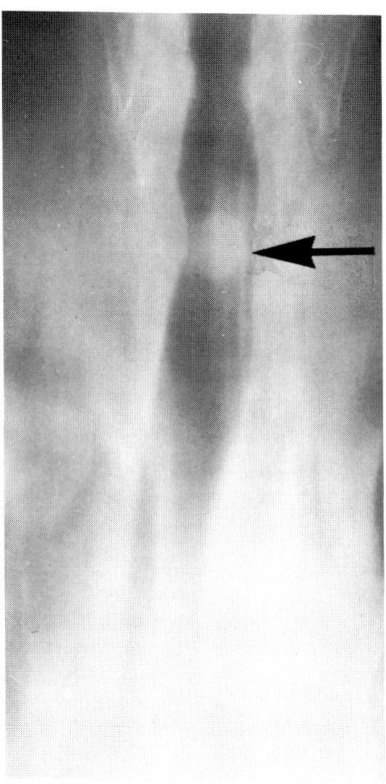

Fig. 5-4. Postintubation granuloma. Tracheal tomogram several months following intubation shows a round soft-tissue shadow (*arrow*). Histologically it represented granuloma secondary to previous tracheal injury. (Courtesy of Dr. Phillip Costello, New England Deaconess Hospital)

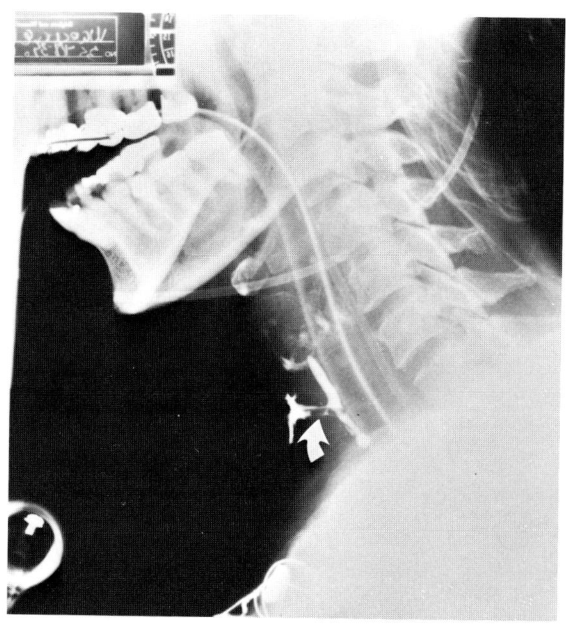

Fig. 5-5. Persistent tracheocutaneous fistula following the removal of a tracheostomy tube. Contrast material shows the fistulous tract (*arrow*). Orotracheal tube is in place.

Complications of PEEP

Patients with acute respiratory failure (ARF) typically ventilate their lungs with small (250–400 ml) tidal volumes without intermittent hyperinflation, or "sighs," and thus develop alveolar collapse and airway closure with consequential hypoxemia. Mechanical ventilation using tidal volumes of 10–15 ml/kg and periodic "sighs" prevents atelectasis and positive end-expiratory pressure (PEEP) and further improves oxygenation in patients with acute respiratory failure, particularly those with adult respiratory distress syndrome (ARDS), pulmonary edema, and atelectasis. A pressure-sensitive valve elevates intrapulmonary pressure at end-expiration, increasing the end-expiratory lung volume (FRC). Thus collapsed airways and underventilated alveoli open, so that arterial oxygenation improves, the work of breathing is decreased, and inspired oxygen concentration can be lowered. Areas of atelectasis open, and interstitial edema returns to the vascular space.

The appearance on the chest x-ray often improves dramatically within hours. This apparent clearing is related to the increased lung volume produced by PEEP and does not necessarily imply physiologic improvement. Pulmonary infiltrates are spread over a larger lung volume, appearing to have regressed, and the diaphragm may appear to be lower. Thus PEEP frequently alters the size or sharpness of pulmonary vessels, the silhouette sign, and the apparent size of the heart and mediastinum. When the patient is weaned, radiographic appearance may deteriorate dramatically because of reduction in lung volume (3,42,67).

Knowledge of ventilator settings is vital in evaluating the severity of infiltration in patients with ARF. It may be necessary on occasion to alter the respirator settings in order to expose comparable films when following the progress of an infiltrate on serial radiographs.

Barotrauma

This topic is discussed in detail elsewhere in Chapter 6.

Five to fifteen percent of patients receiving positive-pressure therapy develop complications of pulmonary barotrauma—pneumothorax, pneumomediastinum, subcutaneous emphysema, or other extraalveolar air collections (37,55,68). Most ventilator-induced barotrauma begins with interstitial pulmonary emphysema (IPE) which occurs when the pressure or relative distention of the alveoli exceeds that in the adjacent interstitium. Alveoli near the pulmonary vessels and interlobular septa rupture, allowing air to dissect along the perivascular sheaths and septa centrally toward the lung hilus and peripherally toward the pleura (65). Air may enter the pleura directly via a preexisting bulla, bleb, pneumatocele, or abscess; thus patients with preexisting lung disease are at a high risk. In the setting of trauma or surgery, the visceral pleura may rupture and communicate with a distal pulmonary airspace.

Extraalveolar air must be recognized promptly to prevent either sudden or progressive respiratory and cardiovascular collapse. Mortality increases significantly with delay in diagnosis (59). Hypertension and cyanosis or increased ventilatory resistance in the presence of a worsening clinical state may herald a pneumothorax. McLoud et al. (43) have found elevation of pulmonary artery pressure to be a useful clinical sign of pulmonary barotrauma. Radiographic examination is usually required to confirm the diagnosis.

It is difficult or impossible to see IPE against a well-aerated lung, but it may become visible when surrounded by parenchymal density in adults with ARDS, extensive pneumonia, edema, hemorrhage, or atelectasis. The direct signs of IPE are subpleural air cysts or bullae, most frequent around the lung hila but best recognized along the inferior or anterior aspects of the lung or fissures (55). Air cysts may coexist with indirect signs of IPE, such as pneumomediastinum and pneumothorax. Indirectly visualized, interstitial air appears as generalized, irregular mottling in the medial half to two-thirds of the lungs, with lucencies occasionally measuring up to 2–3 cm in diameter. IPE changes rapidly and may disappear within one or two days or may progress to subpleural air cyst formation, pneumomediastinum, or pneumothorax. IPE collections are differentiated from air bronchograms in that they are irregular and do not taper. They may also be confused with necrotizing bronchopneumonia and consolidation in a lung with previously existing emphysema. Extensive IPE may make the lung appear better aerated while actually causing further impairment of the lung (65).

Pneumothorax

Pneumothorax is the most frequently recognized manifestation of extraalveolar air in patients on ventilators. Mechanical ventilation tends to perpetuate an air leak once it has developed and often causes a rapid increase in the size and severity of a pneumothorax. Sixty-seven to 97% of pneumothoraces in ventilated patients are under tension (59,68). Because of positive airway pressure used in ventilation, little if any shift of the mediastinum will occur, even in the presence of significant tension. Depression of a hemidiaphragm is a more reliable sign than mediastinal shift (27).

In the supine patient, air rises anteriorly and may not be seen at all or may mimic a pneumomediastinum or pneumopericardium as it accumulates along the medial pleural space. The best places to search are the most ventral portions of the lower thorax along the juxtacardiac area, the lateral chest wall, and the base. With previous pleural scarring, pneumothorax may remain encapsulated at the lung base even in the erect position (27) (Fig. 5-6). When pneumothorax in a supine patient outlines the anterior costophrenic sulcus, an abrupt curvilinear lucency projects over the right or left upper quadrant. The anterior parietal pleural reflection runs laterally from the 7th

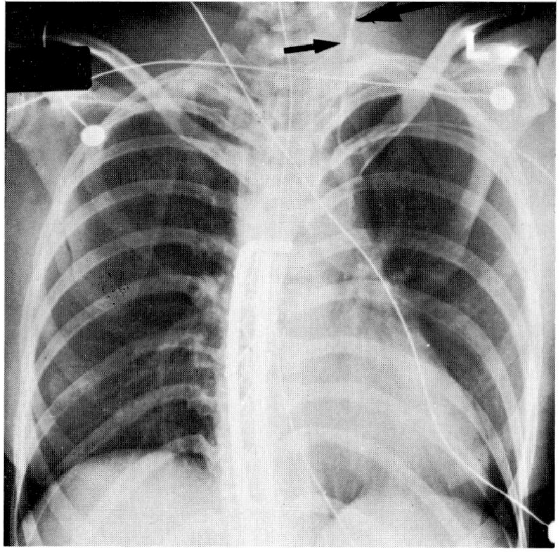

Fig. 5-6. Localized pneumothorax at the lung base (*arrow*). Note also that the central venous pressure line, inserted from the left arm, terminates in the left internal jugular vein (*arrows*).

costal cartilage to the midaxillary line at the level of the 11th rib and is convex inferiorly (52). If lucency of the upper quadrant is seen, the cross-table lateral or decubitus film with the side in question elevated confirms the diagnosis and allows estimation of the side of the pneumothorax. Whenever possible, an upright expiratory radiograph, cross-table lateral or decubitus, should be exposed when pneumothorax is suspected.

The final distribution of free pleural air represents the net result of effects due to gravity, the lung hinge mechanism, and the recoil characteristics of the lung and chest wall (38). Thus the lung normally swings posteromedially when air collects anteromedially, accounting for several useful signs of pneumothorax in the supine patient: visibility of the anterior costophrenic sulcus, hyperlucent lung, paramediastinal lucency, and enhanced sharpness of the ipsilateral mediastinal contour. With further accumulation anteriorly, there may be separation of the lateral surface of the lung from the parietal pleura. Posteromedial pneumothorax has recently been described in the presence of lobar collapse. This unusual distribution illustrates the principle that air tends to accumulate in those parts of the pleural space that overlie collapsed lung. Thus, abnormalities of the pleura such as adhesions may also force air to accumulate in atypcial positions.

Factors that increase the incidence of pneumothorax during continuous ventilatory support in-

clude volume-cycled as opposed to pressure-regulated ventilators; chronic obstructive pulmonary disease; excessive tidal volumes; increased end-expiratory pressures; PEEP; and percutaneous subclavian venipuncture during pressure ventilation (59). Beware of skin folds, bandages, and other artifacts which may mimic a pneumothorax.

Pneumomediastinum

In pneumomediastinum occurring after surgery, trauma, or infection, air may reach the mediastinum by dissecting along tissue planes from the neck or retroperitoneum. However, in the patient on a respirator, the pathway involves alveolar rupture and interstitial air dissection. The radiographs will demonstrate sharp lucencies around the heart and mediastinum and concomitant subcutaneous emphysema (Fig. 5-7). More subtle findings include a crescent of air outlining the aortic knob or descending aorta; a lucent stripe between the lung base and the diaphragm underlining the heart across the midline; or a sharp, lucent line on lateral views outlining the ascending aorta, great vessels, and prevertebral soft tissues. Again, subcutaneous air in the neck or retroperitoneum confirms the diagnosis of pneumomediastinum.

Pneumopericardium

Air enters the pericardium after surgery, trauma, or infection, and presents as a lucent rim around the heart which extends only as high as the great vessels on the upright radiograph. On the supine radiograph, however, pneumopericardium may masquerade as pneumothorax or pneumomediastinum. A lateral decubitus or horizontal-beam lateral film will provide the answer.

Subcutaneous Emphysema

Pulmonary barotrauma or local trauma such as tracheostomy or surgery may produce linear lucencies outlining the tissue planes or bubbles in the soft tissues. In the presence of a thoracostomy drainage tube, increasing subcutaneous air may signal tube malfunction or the development of a bronchopleural fistula.

Extrathoracic Gas

Retroperitoneal extraalveolar air can develop in patients with pneumomediastinum when air dis-

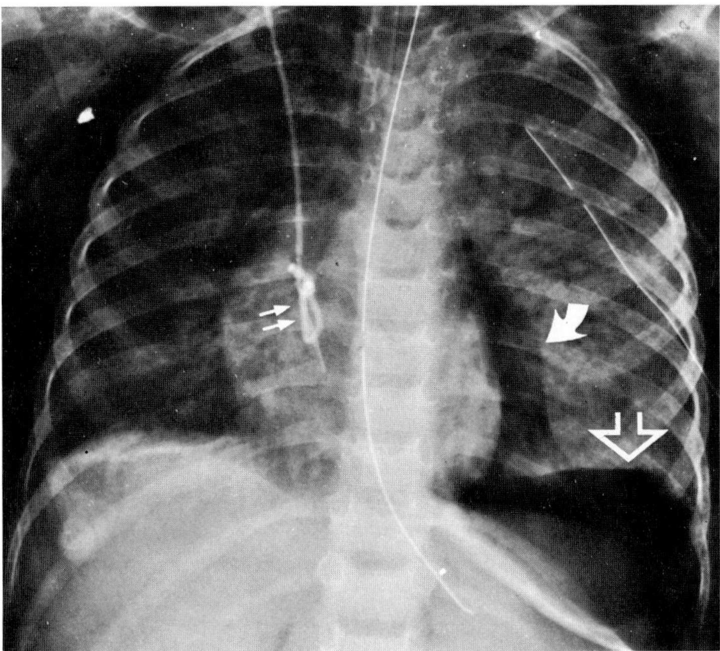

Fig. 5-7. Pneumomediastinum. Five-year old child following extensive abdominal cancer surgery. Patient is on the ventilator. Note pneumomediastinum along the left heart border (*solid arrow*), infrapulmonary pneumothorax (*hollow arrow*), and subcutaneous emphysema. A CVP line is knotted in the right atrium (*double arrows*).

sects downward along fascial planes surrounding the aorta and esophagus (55). Free intraperitoneal air in mechanically ventilated patients is less well understood. It has been postulated that mediastinal and retroperitoneal air dissects along the aorta and mesenteric vessels into the subserosa of the bowel at the point of vascular penetration and ruptures into the peritoneal cavity (55,60,65).

Unnecessary laparotomies have resulted when streaks of gas below the diaphragm are mistakenly attributed to visceral perforation. Retroperitoneal air appears as crescentic collections over the dome and lateral aspects of the liver extending into the flanks. Free intraperitoneal air, on the other hand, is more centrally located, less crescentic, and demonstrates a flat, inferior margin or an air-fluid level. Unlike retroperitoneal air, pneumoperitoneum freely changes with patient position. Clinical history and concomitant pneumomediastinum help to distinguish ventilator-related extraalveolar air from air due to perforation of a viscus.

Chest Tubes

Closed-thoracostomy tubes are used to evacuate pneumothoraces and to drain pleural effusions, particularly empyemas and hemothoraces. The tubes should be anterosuperior for a pneumothorax and posteroinferior for a hydrothorax. Radiographs following tube insertion or manipulation verify position. At times a horizontal-beam lateral radiograph best defines tube position relative to an air or fluid collection. When adhesions or loculations present a problem, ultrasound may guide tube placement. Malfunction of a chest tube may result from kinking, plugging by debris, or inadvertent extrapleural placement. The side hole, usually identified by a discontinuity in the radiopaque stripe, may be a clue to extrathoracic placement.

The tract of a chest tube, once removed, may appear as parallel pleural scars (Fig 5-8). Rarely, entrapment and focal lung infarction caused by chest tube aspiration of pulmonary tissue can be demonstrated (57).

Infection

Endotracheal intubation for mechanical ventilation bypasses or interferes with normal upper airway filters and ciliary activity of the trachea and bronchi and invites colonization of the pharynx and trachea with pathogenic organisms. Purulent

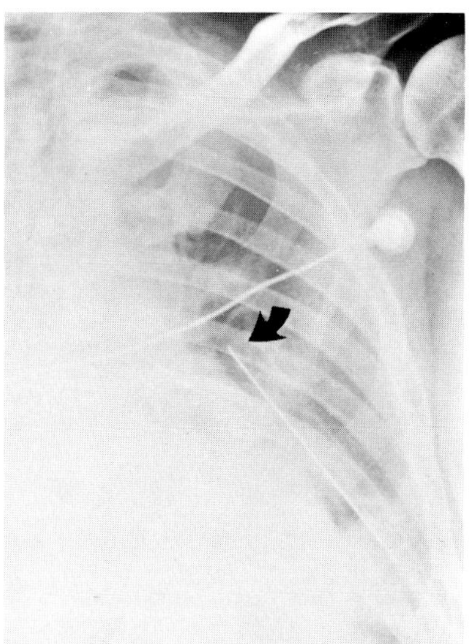
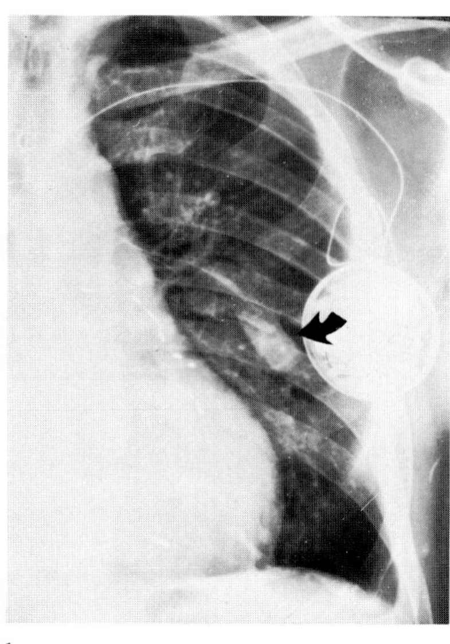

a   b

Fig. 5-8, a and b. Pleural scar from chest tube. a Left-sided chest tube in place (*arrow*). Note left pleural effusion. **b** Same patient five years later. Note pleural scar corresponding to the location of the previous chest tube (*arrow*).

tracheitis or pneumonia ensues in 10%–20% of patients (24). Nosocomial infection in the intensive care setting most often involves gram-negative enteric organisms (4). This subject is discussed elsewhere in this book. Since cultures from the airways are almost always positive due to colonization, a positive sputum culture does not necessarily mean pneumonia. Furthermore, the clinical and radiographic picture may be confounded by atelectasis and retained secretions. Serial gram stains and sputum cultures and occasionally fiberoptic bronchoscopy document changes in the respiratory flora.

Oxygen Toxicity

This complication was recognized by Winter and Smith (66) in 1897. Prolonged exposure to high concentrations of oxygen can produce interstitial and intraalveolar edema, hemorrhage, and hyaline membranes as well as other nonspecific responses similar to those described in acute respiratory failure. Oxygen toxicity is both time- and concentration-dependent. Many patients can tolerate oxygen concentrations of less than 40% over long periods of time without apparent risks, and some patients tolerate concentrations of 60% for sustained periods without apparent damage. In general, patients should be ventilated at the lowest oxygen concentration capable of maintaining an arterial hemoglo-

bin saturation of 90%. In the chronically hypoxemic patient, wisdom may dictate an arterial oxygen concentration in the hypoxemic range. Other maneuvers may serve to increase arterial O_2 tension at a given inspired concentration: optimal ventilatory patterns, fluid restriction, maintenance of electrolyte balance, and the institution of PEEP in the ventilatory cycle. There is no significant toxicity in man breathing pure oxygen for 24 hours or less. Thereféore, oxygen should not be withheld in emergency situations (16,48,66).

Pathologic and radiographic features of oxygen toxicity fall into the category of ARDS and are nonspecific. The radiograph demonstrates a diffuse alveolar or interstitial process. Congestive heart failure, pulmonary edema, aspiration pneumonia, severe infection, lung contusion, pulmonary embolism, and fat emboli produce the same findings.

Cardiovascular Catheters

Central venous pressure (CVP) monitoring via an intravenous catheter simplifies the task of maintaining optimal blood volume in patients in whom multiorgan failure obscures the usual physical signs. CVP measurement directly reflects right atrial pressure, which, in turn, reflects right and

Table 5-2. Complications of Central Vein Catheters

Related to site of approach:

	Common	Uncommon
Subclavian	Pneumothorax	Brachial plexus injury
	Subclavian artery puncture	Arteriovenous fistula
	Air embolus	
Internal jugular	Carotid artery puncture	Phrenic nerve injury
	Air embolus	Thoracic duct laceration
	Pneumothorax	
Arm vein	Infection	
	Catheter movement	

Unrelated to site of approach:

Sepsis
Catheter embolus
Thrombosis
Central vein perforation
   hemo/hydrothorax
   hemo/hydromediastinum

left ventricular end-diastolic pressure and volume. Pressures greater than 15 cm of water suggest cardiac failure, tamponade, or hypervolemia. Pressures below 4 cm of water suggest hypovolemia. Central venous catheters also provide a means for administration of medications and for hyperalimentation, since central veins offer more reliable flow than do peripheral veins, which are more likely to constrict during cardiovascular collapse. (Table 5-2.)

Techniques of placement of central catheters include peripheral venipuncture, with the use of long catheters, internal and external jugular venipuncture, and subclavian puncture by supraclavicular or infraclavicular approaches. The subclavian and internal jugular approaches are most popular because of the relatively constant anatomy and because catheters so used are shorter and cross no moving joints, thus minimizing changes in catheter position after initial placement.

The catheter tip should lie within the true central venous system, between the right atrium and the most proximal venous valves, in order to accurately reflect pressures within the central venous system. The most proximal valves are found in the subclavian vein and in the internal jugular vein approximately 2.5 cm from their junction to form the brachiocephalic vein. The last valve in the subclavian vein is at about the level of the first rib anteriorly (51). Proper position on x-ray is therefore medial to the anterior portion of the first rib at the junction of the brachiocephalic vein and the superior vena cava or within the superior vena cava itself.

After any attempt at catheter placement, successful or not, obtain a radiograph to exclude a pneumothorax, effusion, or hematoma (Fig. 5-9). The rate of pneumothorax at the time of insertion is 1.2%–10% (63), and prospective studies have shown that approximately one-third of CVP catheters are incorrectly placed at the time of initial insertion. The most common aberrant locations include the internal jugular vein (Fig. 5-6), azygos vein (Fig. 5-10), right atrium or right ventricle, or various extrathoracic locations (Fig. 5-11), including the upper extremities or the hepatic veins (15,24,40).

Catheter malposition can cause dangerous mechanical complications as well as unreliable CVP readings. The catheter tip can perforate the right atrium, and rapidly fatal cardiac tamponade may develop with continued infusion of fluid through the catheter into the pericardial space following perforation (14). Right ventricular position of the catheter can induce cardiac arrhythmias or perforation. Perforation is more likely with the use of a rigid catheter, which can puncture an area of weakened myocardium. With ectopic CVP catheters, potentially toxic substances such as hyperalimentation solutions may infuse into the heart or mediastinum. Fluid infusion through a catheter that has perforated into the mediastinum or pleura may result in radiographic findings identical with those of intrathoracic hemorrhage. Mediastinal widening with occasional obscuration of the aortic knob and widening of the paramediastinal lines, tracheal displacement, and the left apical cap sign may mimic an aortic laceration from blunt deceler-

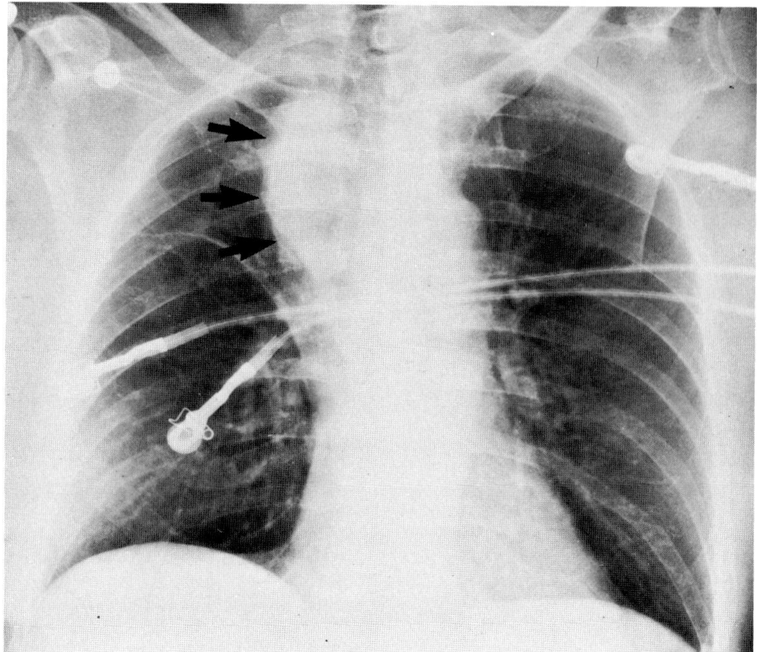

Fig. 5-9. Postcatheterization hematoma. Radiograph obtained following an attempted placement of a central venous line in the right subclavian vein. Note the large paratracheal hematoma (*arrows*), which was not present previously. (Courtesy of Dr. Phillip Costello, New England Deaconess Hospital)

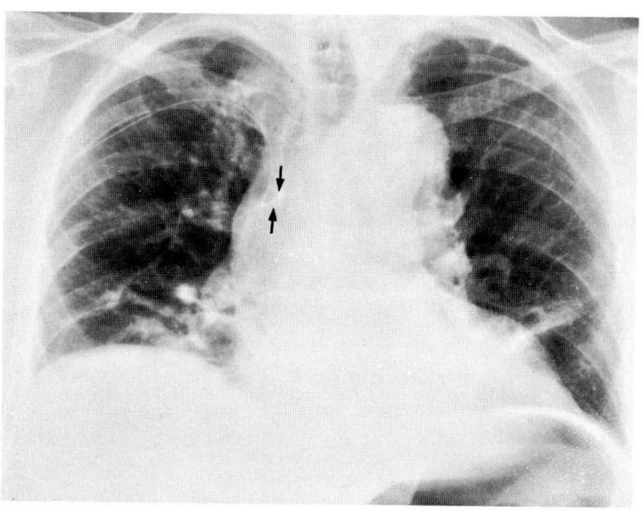

a

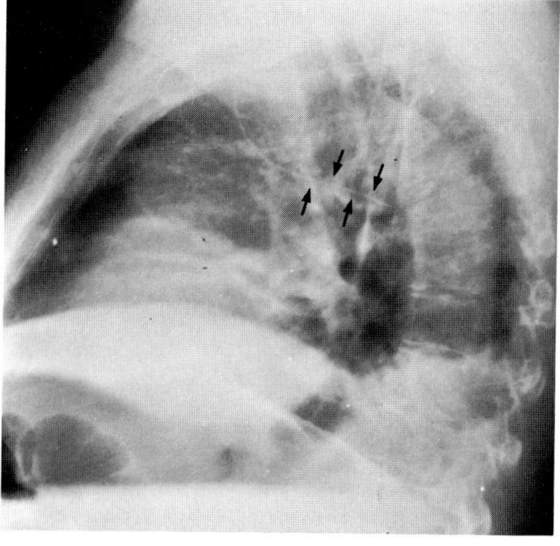

b

Fig. 5-10, a and b. Central venous pressure line terminating in the azygos vein (*arrows*). Note in **b** the posterior orientation of the azygos arch.

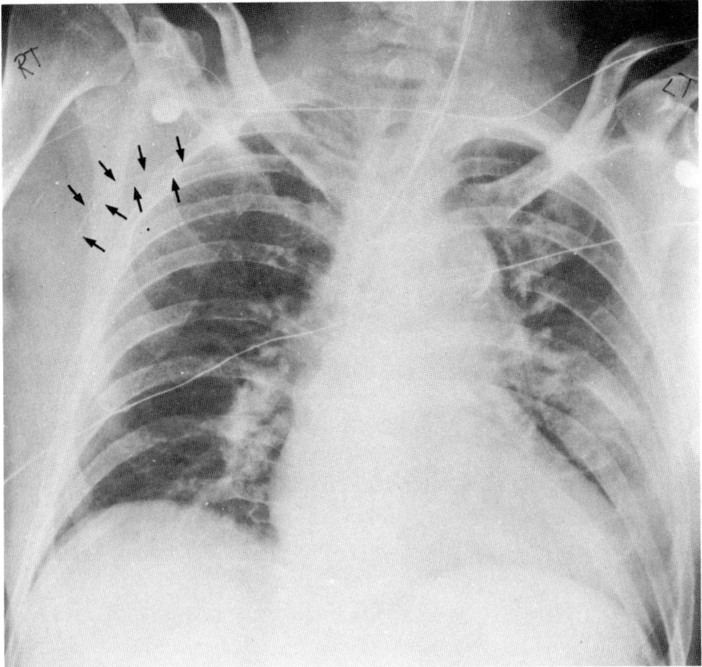

Fig. 5-11. Central venous line inserted from the right arm terminates in one of the thoracic wall veins (*arrows*). (Courtesy of Dr. Paul Spirn, Massachusetts General Hospital)

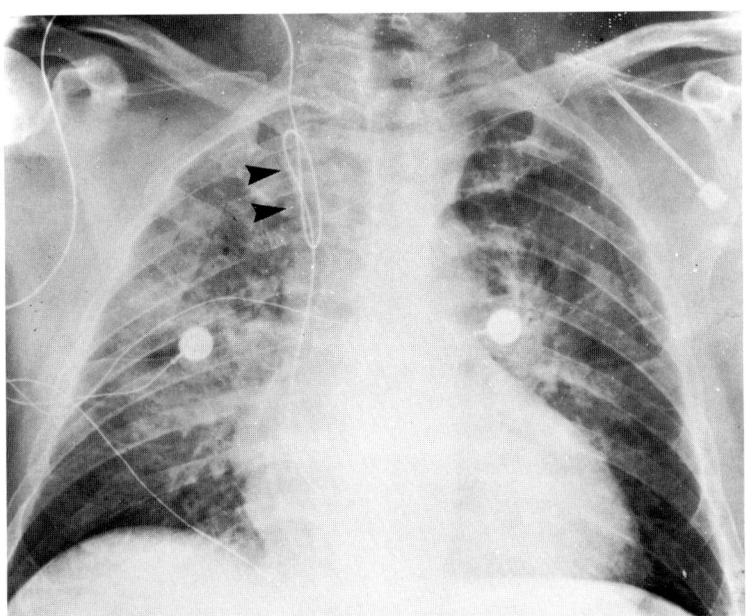

Fig. 5-12. Knotted CVP catheter (*arrows*) **in superior vena cava.** (Courtesy of Dr. Paul Spirn, Massachusetts General Hospital)

ation chest injury (29). Thoracentesis or injection of a small amount of contrast will confirm aberrant catheter placement.

Intravascular catheters may fracture if withdrawn with a cutting needle still in the vessel, and fractures can occur within the venous system at points of stress. They may detach from their hubs, lodging in the vena cava, the right heart, or in the pulmonary artery, with resulting thrombosis, infection, or perforation (15,40). Occasionally catheters may become knotted within the vascular system (Fig. 5-7, 5-12). Rescue operations can be performed nonoperatively via a snare inserted percutaneously into the femoral vein under fluoroscopy (24,31).

Certain complications of CVP catheters such as thrombosis or infection may not be related to insertion but evolve from the presence of an intravascular foreign body. A retained central venous pressure catheter has been reported as a cause of superior vena cava syndrome, confirmed by CT scan (35).

Flow-Directed Pulmonary Artery Catheters

CVP catheters reflect left-sided cardiac pressures only indirectly, assuming that right- and left-sided pressures will vary in the same magnitude and direction. However, in multiorgan system failure or injury, there is no predictable correlation. Pulmonary capillary wedge (PCW) pressure is a more direct index of left atrial pressure. (Table 5-3.)

The Swan-Ganz catheter, introduced in 1970,

is equipped with a lumen for recording pressures and for withdrawing pulmonary arterial blood samples, a smaller lumen used to inflate a balloon with gas, and a third lumen positioned to open into the right atrium when the tip of the catheter is placed within the pulmonary artery. A thermistor approximately 4 cm from the catheter tip permits thermodilution cardiac output determination (9).

The catheter is introduced via antecubital, jugular, or subclavian vein and is advanced through the right side of the heart into the pulmonary artery 2–3 inches distal to the bifurcation of the main pulmonary artery. The balloon is then inflated, causing the catheter to float into the "wedge" position. With deflation, the tip recoils into the pulmonary artery.

There are risks associated with insertion such as arterial puncture, pneumothorax, infection, and thrombosis at the insertion site (8). Too much slack in the catheter may allow distal migration. The morbidity associated with the flow-directed balloon-tipped catheter is estimated at 7.2% (18) and results primarily from pulmonary infarction (Fig. 5-13) distal to the catheter tip when it occludes the pulmonary artery or from thrombosis about the catheter tip (44). The balloon should be inflated only during pressure measurement, to lessen the risk of obstruction of a major pulmonary artery and significant infarction (Fig. 5-14). The balloon is identified on the radiograph as a 1-cm rounded lucency located at the catheter tip and should never be seen on routine films. Passage of the Swan-Ganz catheter to the right side of the heart is associated with tachyarrhythmias and, infrequently, knotting of the catheter and balloon rupture (46).

Table 5-3. Complications of Flow-Directed Pulmonary Artery Catheters

Complication	Cause
Arrhythmias	Ventricular irritation
Pulmonary infarction	Persistant arterial occlusion by catheter or balloon; catheter-induced thromboembolism
Pulmonary artery perforation	Balloon inflation following distal migration of catheter tip
Intracardiac knotting	Rapid insertion; right ventricular dilatation
Marantic endocarditis	Prolonged catheter placement
Sepsis	Prolonged catheter placement

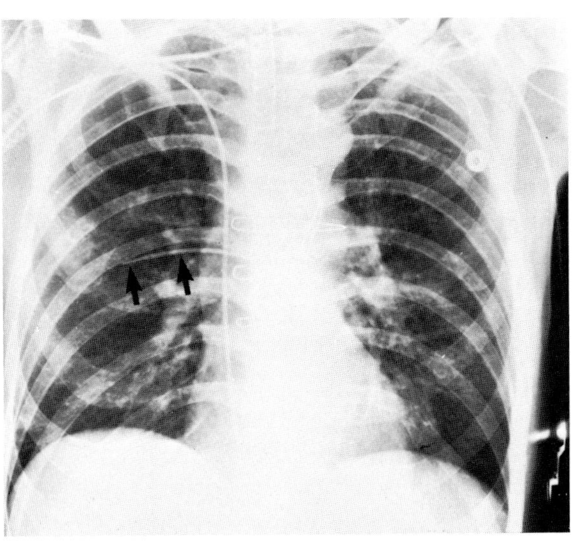

a

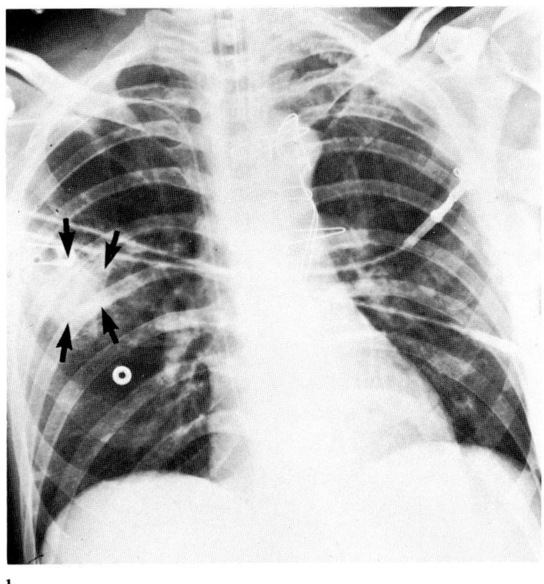

b

Fig. 5-13, a and b. Postcatheterization infarction. a Swan-Ganz catheter terminates distally in the superior division of the right pulmonary artery (*arrows*). **b** Four days later the line has been removed and there is a round opacity (*arrows*) in the same location attributed to infarction. (Courtesy of Dr. Phillip Costello, New England Deaconess Hospital)

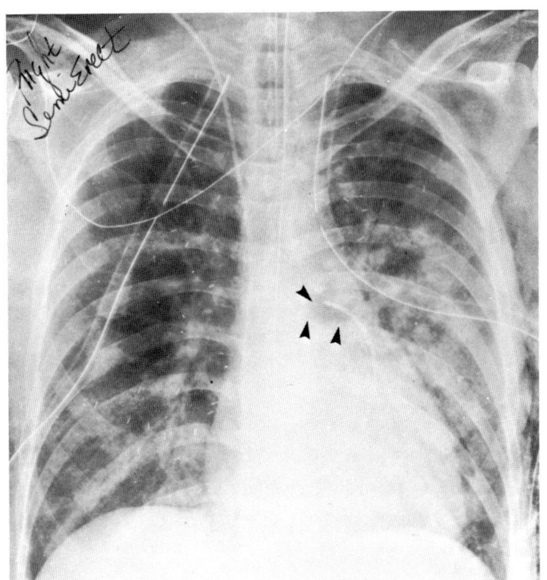

Fig 5-14. Inflated balloon in the main pulmonary artery (*arrows*). It should never be seen on the film, which should not be taken during pressure measurement. (Courtesy of Dr. Paul Spirn, Massachusetts General Hospital)

Cardiac Pacemakers

Complications associated with pacemakers are discussed elsewhere in this volume.

Intraaortic Counterpulsation Balloon

The intraaortic counterpulsation balloon (IACB) was introduced in the 1960s for the treatment of cardiogenic shock, and this continues to be a major indication for its use. Patients in cardiogenic shock following myocardial infarction may be stabilized by the use of the IACB prior to coronary artery bypass surgery. The IACB may be used preoperatively in high-risk patients, in the immediate postoperative period, and in patients who otherwise could not be weaned from cardiopulmonary bypass (32).

The IACB is a large catheter introduced into the common femoral artery. It is advanced retrograde and positioned in the upper descending thoracic aorta. The balloon extends for approximately 26 cm surrounding the distal end of the catheter. It is distended with about 40 ml of gas during diastole and forcibly deflated during systole, timed by the ECG. Mechanical circulatory assistance with the IACB increases perfusion of the coronary arteries and oxygen delivery to the myocardium during diastole. On the radiograph, the catheter tip should be between the level of the left mainstem bronchus inferiorly and the level of the aortic arch superiorly, just distal to the left subclavian artery (32).

Insertion of an excessively long catheter can result in obstruction of the left subclavian artery or in aortic tear, with subsequent dissection of the origin of the subclavian artery. If the balloon is too high in the aortic arch, there is increased risk of cerebral embolism. Atherosclerosis of the abdominal aorta sometimes precludes proper positioning. If the balloon is positioned too distally, counterpulsation is less effective, and the balloon may obstruct major abdominal vessels. With change of patient position from recumbent to sitting, the balloon may move cephalad 1–4.5 cm. Thus, frequent radiographic checks are recommended. Further risks include aortic dissection, which may be detected when there is loss of definition of the descending thoracic aorta on the chest radiograph; destruction of platelets and red blood cells; balloon rupture with gas embolization; arterial insufficiency in the catheterized leg; and occasional ventricular rupture, probably secondary to underlying myocardial infarction (32,56).

Cardiopulmonary Resuscitation

Cardiopulmonary resuscitation, or CPR, was successfully used before 1960 and is now a standardized and widely applied technique in the initial management of cardiopulmonary arrest. Excessive and misplaced compression may cause chest trauma such as rib fractures with fat emboli, sternal fracture, costochondral separation, and flail chest. Compression over the xiphoid process may cause liver laceration, and overly zealous compression may cause trauma to the heart and other mediastinal organs (11,41). Patients should be ob-

served after resuscitation for signs of pulmonary parenchymal contusion, laceration, or atelectasis; hemothorax, pneumothorax, mediastinal hemorrhage, pneumomediastinum; and sternal and rib fractures.

Cardiopulmonary Disorders

This section will review briefly some of the cardiopulmonary complications most often seen in the ICU.

Atelectasis

Atelectasis is often associated with general anesthesia and is most often seen following thoracic or upper abdominal surgery, particularly in patients with preexisting lung disease, in smokers, and in obese and elderly patients. The incidence increases with prolonged anesthesia time (21).

At 24–48 hours postoperatively, the radiographic findings range from elevation of the diaphragm to linear or discoid atelectasis and to segmental or lobar consolidation with volume loss. The radiographic pattern of left lower lobe infiltration and atelectasis following cardiac surgery was recently analyzed by Benjamin et al. (5) and was shown to be related to topical cooling of the heart with ice, which paralyzes the phrenic nerve, and to direct surgical trauma to the left lower lobe. When atelectasis persists beyond the third or fourth postoperative day, pneumonia is a possibility.

Aspiration

Aspiration is associated with vomiting, tracheostomy and intubation, nasotracheal intubation, anesthesia, and central nervous system depression. Within two to four hours after aspiration, the chest x-ray may disclose an infiltrate. The most common sites of infiltration are the lung bases and perihilar areas. Bilaterally symmetric and diffuse infiltrates may mimic congestive heart failure. The radiograph usually clears within several days, and an increase in an infiltrate after the third or fourth day usually signifies superinfection with gram-negative organisms (4,6,24,47,58).

Pneumonia

The diagnosis is made on clinical grounds (fever and leukocytosis) and is supported by a stable or progressive infiltrate on chest x-ray. The sputum may not be diagnostic because of colonization of the upper respiratory tract with gram-negative organisms. The radiographic appearance may be complicated by chronic obstructive pulmonary disease (COPD) and congestive heart failure. As a general rule, infiltrates due to infection appear later and progress more slowly than those due to aspiration or atelectasis.

Pulmonary Edema

The usual indicators of congestive heart failure (CHF)—upper lobe pulmonary vascular redistribution, interstitial edema, perihilar haze, peribronchial edema, and alveolar infiltrates—are unreliable on a portable radiograph. Upper lobe redistribution is a normal finding in the supine patient. However, when upright, six-foot target-to-film distance chest x-rays are available, it may be possible to make a radiographic diagnosis of CHF in the ICU (7).

Pulmonary edema may have an atypical distribution because of the effects of gravity in the bedridden patient and because edema does not accumulate in underperfused areas, as in patients with COPD or pulmonary embolism. ICU patients are subject to noncardiac pulmonary edema without the changes of redistribution, pulmonary hypertension, and cardiomegaly, for example, in uremia, aspiration, sepsis, allergic reaction, fluid overload, and neurogenic disorders (4,6,28,54).

Respiratory Distress Syndrome

Adult respiratory distress syndrome (ARDS) or acute respiratory failure due to noncardiogenic pulmonary edema may be secondary to shock, sepsis, trauma, viral infections, and other disorders. The radiograph is at first normal, followed in 24–36 hours either by continuation of the normal or by interstitial perihilar edema. By this time, the patient has developed tachypnea, dyspnea, cyanosis, and hypoxia, and over the next 24–48 hours there is a further fall in oxygen saturation. The radiographic pattern changes to one of patchy, ill-defined alveolar infiltrates, then to confluent,

bilateral alveolar densities. Initially, the radiographic pattern may mimic massive pulmonary embolism, which can be excluded by lung scan. CHF is excluded by means of pulmonary capillary wedge pressure and by the absence of cardiomegaly. When the radiographic pattern stabilizes, it is most suggestive of ARDS. A secondary process such as infection or barotrauma may follow (20,48,53).

Pleural Effusions

Pleural effusions are so common in the postthoracotomy patient as to be considered normal. Larger-than-expected effusions may be due to hemorrhage or infection and may become loculated. Pleural effusion lasting until the third postoperative day may signal the postpericardiotomy syndrome and may be accompanied by pericardial effusions and pulmonary infiltrates (34). Pleural effusions have been found in 60% of patients after upper abdominal surgery and in 34% after lower abdominal surgery. Effusions due to subdiaphragmatic abscesses rarely appear until the second postoperative week (22).

Mediastinal Widening

Postthoracotomy widening of the mediastinum is attributable to hemorrhage or edema but rarely necessitates reoperation. Katzberg et al. found that those patients requiring reexploration had at least a 60% increase in width of the mediastinum. Other signs of mediastinal bleeding include obscuration of the aortic knob and loss of sharpness of the aortic contour, displacement of the trachea to the right, downward displacement of the left mainstem bronchus, and pleural effusion, usually on the left (36).

Pulmonary Embolism

Pulmonary embolism is usually a late complication of surgery and is difficult to diagnose on the chest radiograph. Findings may include infiltrates, atelectasis, elevation of the diaphragm, pleural effusion, and local hyperlucency. Perfusion lung scan is likely to be positive in the postoperative period because of other cardiopulmonary disorders. Pulmonary angiography may be necessary for a definitive diagnosis.

References

1. Abramson N, Ward K, Grenvik A, et al: Adverse occurrences in intensive care units. JAMA 244:1582–1584, 1980.
2. Adams FG: A simplified approach to the reporting of intensive therapy unit chest radiographs. Clin Radiol 30:219–226, 1979.
3. Altman AR, Johnson TH: Roentgenographic findings in PEEP therapy. JAMA 242:727–730, 1979.
4. Bartlett JG, Gorbach SL: The triple threat of aspiration pneumonia. Chest 68:560–566, 1975.
5. Benjamin JJ, et al: Left lower lobe atelectasis and consolidation following cardiac surgery: the effect of topical cooling on the phrenic nerve. Radiology 142:11–14, 1982.
6. Cameron JL, Reynolds J, Zuidema GD: Aspiration in patients with tracheostomies. Surg Gynecol Obstet 136:68–70, 1973.
7. Chait A, et al: The bedside radiograph in the evaluation of incipient heart failure. Radiology 105:563–566, 1972.
8. Chastre J, et al: Thrombosis as a complication of pulmonary-artery catheterization via the internal jugular vein: prospective evaluation by phlebography. N Engl J Med 306:278–280, 1982.
9. Chatterjee K, Swan HJC, Ganz W, Gray R, Loebel H, Forrester JS, Chonette D: Use of a balloon-tipped flotation electrode catheter for cardiac monitoring. Am J Cardiol 36:56–61, 1975.
10. Ching NPH, Ayres SM, Spina RC, Nealon TF: Endotracheal damage during continuous ventilatory support. Ann Surg 179:123–127, 1974.
11. Clark DT: Complications following closed chest cardiac massage. JAMA 181:127–129, 1962.
12. Conrardy PA, Goodman LR, Lainge F, Singer M: Alteration of endotracheal tube position: flexion and extension of the neck. Crit Care Med 4:8–12, 1976.
13. Cullen DJ: Results and costs of intensive care. Anesthesiology 47:203–216, 1977.
14. Dane TEB, King EG: Fatal cardiac tamponade and other mechanical complications of central venous catheters. Br J Surg 62:6–10, 1975.
15. Deitel M, McIntyre JA: Radiographic confirmation of site of central venous pressure catheters. Can J Surg 14:42–52, 1971.
16. Deneke SM, Fanburg BL: Normobaric oxygen toxicity of the lung. N Engl J Med 303:76–86, 1980.
17. Eaton RJ, Senior RM, Pierce JA: Aspects of respiratory care pertinent to the radiologist. Radiol Clin North Am xi:93–107, 1973.
18. Foote GA, Schobel SI, Hodges M: Pulmonary complications of the flow-directed balloon-tipped catheter. N Engl J Med 290:927–931, 1974.
19. Frank L, Massaro D: Oxygen toxicity. Am J Med 69:117–126, 1980.
20. Gobein RP, Reines DH, Schobel SI: Localized tension pneumothorax: unrecognized form of barotrauma in adult respiratory distress syndrome. Radiology 142:15–19, 1982.
21. Goodman LR: Postoperative chest radiograph: I. Alterations after abdominal surgery. AJR 134:533–541, 1980.
22. Goodman LR: Postoperative chest radiograph: II. Alterations after major intrathoracic surgery. AJR 134:803–813, 1980.
23. Goodman LR, Conrardy PA, Laing F, Singer MM: Radiographic evaluation of endotracheal tube position. AJR 127:433–434, 1976.
24. Goodman LR, Putman CE: Intensive Care Radiology. St Louis: CV Mosby Co, 1978.
25. Goodman LR, Putman CE: The acute care unit: radiographic considerations. In Teplich JG, Haskin ME (eds): Surgical Radiology, vol I. Philadelphia: WB Saunders Co, 1981.
26. Greenbaum DE, Marschall KE: The value of routine daily chest x-rays in intubated patients in the medical intensive care unit. Crit Care Med 10:29–30, 1982.
27. Greene R, McLoud TC, Stark P: Pneumothorax. Semin Roentgenol 12:184–196, 1977.
28. Harrison MO, Conte PJ, Heitzman ER: Radiological detection of clinically occult cardiac failure following myocardial infarction. Br J Radiol 44:265–272, 1971.
29. Hewes RC, Smith DC, Lavine MH: Iatrogenic hydromediastinum simulating aortic laceration. AJR 133:817–820, 1979.
30. Hilberman M: The evolution of intensive care units. Crit Care Med 3:159–165, 1975.
31. Hipona FA, Sciammas FD, Hublitz UF: Nonthoracotomy retrieval of intraluminal cardiovascular foreign bodies: clinical and experimental aspects. Radiol Clin North Am 9:583–595, 1971.
32. Hyson EA, Ravin CE, Kelley MJ, Curtis A McB: Intraaortic counterpulsation balloon: radiographic considerations. AJR 128:915–918, 1977.
33. James AE, MacMillan AS, Eaton SB, Grillo HC: Roentgenology of tracheal stenosis resulting from cuffed tracheostomy tubes. AJR 109:455–466, 1970.
34. Kaminsky ME et al: Postpericardiotomy syndrome. AJR 138:503–508, 1982.
35. Kanada DJ, Jung RC, Ishihara S: Superior vena cava syndrome due to a retained central venous pressure catheter. Chest 75:734–735, 1979.
36. Katzberg RW, Whitehouse GH, de Weese JA: The early radiologic findings in the adult chest after cardiopulmonary bypass. Cardiovasc Radiol 1:205–215, 1978.
37. Kumar A, Pontoppidan H, Falke KJ, Wilson RS, Laver MB: Pulmonary barotrauma during mechanical ventilation. Crit Care Med 1:181–186, 1973.
38. Lams PM, Jolles H: The effect of lobar collapse on the distribution of free intrapleural air. Radiology 142:309–312, 1982.
39. MacMillan AS, James AE, Stitik FP, Grillo HC: Radiological evaluation of post-tracheostomy lesions. Thorax 26:696–703, 1971.
40. McGoun MD, Benedetto PW, Greene BM: Complications of percutaneous central venous catheterization: a report of two cases and a review of the literature. Johns Hopkins Med J 145:1–6, 1979.
41. McIntyre KM, Parisi AF, Benfari R, Goldberg AH, Delan JE: Pathophysiologic syndromes of cardiopulmonary resuscitation. Arch Intern Med 138:1130–1133, 1978.

42. McLoud TC, Barash PG, Ravin CE: PEEP: radiographic features and associated complications. AJR 129:209–213, 1977.
43. McLoud TC, Barash PG, Ravin CE, Mandel SD: Elevation of pulmonary artery pressure as a sign of pulmonary barotrauma (pneumothorax). Crit Care Med 6:81–84, 1978.
44. McLoud TC, Putman CE: Radiology of the Swan-Ganz catheter and associated pulmonary complications. Radiology 116:19–22, 1975.
45. Ovenfors C, Hedgcock MW: Intensive care unit radiology: problems of interpretation. Radiol Clin North Am 16:407–439, 1978.
46. Pace NL: A critique of flow-directed pulmonary arterial catheterization. Anesthesiology 47:455–465, 1977.
47. Pavlin EG, Van Nimwegan D, Hornbein TF: Failure of a high-compliance low-pressure cuff to prevent aspiration. Anesthesiology 42:216–219, 1975.
48. Pontoppidan H, Geffin B, Lowenstein E: Acute respiratory failure in the adult (second of three parts). N Engl J Med 287:743–752, 1972.
49. Pontoppidan H, Laver MB, Geffin B: Acute respiratory failure in the surgical patient. Adv Surg 4:163–254, 1970.
50. Pontoppidan H, Wilson RS, Rie MA, Schneider RC: Respiratory intensive care. Anesthesiology 47:96–116, 1977.
51. Ravin CE, Putman CE, McLoud TC: Hazards of the intensive care unit. AJR 126:423–431, 1976.
52. Rhea JT, van Sonnenberg E, McLoud TC: Basilar pneumothorax in the supine adult. Radiology 133:593–595, 1979.
53. Rinaldo JE, Rogers RM: Adult respiratory distress syndrome: changing concepts of lung injury and repair. N Engl J Med 306:900–909, 1982.
54. Robin ED, Cross CE, Zelis R: Pulmonary edema. N Engl J Med 288:239–246, 292–304, 1973.
55. Rohlfing BM, Webb WR, Schlobohm RM: Ventilator-related extraalveolar air in adults. Radiology 121:25–31, 1976.
56. Scheidts et al: Intraaortic balloon counterpulsation in cardiogenic shock: report of a cooperative clinical trial. N Engl J Med 288:979–984, 1973.
57. Stahly TL, Tench WD: Lung entrapment and infarction by chest tube suction. Radiology 122:307–309, 1977.
58. Stark P: Inadvertent nasogastric tube insertion into the tracheobronchial tree: a hazard of new high-residual volume cuffs. Radiology 142:239–240, 1982.
59. Steier M, Ching N, Roberts EB, Nealon TF: Pneumothorax complicating continuous ventilatory support. J Thorac Cardiovasc Surg 67:17–23, 1974.
60. Summers B: Pneumoperitoneum associated with artificial ventilation. Br Med J 1:1528–1530, 1979.
61. Tabrisky J, Herman MW, Torrance DJ, Hieshima GB: Mobile 240 kVp phototimed chest radiography. AJR 135:295–300, 1980.
62. Trunet P, LeGall J-P, Lhoste F, et al: The role of iatrogenic disease in admissions to intensive care. JAMA 244:2617–2620, 1980.
63. Tuddenham WJ: Iatrogenic lesions of the lungs. *In* Teplick JG, Haskin ME (eds): Surgical Radiology, vol II. Philadelphia: WB Saunders Co, 1981.
64. Weber AL, Grillo HC: Tracheal stenosis: an analysis of 151 cases. Radiol Clin North Am 16:291–308, 1978.
65. Westcott JL, Cole SR: Interstitial pulmonary emphysema in children and adults: roentgenographic features. Radiology 111:367–378, 1974.
66. Winter PM, Smith G: The toxicity of oxygen. Anesthesiology 37:210–241, 1972.
67. Zimmerman JE, Goodman LR, Shahvari MBG: Effect of mechanical ventilation and positive end-expiratory pressure (PEEP) on chest radiograph. AJR 133:811–815, 1979.
68. Zwillich CW, Pierson DJ, Creagh CE, Sutton FO, Schatz E, Petty TL: Complications of assisted ventilation: a prospective study of 354 consecutive episodes. Am J Med 57:161–170, 1974.

6 Barotrauma

Jack L. Westcott
and Solon Cole

Although the use of mechanical ventilation has improved the management and survival of patients with acute respiratory failure (1–5), it has become evident that serious and even fatal complications may result from both the effects of mechanical ventilation and the use of supplemental oxygen (6–15). Some of the alleged deleterious effects are difficult to distinguish from pathologic changes secondary to the underlying pulmonary disorder. However, many are clearly recognizable, and the radiologist has an important role to play in the recognition, treatment, and prevention of these complications. The major adverse effects of positive pressure breathing (PPB) may be divided into the following categories: (a) complications due to the endotracheal or tracheostomy tube, (b) physiologic effects on cardiac output and the amount of water in the lungs, (c) lung trauma secondary to high inspiratory pressures, and (d) the effects of supplemental oxygen. The emphasis on the complications of PPB in this chapter is not intended to detract from the value of assisted ventilation. Patients in whom complications develop are usually those who have severe respiratory failure, and most of these patients would have died prior to the use of ventilatory support.

PPB may cause significant changes in the size of the heart, the appearance of the pulmonary vasculature, and the amount of water in the lungs. We have not been able to find any convincing evidence that indicates that PPB by itself leads to a clearing of pulmonary edema. However, since the air:fluid ratio increases with increased lung volume, the lungs always *look* clearer when the patient is placed on PPB, whether the underlying disorder is pneumonia, ARDS,* or edema associated with pulmonary venous hypertension. Therefore, the chest x-ray may show marked improvement despite the presence of significant residual disease (Figs. 6-1, and 6-14). PPB may actually contribute to the development of pulmonary edema; in some patients, sodium and water retention and pulmonary edema have occurred during therapy with continuous positive pressure breathing (CPPB) and especially positive end-expiratory pressure (PEEP). The mechanisms are not entirely known, but several investigators (16–19) have shown that antidiuretic hormone secretion may be increased and glomerular filtration decreased during treatment with CPPB (16,17). Unlike the edema associated with ARDS, this responds well to diuretics and sodium restriction (18,20).

The heart and pulmonary vessels may also show significant changes following the institution and cessation of CPPB. The heart frequently appears smaller during PPB (Fig. 6-1). Part of this effect is probably due to better lung expansion, but part may be real, since CPPB and especially PEEP frequently cause a decrease in cardiac output (21,22,23). One possible mechanism is that increased intrathoracic pressure interferes with venous return to the heart. Another is that proposed by Jardin et al. (24), who used echocardiography to study patients receiving PEEP. They demonstrated that there was right ventricular enlargement, leftward deflection of the interventricular

---

* In this chapter, the various types of noncardiogenic pulmonary edema will be designated as acute respiratory distress syndrome (ARDS).

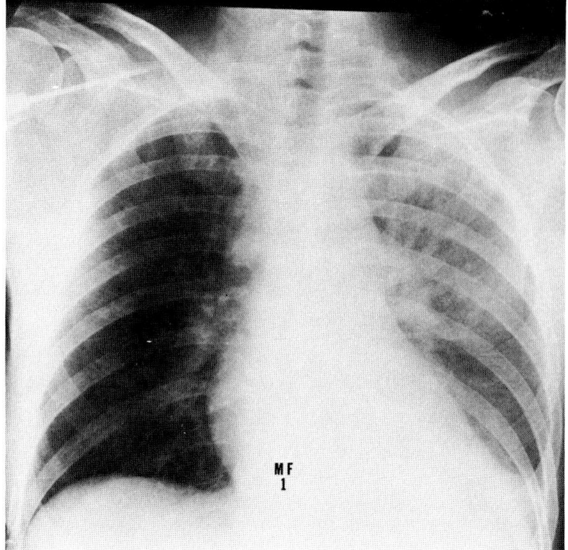

a

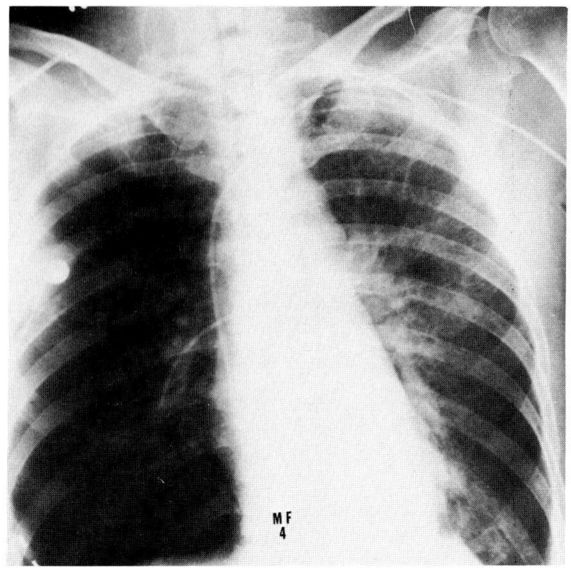

b

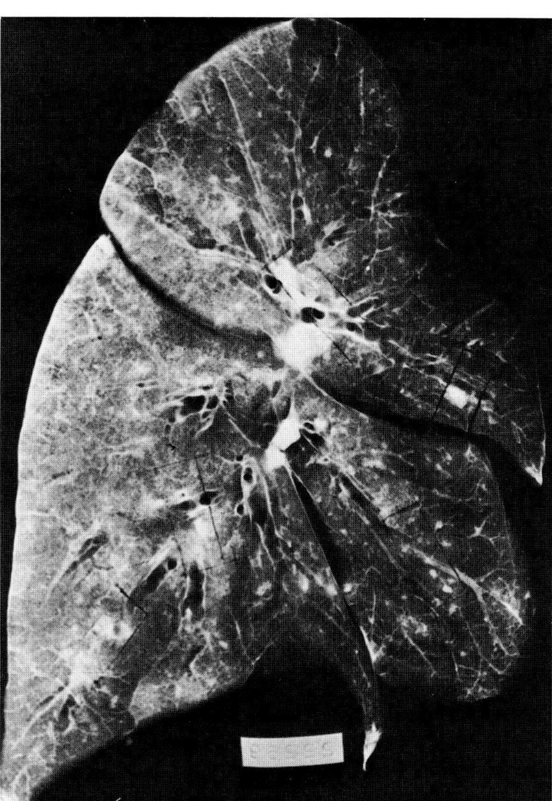

c

Fig. 6-1, a–c. Fifty-seven-year-old woman with known metastatic breast cancer and acute respiratory failure. a Chest x-ray revealed a pulmonary edema pattern (worse on the left) and probable mediastinal lymphadenopathy. She was treated with PEEP and 50% oxygen. b Chest x-ray on the following day appears improved. Although the lungs are well expanded and the right lung appeared clear, she remained severely hypoxemic. She subsequently developed hypotension and died later the same day. c A sagittal postmortem radiograph of the fixed inflated right lung shows extensive metastatic disease and extensive pulmonary edema despite the relatively normal radiographic appearance of the right lung prior to death. Microscopic examination revealed diffuse metastatic breast cancer in both lungs with lymphangitic spread, neoplastic invasion of the pulmonary vessels, tumor thromboemboli in the small pulmonary arteries and veins, and pulmonary edema.

septum, and a decrease in left ventricular size presumably as a result of increased pulmonary vascular resistance induced by PEEP. Ovenfors (25) performed pulmonary angiography in dogs receiving PPB and demonstrated a significant decrease in the size of the pulmonary arteries and veins. The corollary of these findings is that a decrease in heart and pulmonary vessel size does not necessarily indicate improvement in patients with congestive heart failure (CHF). Conversely, an increase in cardiac and pulmonary vessel size following cessation of CPPB does not by itself indicate CHF.

The most serious complications of mechanical ventilation are (a) air-leak phenomena, i.e., interstitial pulmonary emphysema (IPE) and its sequelae, and (b) oxygen toxicity. The remainder of this chapter will be devoted to the first of these entities. The material presented here will be based on previous investigations in addition to our own observations made in patients (26) and experimental animals (27). Our pathologic data were derived from an autopsy study using radiologic-pathologic correlations of fixed inflated lungs from approximately 75 patients who died of acute respiratory failure (ARF), all of whom were treated with CPPB, and from an animal study (using pigs) designed to assess the pulmonary effects of PPB in the absence of supplemental oxygen (27).

Interstitial Pulmonary Emphysema (IPE)

The mechanisms responsible for IPE have been reported on many occasions (9,25–39), but the most complete investigations remain those by Macklin (37) and Macklin and Macklin (38). They showed that IPE occurs when the pressure or relative distention of the airspaces exceeds the tension in the adjacent perivascular connective tissues and interlobular septa. When the alveolar:interstitial pressure gradient exceeds a certain critical level (see later), rupture of alveoli immediately adjacent to the interlobular septa and the perivascular connective tissues permits air to enter the interstitium (Figs. 6-4c and 6-5g). The air then dissects along the vascular sheaths and interlobular septa centrally to the hilum and peripherally to the pleura (Figs, 6-3, 6-4a, 6-5e, 6-5h, 6-5i, 6-8d, 6-11). IPE

has not been observed in the alveolar septal walls nor bronchi (Fig. 6-4d). According to Macklin (37), there is no gradient between alveoli and bronchi, and peribronchial air dissection does not occur. Multiple areas of alveolar rupture must occur in order to produce clinically significant IPE.

On gross examination of the lungs, most of the perivascular air collections are too small to be seen with the naked eye, but in the interlobular septa and at the junctions of the septa and visceral pleura, the air may form visible bubbles, clefts, and cystlike spaces (Fig. 6-3). In infants, the interstitial air usually is more extensive in the upper lobes and usually extends into the lung periphery (Figs. 6-11 and 6-14). In older children and adults, IPE is more extensive in the medial, anterior, and basal portions of the lungs than it is laterally and posteriorly (Figs. 6-5 and 6-8). The interlobular septa are more numerous in these areas (40), and they are more loosely held together, presumably because the lobules in these areas are required to undergo the most extensive changes in size and shape during respiratory and cardiac motion (41). This loose arrangement of the lobules probably offers less resistance to air dissection and may account for the tendency of IPE to be most extensive medially, anteriorly, and along the diaphragmatic surfaces. Perivascular air dissection is usually more extensive around the pulmonary veins and lymphatics than it is around the arteries (Fig. 6-11d).

Subpleural blebs or air cysts are formed by the continued dissection of air from the interlobular septa into the contiguous subpleural connective tissues (Figs. 6-2, 6-4b, 6-6, 6-7, 6-15). The size of the potential subpleural space allows the subpleural air collections to achieve a much larger size than in the interior of the lung. The air cysts are most common along the medial, inferior, and anterior portions of the lungs, but they are also commonly seen along the fissures. Occasionally (particularly in infants) they may be seen laterally and posteriorly as well. The cysts appear as small pleural "blisters" measuring less than 1 cm in diameter (Fig. 6-3), but occasionally they are much larger. The largest that we have observed pathologically measured 8 cm (Fig. 6-6), but there are reports of giant air cysts measuring up to the size of an entire lung (31).

There are many causes of IPE, and a partial listing includes coughing, straining, blunt chest trauma, forceful inhalation during anesthesia or

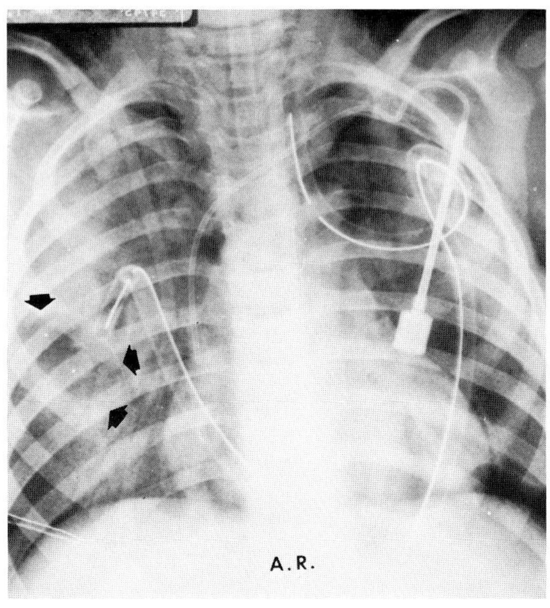

a

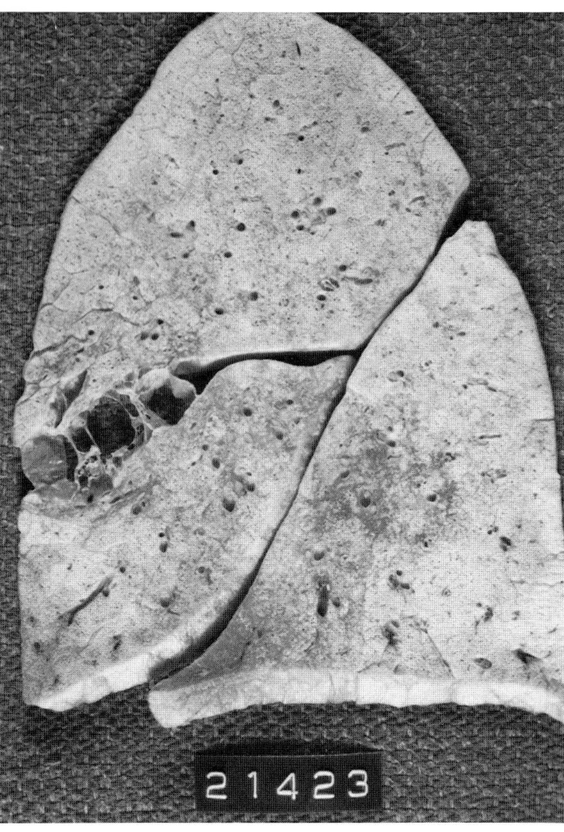

b

Fig. 6-2, a and b. Three-year-old male with near drowning. a Portable chest roentgenogram on ninth day (shortly before death) reveals pulmonary consolidation, a left pneumothorax, and pneumomediastinum. There is a rounded radiolucent area in the lateral aspect of the right lung (*arrows*), which is not well seen in the reproduction. **b** Postmortem sagittal section of the outer third of the right lung reveals dissecting subpleural air cysts adjacent to the minor fissure. There are linear collections of IPE in some of the interlobular septa of the anterior segment of the upper lobe. Except for a few spared lobules posteriorly, there is consolidation (pneumonia) of the entire right lung.

resuscitation, skin diving, and various "air-block" syndromes such as asthma, bronchiolitis, and mucous plug or foreign body (13,25,28,29,31,32, 37,38,41–48). They all have in common a temporary or sustained increase in alveolar pressure leading to alveolar wall rupture. IPE has also been reported with viral and bacterial pneumonias, tuberculosis, hyaline membrane disease, and atelectasis. However, in a hospital setting, the vast majority of cases of IPE are caused by PPB, and IPE may result from PPB even in the absence of underlying pulmonary disease (8,10,14,25–28,34,37,38,44–46).

The peak inspiratory pressures and the elapsed time on the respirator are both important factors for determining the development of IPE and its severity. Using intermittent positive pressure breathing (IPPB) in dogs, Ovenfors (25) found that grossly visible IPE occurred regularly with peak inspiratory pressures between 30 and 35 cm water. At 25 cm peak pressure, IPE was not observed grossly, but it was present microscopically if the IPPB was continued for 12 hours or more. Marcotte et al. (45) found that IPE occurred at slightly lower peak pressures (20–25 cm) in cats. Using pigs, we were able to consistently produce extensive IPE at pressures of 25–50 cm but not below 25 cms H_2O (27). The interstitial air was most extensive in those pigs ventilated at the highest pressures. The inspiratory pressures required to produce IPE in humans are not exactly known, but it probably occurs at approximately the same

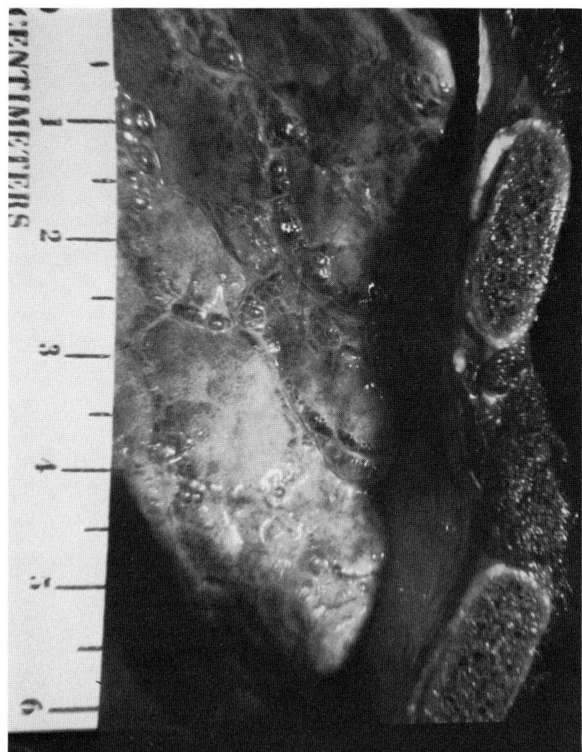

Fig. 6-3. Postmortem in situ appearance of the lingula of a 20-year-old patient with fatal head injury who had received PPB. Autopsy revealed extensive IPE. The interstitial air collections have dissected peripherally to the pleural surface and are seen especially well at the junctions of the interlobular septa and visceral pleura.

levels as in experimental animals (20–25 cm H_2O) (28,47,48,51,52).

Factors other than the peak pressures and elapsed time on PPB are also important. Although IPE may occur at any age, susceptibility to its development seems to vary inversely with increasing age. The vast majority of severe cases have been reported in infants, children, and adults under 40. The perivascular and septal connective tissues are more easily separated and probably more easily dissected by interstitial air in the lungs of young patients than in those of older people.

The underlying pulmonary disorder also influences the susceptibility to the development of IPE. Lenaghan et al. (46) found that dogs with interstitial edema associated with hemorrhagic shock developed IPE at much lower inspiratory pressures than those required to produce it in normal dogs. IPE is frequently florid in newborns (Figs. 6-11, 6-14–16), probably because the interstitial tissues are more edematous and the lobules more loosely

held together than in adults. Patients with ARDS who are receiving PPB very commonly develop IPE, but it appears to be less common in patients with CHF (possibly because the elevated intervascular pressure tends to diminish the alveolar: interstitial pressure gradient). Both viral and bacterial pneumonias markedly increase the susceptibility to IPE, probably because interstitial edema and alveolar wall destruction facilitate interstitial air dissection. IPE and subpleural air cysts may be associated with necrotizing pneumonias in the absence of PPB and are especially likely to occur with gram-negative, staphylococcal, and necrotizing viral pneumonias (31,37,38) (Table 6-1).

The incidence of IPE in patients receiving PPB is unknown because it frequently is undetectable clinically and radiographically. However, the presence of pneumomediastinum (PM) and pneumothorax (PTX) is presumptive evidence for IPE, whether it can be demonstrated or not. It is also probable that IPE is present if the pressures used for assisted ventilation exceed 25 cm water. However, if the maximum pressure used is less than 30 cm water, IPE is almost always mild and is usually radiographically invisible. Grossly visible IPE and serious sequelae seldom occur unless peak pressures exceed 45–50 cm water.

When IPE is very extensive, it can sometimes be radiographically visible without any underlying pulmonary disease, but it usually becomes visible only in those conditions in which the lungs become radiopaque (pneumonia, edema, hemorrhage, or atelectasis). The most severe and most obvious cases of IPE occur in premature infants (10, 32,33,49–52) (Figs. 6-11, 6-14–16). The direct signs of IPE are (a) subpleural air cysts and (b) direct visualization of the interstitial air collections, including visualization of perivascular air (26).

Air cysts may be seen along with other signs of IPE, but they are sometimes the only evidence of dissecting interstitial air. The cysts are anatomically most frequent around the lung hilus, but radiographically they are most easily recognized in other locations, particularly along the inferior or anterior aspects of the lungs or along the fissures (26). The cysts may spontaneously resolve, fill with fluid, or become secondarily infected. They characteristically change in size rapidly. Rohlfing et al. (48) have reported that their appearance frequently heralds the development of other air-leak compli-

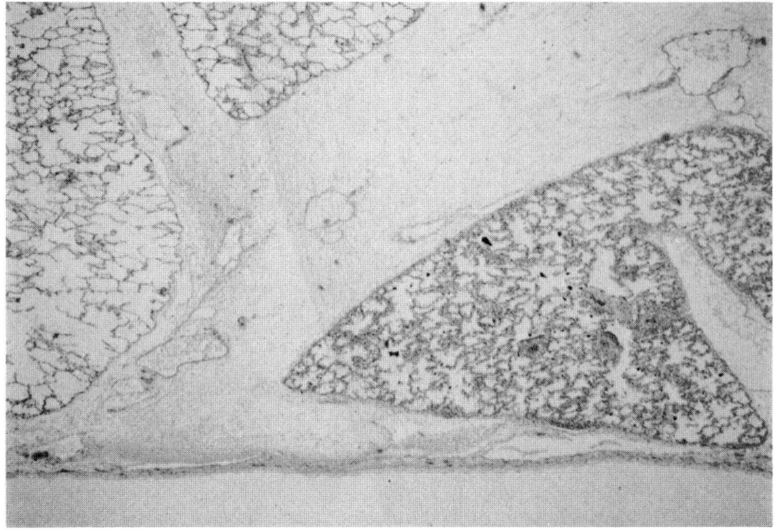

a

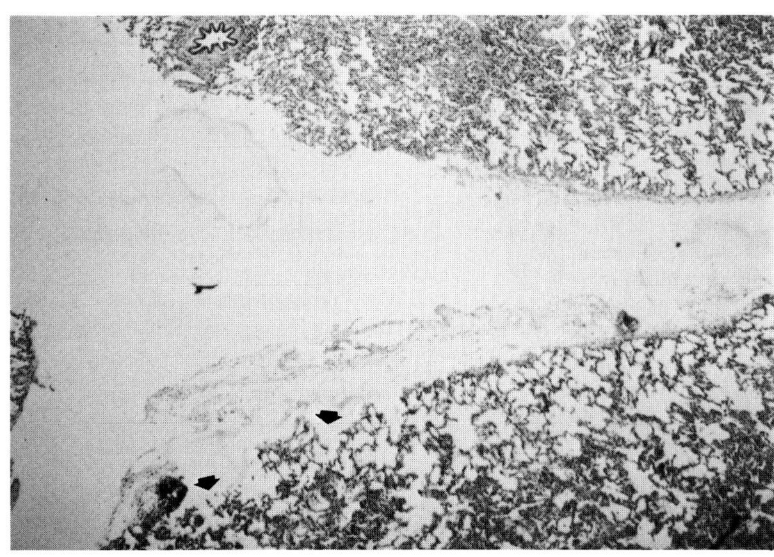

b

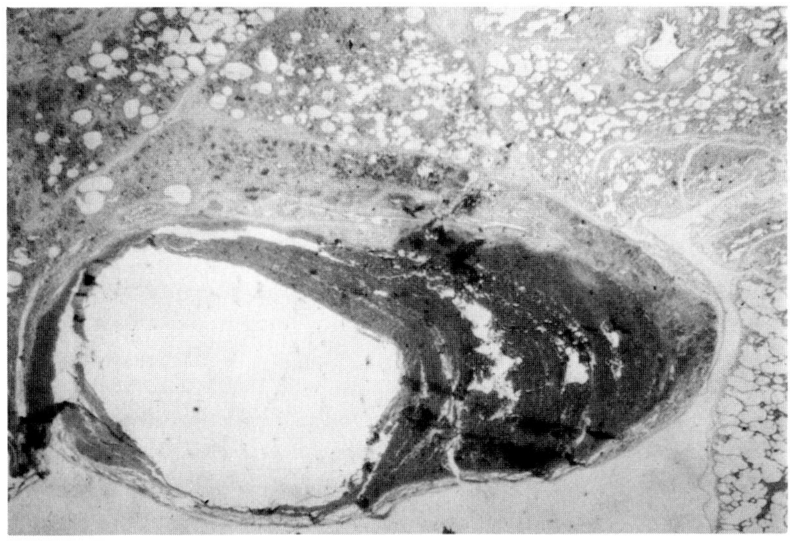

c

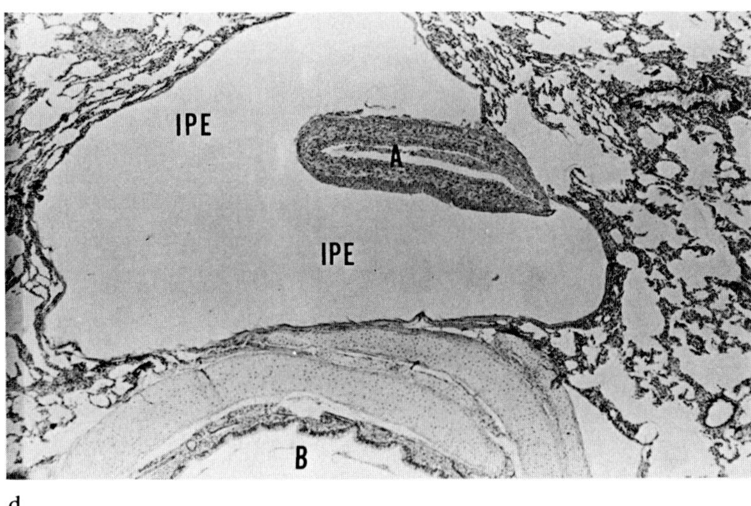

d

Fig. 6-4, a–d. Photomicrographs of lung sections taken from a pig ventilated with room air with IPPB at peak pressures of 30 cm H_2O for 55 hours. **a** The interlobular septum has been markedly widened by IPE, and air has dissected the subpleural connective tissues, causing separation of the marginal alveoli from the pleural surface. There is edema throughout the area of air dissection. **b** Another section shows marked enlargement of the interlobular septa due to the presence of interstitial air. There are several ruptured marginal alveoli (*arrows*). **c** Another section reveals extensive hemorrhage in the wall of an interstitial subpleural air cyst. **d** There is extensive IPE causing complete collapse of an artery (A). There is no dissection of air around the bronchus (B) except where it is immediately adjacent to the involved artery.

Table 6-1. Deleterious Effects of Interstitial Pulmonary Emphysema

   I. Air-leak phenomena
      A. Pneumomediastinum
      B. Pneumothorax
      C. Pneumopericardium
      D. Air embolism
      E. Pneumoperitoneum
  II. Hemodynamic effects (due to arterial and venous compression)
      A. Diminished cardiac output, hypotension, shock
      B. Acute cor pulmonale
      C. Pulmonary edema
 III. Changes in pulmonary function
      A. Increased stiffness of lungs
      B. Atelectasis and hypoxemia
 IV. Secondary infection of the interstitial and subpleural cysts
  V. Secondary changes in pulmonary morphology (? due to mechanical damage from air dissection)
      A. Edema
      B. Hemorrhage
      C. Fibrosis
      D. Hyaline membranes

cations such as pneumothorax or pneumopericardium. The sudden disappearance of an air cyst frequently coincides with the appearance of extraalveolar air in another location (48,53). Although spontaneous resolution is the rule, air cysts may persist for weeks or months, and they sometimes expand to a point where they may cause severe respiratory compromise (53–58) (Figs, 6-15 and 16). Although the mechanism of their formation is different, we believe that subpleural air cysts associated with CPPB probably represent the same entity as posttraumatic pneumatoceles and hematomas.

When IPE is radiographically visible, it is seen as radiolucent bubbles and linear clefts varying in size from 1 to several millimeters in diameter (8,10,51). IPE is usually easier to detect in infants because it is more extensive and probably because the water content of infant lungs increases the background density and makes the interstitial air more visible. In infants, IPE is characteristically diffuse. The upper lobes are usually (but not invariably) more extensively involved than the lower lobes (Figs. 6-11, 6-14, 6-15). Marked hyperinflation of the lungs usually occurs when IPE becomes extensive. In adults, the lateral third of the lungs is usually relatively spared both radiologically and pathologically (Figs. 6-5 and 6-8). The central portions of the lungs, therefore, appear more radiolucent than the periphery. When IPE is visible radiologically in adults, it is usually seen as a generalized, irregular, radiolucent mottling in the medial one-half to two-thirds of the lungs (26) (Figs. 6-5a, 6-5b, 6-7b, 6-8b). However, in some patients, the bubbles and clefts of interstitial air are much larger and are seen as discrete radiolucent pockets measuring up to 2–3 cm or more in diameter (Fig. 6-7c–e). Frequently, IPE is localized or at least best visualized in one area, usually at the lung bases.

Another diagnostic sign of IPE is the visualization of perivascular air (8,25,26). Ovenfors (25) described this finding in several patients who almost certainly had IPE (although pathologic confirmation was not obtained) and also in dogs with experimentally produced IPE. The air is seen as a radiolucent halo around axially projected vessels and as radiolucent streaks adjacent to longitudinally projected vessels (Figs. 6-4, 6-7b, 6-8). Although visualization of perivascular air is a highly specific sign of IPE, it is less often visualized radiographically than are the subpleural air cysts and mottled radiolucencies.

IPE characteristically changes rapidly. Frequently, it appears and disappears within several hours. Persistent IPE (PIPE) for several days frequently indicates irreversibility. When PIPE is confined to one or more lobes, it frequently results in a form of lobar emphysema sometimes requiring surgical removal (54–57). Diffuse bilateral PIPE (Fig. 6-16) usually follows the use of high concentrations of oxygen as well as high ventilator pressures and is much more ominous. Stocker and Madewell (57) studied 12 infants with the diffuse form of PIPE; 11 patients developed signs of bronchopulmonary dysplasia (BPD), and all 12 infants died. Infection may also delay the clearing of IPE; if the interstitial air collections and air cysts become secondarily infected, they may persist with very little change for days or weeks.

Differentiation of IPE from an air bronchogram may be difficult, especially in patients receiving PPB in whom the airways are often distended. IPE collections tend to be more numerous, more haphazardly oriented, and more irregular than air-filled bronchi.

It may be difficult to distinguish between IPE and necrotizing bronchopneumonia. The mottling of IPE usually appears rapidly at a time when

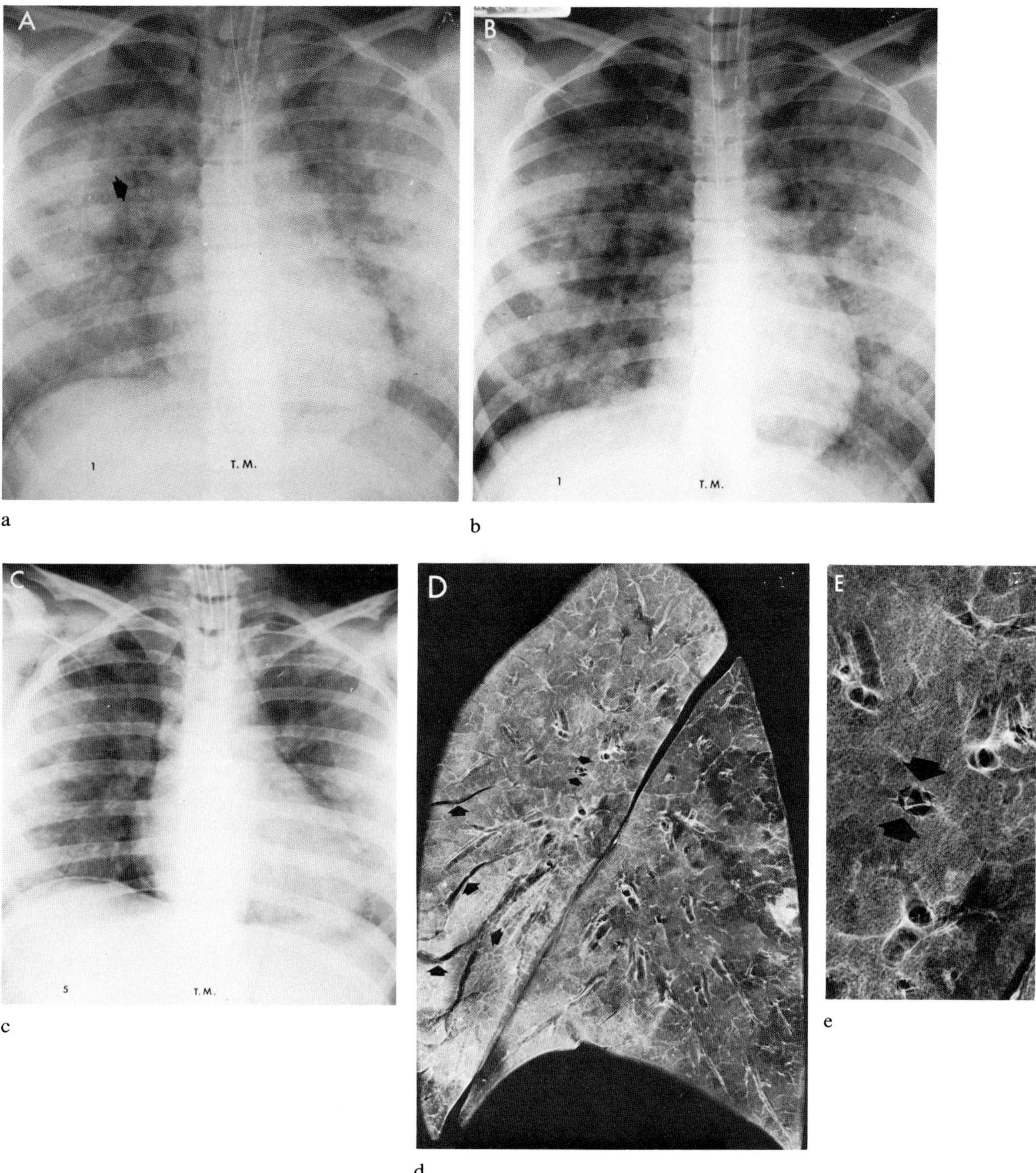

Fig. 6-5, a–j. **A 22-year-old woman with adenovirus pneumonia and acute respiratory failure (ARF) treated with CPPB from admission to death five days later.** Admission chest x-ray done earlier the same day showed diffuse interstitial edema. **a** Chest x-ray after tracheal intubation and institution of CPPB and O$_2$ therapy. The lungs show a pulmonary edema pattern. There are round and linear mottled radiolucencies in the medial third of both lungs. The predilection of IPE for the inner portions of the lungs probably accounts for the difference in density between the inner and outer portions. Right upper lobe arrow points to probable perivascular air around a pulmonary vessel. **b** Repeat radiograph on same day shows an increase in the size and extent of the mottled radiolucencies particularly on the right. **c** On the fifth day, the IPE is almost cleared. Mediastinal, soft-tissue, and extraperitoneal air is still present. Although respiratory function was improved, she has suffered severe hypoxemic brain damage and died later the same day. **d** Radiograph of a sagittal section taken from midportion of left lung reveals numerous dissecting clefts of air in the interlobular septa which are best seen anteriorly in both the upper lobe and lingula. (*arrows*) Apposed arrows show dissected air causing partial collapse of a pulmonary vein. **e** Close-up of vein shown in D. Air has dissected the vein wall away from the surrounding lung.

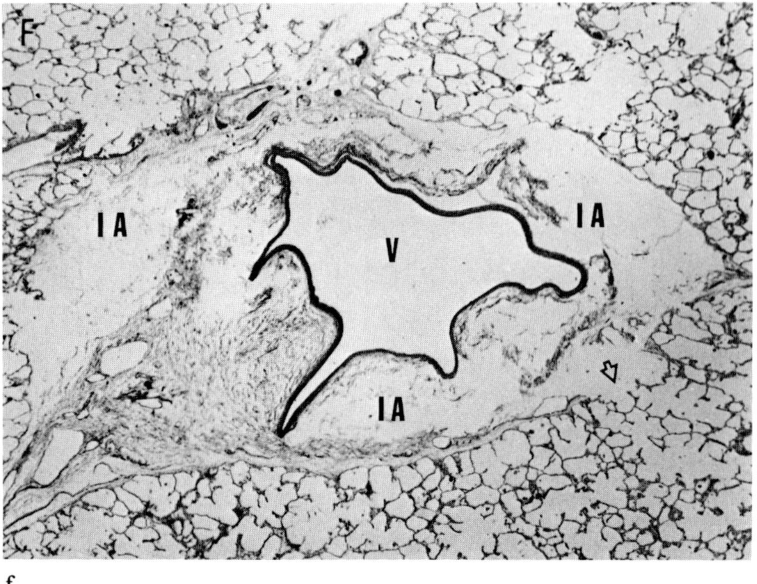

f

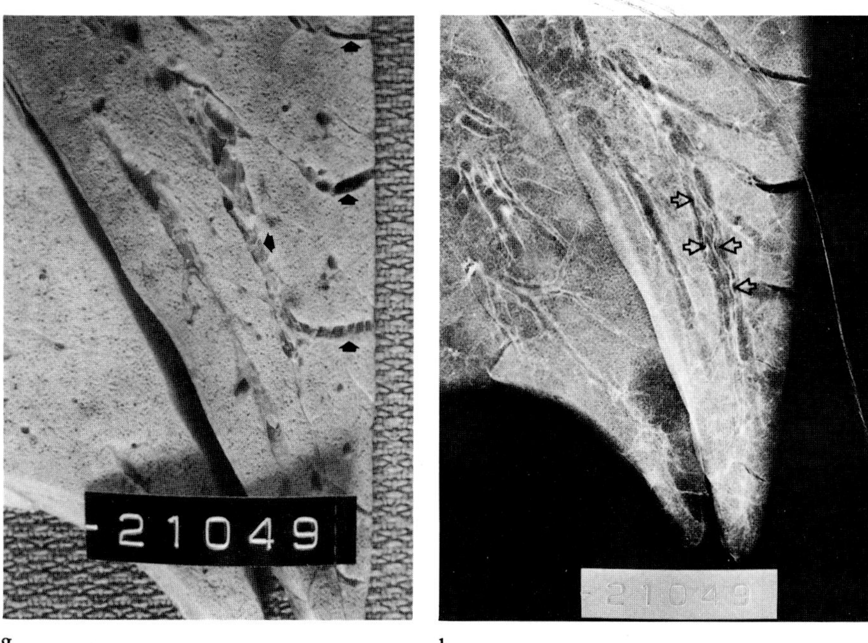

g   h

Fig. 6-5. (cont.) **f** Microscopic section through the collapsed vein. The interstitial air (IA) has dissected the perivascular connective tissues, collapsed the vein (V), and separated it from the surrounding lung. There is rupture of the walls of several perivascular marginal alveoli (*arrow*). **g, h** Close-up photograph and radiograph of a section of inflated lung shows IPE separating the connective tissues of the interlobular septa of the lingula (*closed arrows*). A long segment of a vein in one of the septa shows varying degrees of collapse from the surrounding IPE (*open arrows*).

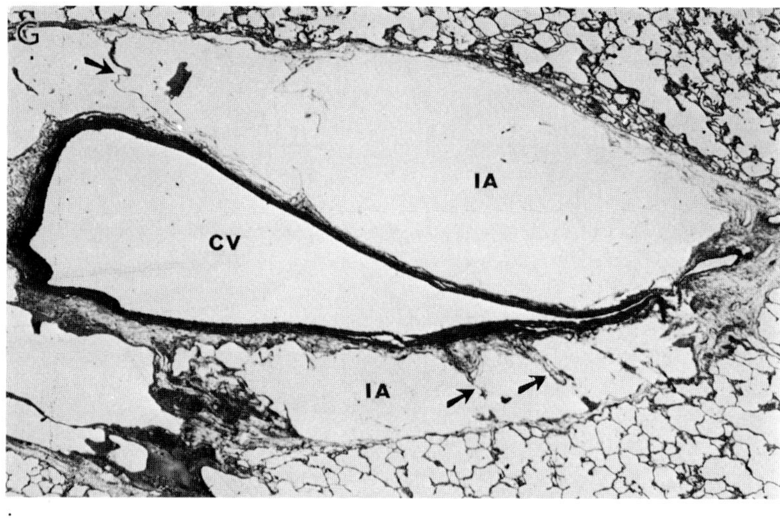

i

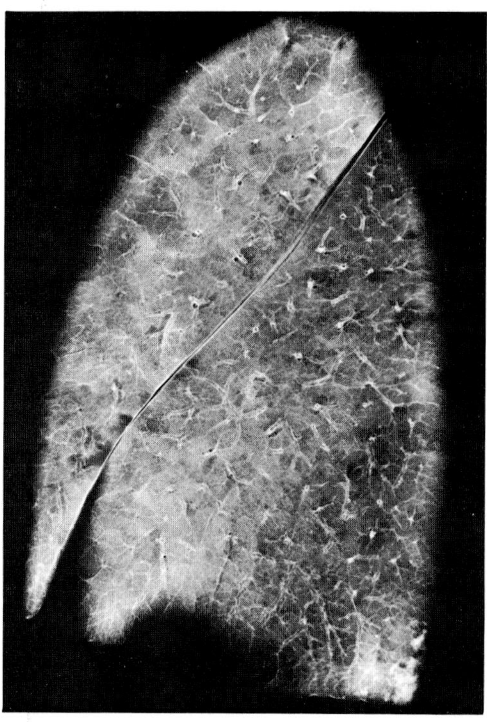

j

Fig. 6-5. (cont.) **i** Microscopic section taken obliquely through a collapsed vein (CV) within an interlobular septum reveals extensive surrounding interstitial air (IA). Small vascular branches (*arrows*) are seen connecting the vein wall to the surrounding lung parenchyma. Rupture of the small branches may account for the interstitial hemorrhage which is frequently observed accompanying IPE. **j** Radiograph of a sagittal section taken through the lateral portion of the left lung reveals diffuse consolidation (predominantly edema), but there is no demonstrable IPE. On the standard chest x-rays, there was also relative sparing laterally.

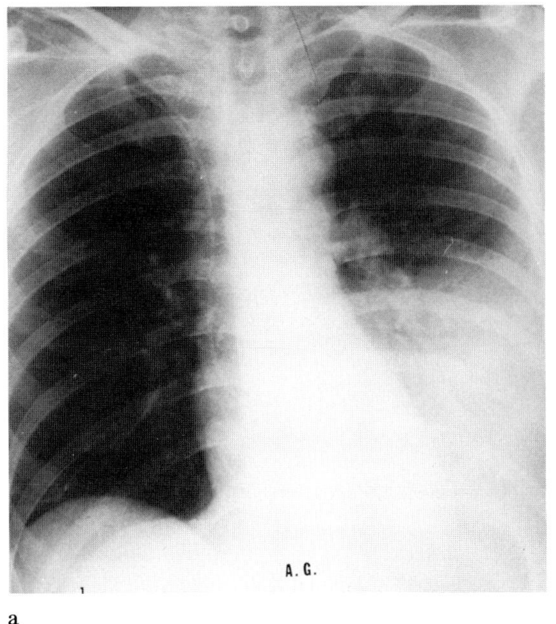

a

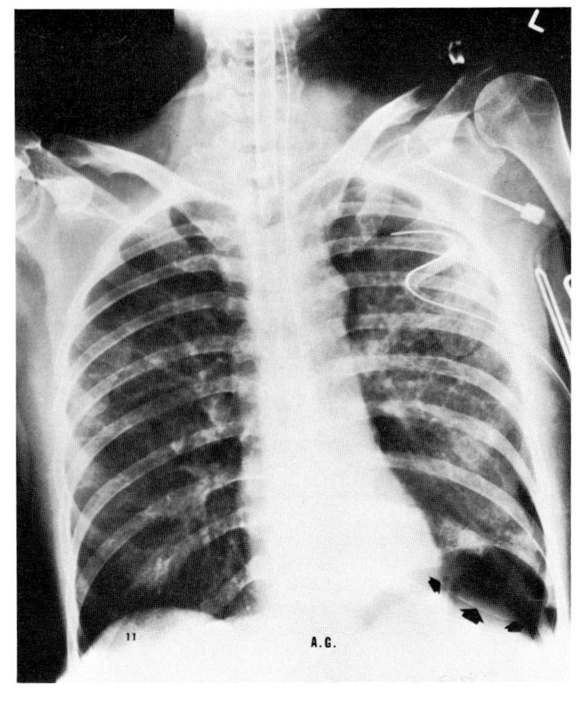

c

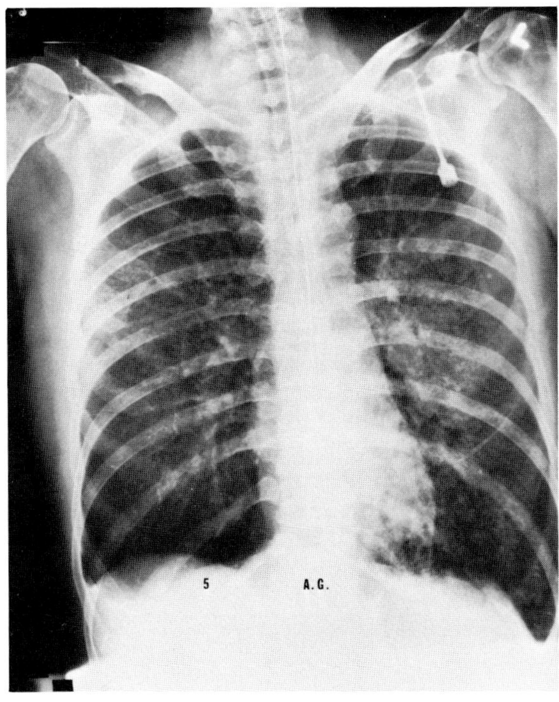

b

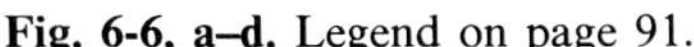

Fig. 6-6, a–d. Legend on page 91.

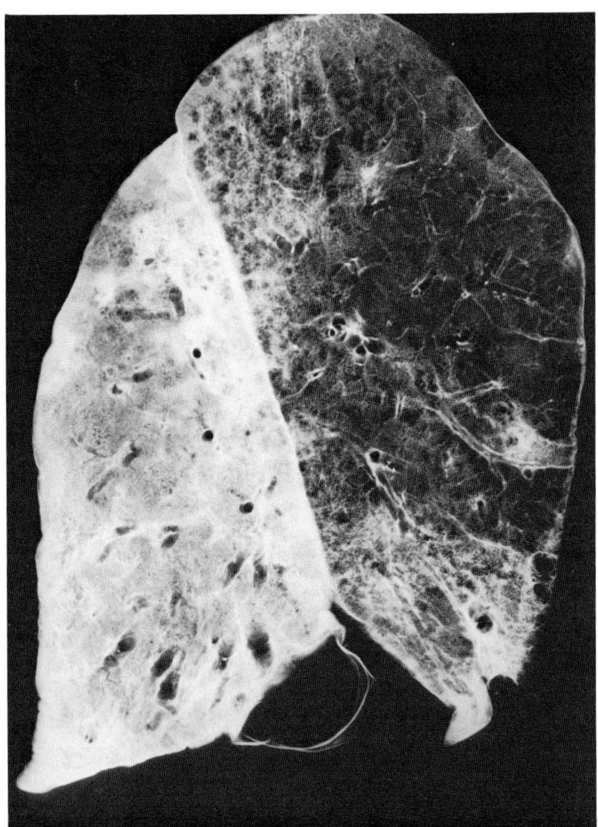

d

the lungs are diffusely consolidated. IPE usually changes faster than the gram-negative pneumonias and is usually followed or accompanied by other signs of air dissection, such as PM and PTX; however, IPE and pneumonia often coexist, and persisting IPE should strongly suggest the presence of associated infection (26) (Table 6-2).

At times, IPE may be difficult to distinguish from consolidation in a lung with previously existing emphysema. However, most cases of IPE are seen in a younger age group, and IPE is characteristically most extensive in the central and lower portions of the lungs in contrast to emphysema, which is usually most severe in the upper lobes (26).

The diagnosis of IPE may be supported in some patients by indirect signs. Localized inversion of the diaphragm may accompany the appearance of subpleural air cysts, and some patients with IPE exhibit a localized area of radiolucency immediately above the diaphragm. We were not able to demonstrate these areas pathologically and are not certain whether they represent subpleural air cysts that resorbed, localized areas of hyperexpanded lung, or possibly examples of inferior pneumothorax.

IPE may cause several deleterious effects which may be grouped into the following categories: (a) air-leak phenomena, (b) hemodynamic alterations, (c) changes in pulmonary function, (d) secondary infection, and (e) secondary changes in pulmonary morphology.

Air-Leak Phenomena

Soft-tissue air dissection, pneumomediastinum (PM), pneumothorax (PTX), pneumopericardium (PP), air embolism (AE), extraperitoneal air dissection, and pneumoperitoneum are the most readily identifiable sequelae of IPE. Once interstitial air dissection is initiated, it may increase rapidly in the lung and extend along the continuous connective-tissue fascial planes to the mediastinum, opposite lung, neck, retroperitoneal tissues, chest and abdominal wall, as well as into the extremities. As long as the pressure at the sites of alveolar rupture is maintained at high enough levels to maintain a positive alveolar:interstitial pressure gradient, air dissection will continue. The connective tissue planes are continuous and appear to offer no significant resistance to air dissection.*

Pneumothorax

Pneumothorax PTX) is common in patients who require high pressures to maintain satisfactory oxygenation, and it is a major cause of morbidity and mortality (Fig. 6-11). Because of the rapidity with which pneumothorax may develop, a high index of suspicion should be maintained in patients who are receiving PPB. A pneumothorax does not have to occupy a large volume to be under tension in patients with noncompliant lungs, and pneumo-

Table 6-2. Radiologic Features of Interstitial Pulmonary Emphysema

---

I. Direct signs of IPE
  A. Mottled radiolucencies in central parts of lungs
  B. Larger spaces in interlobular septa
  C. Perivascular air
  D. Subpleural air cysts
II. Indirect
  A. Pneumomediastinum, pneumothorax, soft-tissue air, and other air-leak phenomena
  B. Radiolucent zone above diaphragms

---

* One exception occurs in infants where significant tension pneumomediastinum frequently occurs without decompression of air into the neck.

Fig. 6-6, a–d. A 51-year-old woman with pneumonia, sepsis, and ARDS who received CPPB throughout her illness. a A portable chest x-ray on day 1 reveals left lower lobe pneumonia. **b** On day 5, mottled circular and linear radiolucencies have developed in the left lower lobe. **c** On day 11, a large subpleural air cyst appeared along the inferior surface of the left lower lobe (*arrows*). There is also a left pneumothorax. The subpleural air cyst and mottled left lower lobe "cavities" persisted until the patient's death on the 25th day. **d** Radiograph of a midsagittal section of the left lung. The large subpleural air cyst is seen along the anteroinferior aspect of the left lower lobe. Microscopic examination revealed thickening of the wall of the subpleural cyst due to acute and chronic inflammation. There were also infected "cysts" in the posterior basal segment of the left lower lobe and extensive pneumonia of the entire left lower lobe.

                                        J. L. Westcott and S. Cole

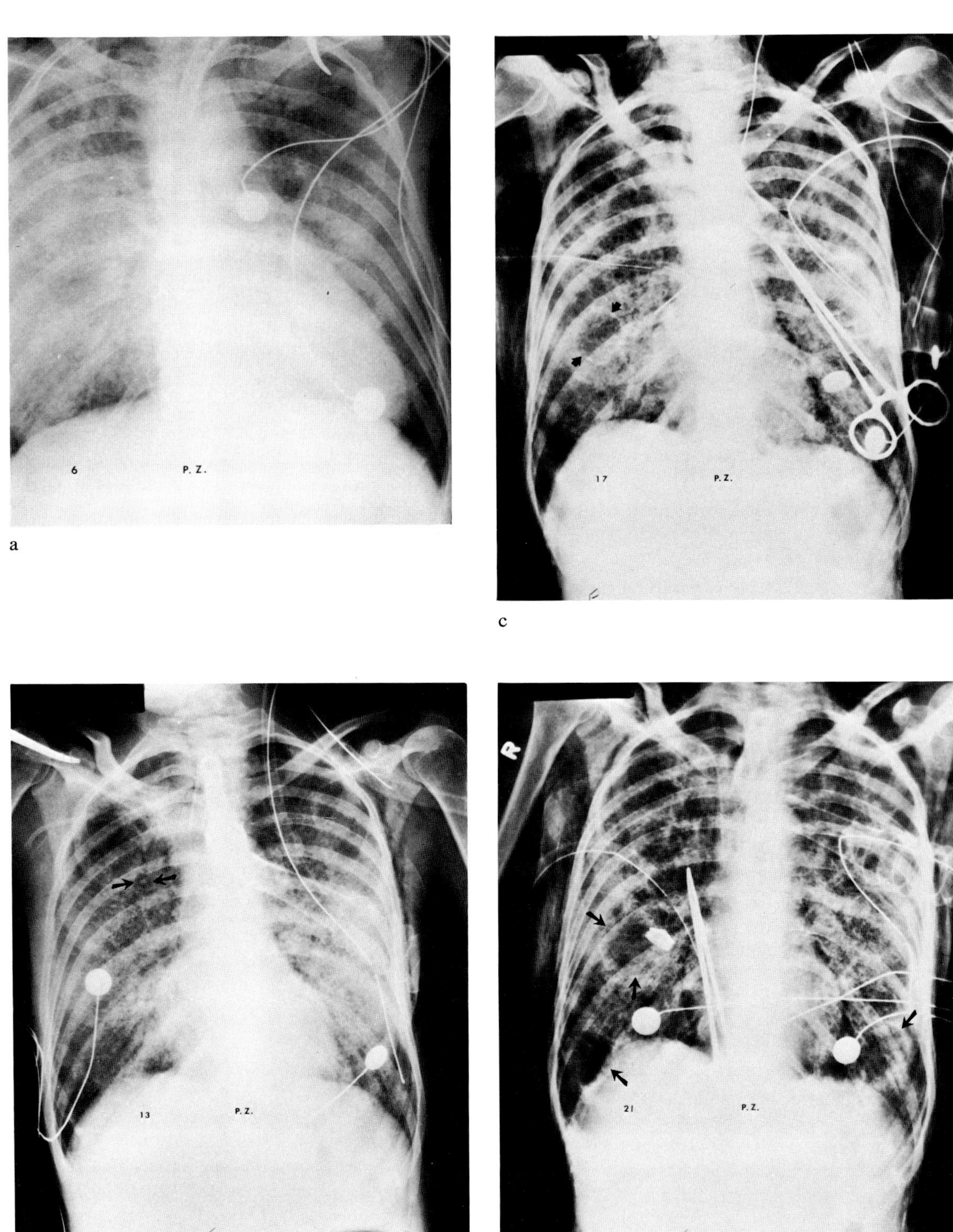

Fig. 6-7. Legend on page 93.

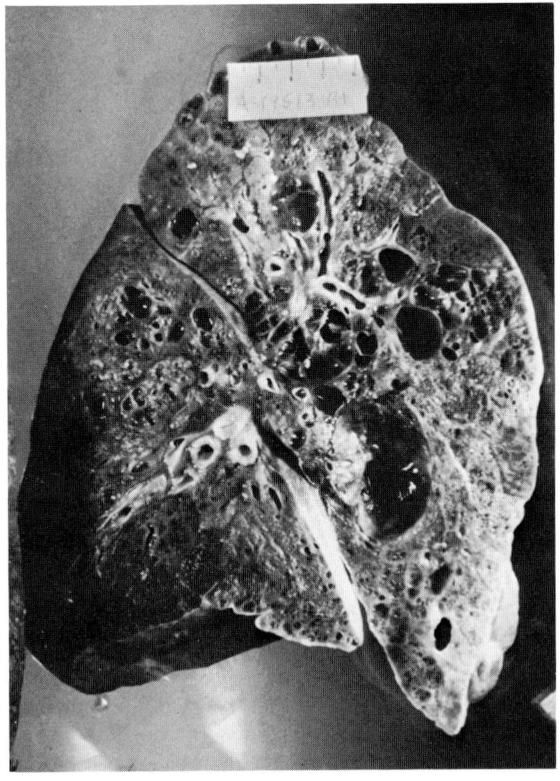

e

Fig. 6-7, a–e. A 34-year-old woman with postoperative ARDS, pneumonia, and gram-negative sepsis treated with antibiotics, CPPB, and supplemental O₂. a On the 6th postoperative day, there is diffuse consolidation of both lungs. There is a relatively clear area above the medial right diaphragm. **b** On the 13th day there are diffuse mottled circular radiolucencies in the medial two-thirds of both lungs. There is a round radiolucency in the right upper lobe (*arrows*) with a central opacity, which probably represents a large perivascular air collection. One day earlier, the patient developed sudden severe respiratory distress and cyanosis which could not be relieved by oxygen and which were followed by cardiac arrest. These events seemed to occur at the same time that extensive IPE was visualized radiographically. **c** By day 17, the IPE has progressed markedly. There are various-sized cystic areas throughout both lungs, and a large air cyst is seen in the right lung (*arrows*). **d** Portable chest x-ray on day 21 reveals very extensive IPE: the lungs appear to be largely replaced by large and small cystic airspaces. The patient had severe respiratory insufficiency at this time, and she died 10 days later without any significant further radiographic changes. **e** Photograph of the sectioned right lung at autopsy reveals large and small cystic spaces throughout the right lung. Microscopic study confirmed the presence of extensive IPE, acute and chronic inflammation, interstitial edema and hemorrhage, and infection of many of the air cysts.

thorax may be especially difficult to detect in patients who are supine. It is usually impossible to determine the site of pleural rupture in patients with PTX even at postmortem examination.† Macklin (37) believed that pneumothorax results from rupture of the delicate mediastinal pleura because it is not as thick and tough as the visceral pleura. However, pneumothorax secondary to rupture of pulmonary subpleural air cysts have been reported by numerous authors (7,28,36,44,59). According to Fleming and Bowen (7), when a leak from a pulmonary subpleural cyst occurs, the cyst is usually infected. In their series of 128 patients with ARF, 19 (15%) developed PTX; and of those 19, 17 (89%) had an associated gram-negative or staphylococcal pneumonia. Our own experience is much more limited, but we have examined the lungs postmortem in 9 patients who had developed episodes of tension PTX. In 6 patients, the cause of the pneumothorax could not be identified, but in 3, the pneumothorax was due to rupture of an infected subpleural air cyst. Regardless of the site of rupture, PPB can rapidly convert an ordinary pneumothorax into tension pneumothorax, resulting in the death of the patient (4,7,44,59). Tension PTX is especially common in patients who have other large extraalveolar air collections (subpleural air cysts, pneumomediastinum, pneumopericardium, etc.).

Pneumomediastinum

Pneumomediastinum (PM) by itself is usually an incidental finding, but when it occupies a large volume, it may diminish total lung capacity, compress and displace the heart and great vessels, and diminish venous return and cardiac output (25, 34,37,38,52). (See hemodynamic effects later and Figs. 6-9 and 6-10.) PM is usually the first radiographic sign indicating that alveolar rupture and

---

† Pneumothorax associated with interstitial emphysema obviously does not include the syndrome of spontaneous pneumothorax, which almost always results from direct rupture of apical subpleural cysts or blebs.

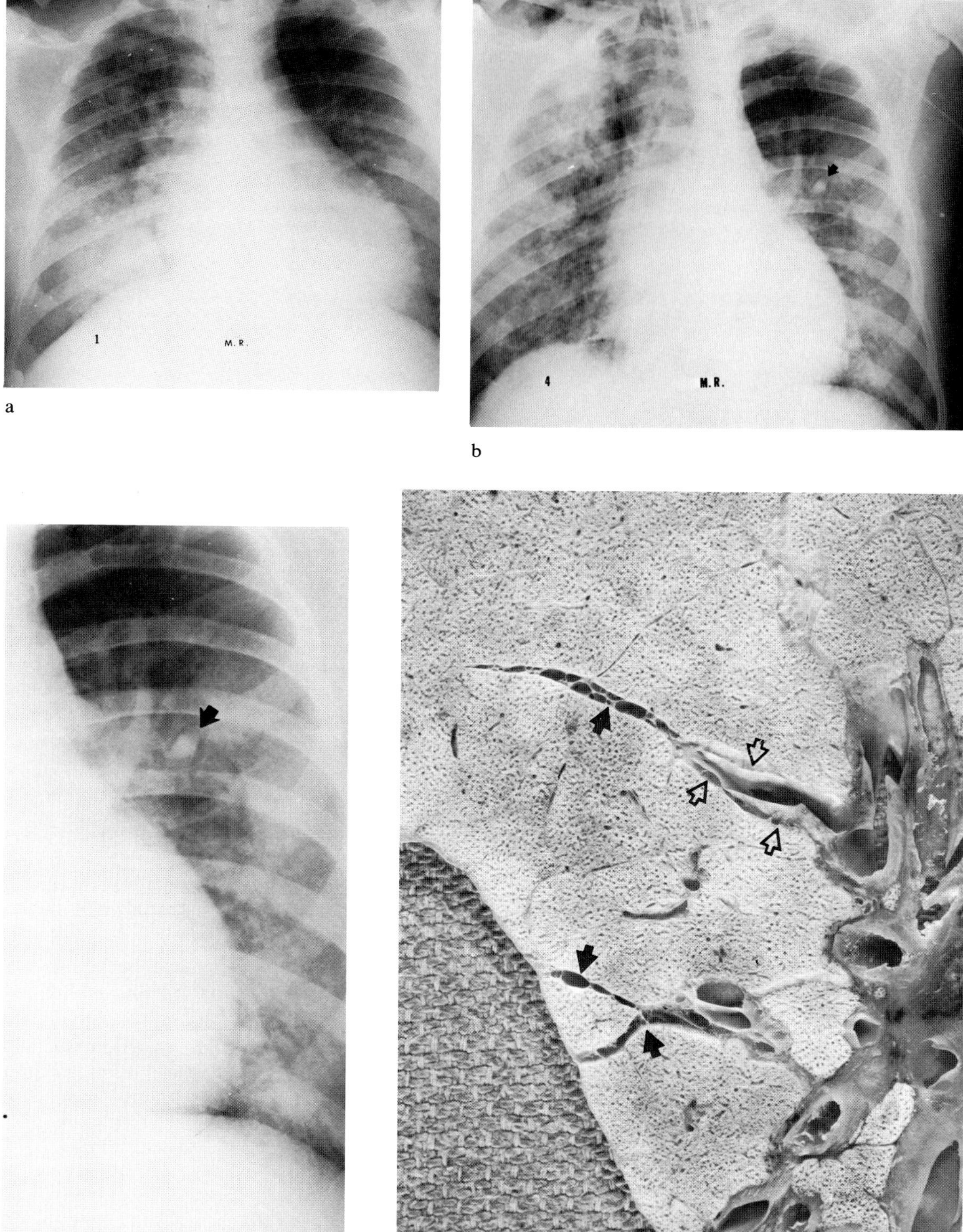

Fig. 6-8, a–d. A 34-year-old man with aortic stenosis, pneumonia, and gastrointestinal bleeding. a Portable chest roentgenogram on day one reveals pneumonia and/or pulmonary edema which is most marked on the right. **b, c** On the fourth day, there is more consolidation of the lungs, but there is now radiolucent mottling of the inner halves of both lungs, which is best seen on the right. There is a clear zone just above the medial right diaphragm. There is perivascular air around a large vessel in the left upper lobe (*arrow*). The patient died later the same day. **d** Photograph of a section through the medial portion of the upper lobe of the fixed inflated left lung reveals interstitial air in the interlobular septa (*closed arrows*) with air dissection around the vein draining the anterior segment of the left upper lobe (*open arrows*).

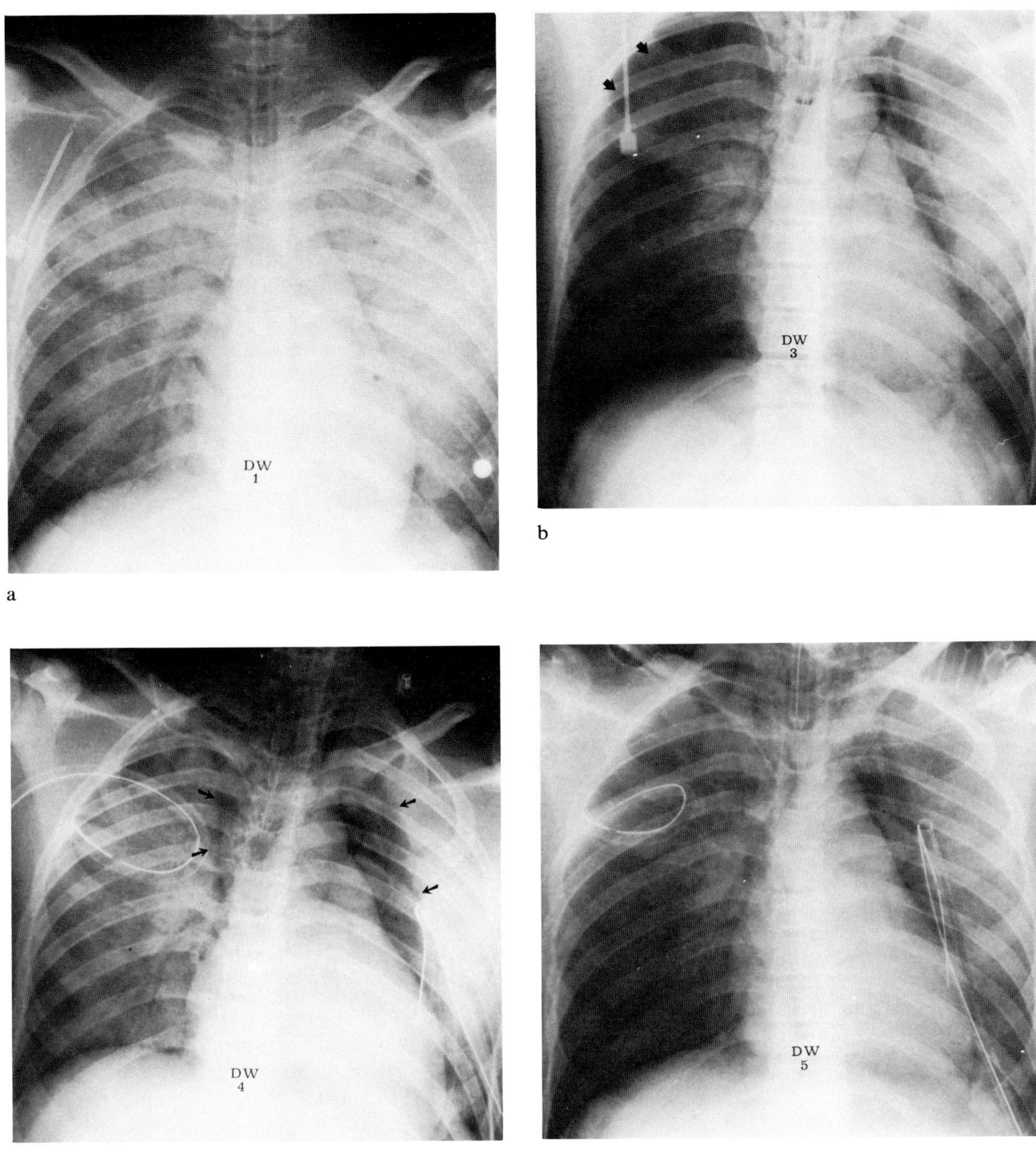

Fig. 6-9, a–d. Tension pneumomediastinum in a 14-year-old boy following head trauma. a Inital chest x-ray revealed diffuse pulmonary edema. **b** Four hours later, following institution of PEEP, the arterial pO_2 was 59 mm Hg on 40% O_2. Chest x-ray revealed partial clearing of the right-sided edema, a small right pneumothorax (*arrows*), and mediastinal emphysema. **c** Respiratory distress worsened over the next two hours. FiO_2 was increased to 100%, but the pO_2 remained between 70 and 75 mm Hg. A chest x-ray revealed increasing mediastinal emphysema, particularly on the left (*arrows*). Both lungs show increased opacity, suggesting that there is edema secondary to tension pneumomediastinum. **d** Two hours later a tracheostomy was performed. Upon incision of the pretracheal soft tissues there was a distinct loud hiss of escaping air. There was a dramatic and rapid improvement in the patient's respiratory status. Dyspnea quickly subsided, and the pO_2 increased from 74 to 290 mm Hg (100% FiO_2). The chest x-ray, done immediately following the tracheostomy, still shows pneumomediastinum, but it is much smaller, and there is marked clearing of the pulmonary edema.

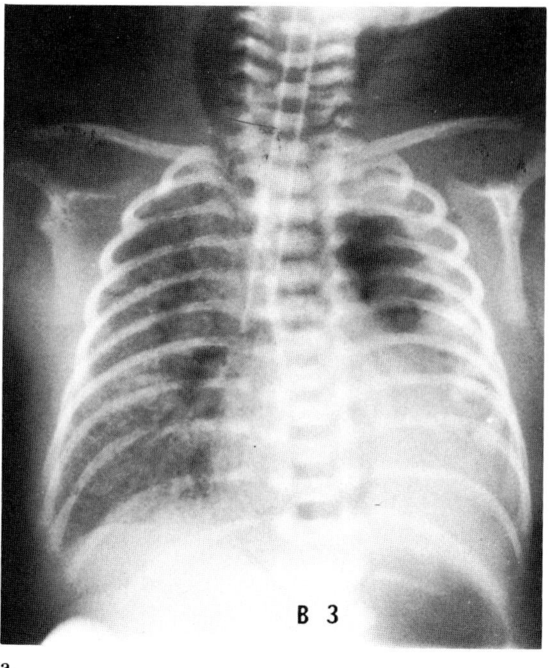

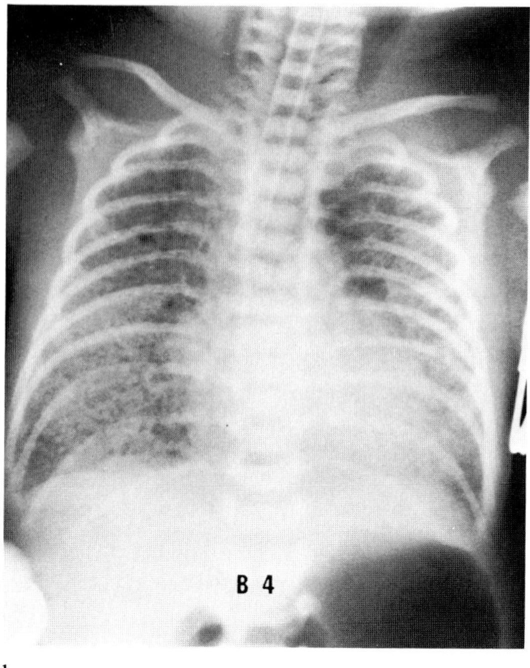

a
b

Fig. 6-10, a and b. Premature infant with RDS receiving CPPB and supplementary O₂; increasing respiratory insufficiency. a Chest x-ray on day 3 reveals bilateral IPE, a large pneumomediastinum (PM), and a dense left lung possibly secondary to vascular compression. The pneumomediastinum has been partially decompressed into the neck. An endotracheal tube is in the right mainstem bronchus. **b** Chest x-ray 12 hours later. Improvement occurred following withdrawal of the endotracheal tube from the right bronchus into the trachea and by decreasing the peak inspiratory pressures. The lungs still show extensive IPE, but the pneumomediastinum and marked opacity of the lungs have improved.

IPE have occurred. Tension PM is more likely to occur in infants because air does not escape as readily into the neck from the mediastinum as it does in adults.

Pneumopericardium

Pneumopericardium (PP) is a rare complication of PPB and occurs usually in infants (14,15,60–64) (Fig. 6-12). To our knowledge, no *well-documented* cases have occurred in adults as a result of PPB alone. The exact site of entry of air into the pericardial sac is uncertain. In those cases that have come to autopsy there has been no obvious source of the PP. Although congenital pericardial defects have been mentioned as a possible cause, none have been documented. Possibly, PP results from dissection of mediastinal air along the peri-

vascular sheaths of the blood and lymphatic vessels supplying and draining the pericardium with eventual rupture into the pericardial sac. PP may at times be diagnosed clinically by the presence of a pericardial rub or "crunch," muffled heart sounds, and evidence of cardiac tamponade, but definitive diagnosis is almost always radiologic. PP does not always cause ill effects, but if the pericardial air is under tension, rapid and fatal cardiac tamponade may occur. In those infants who have no signs of tamponade, conservative measures alone may be effective (62,64). Conservative treatment consists of (a) substituting 100% oxygen in the inspired air to increase the absorption of the air leak, and (b) decreasing the peak pressures used for mechanical ventilation if possible to diminish the forces driving air into the pericardial sac. However, such conservative measures by themselves are not always effective, and if there is radiographic or clinical evidence of tamponade,* immediate pericardiocentesis should be performed. Despite such measures, the mortality rate for PP is high, and in most reported series, it exceeds 50%. Brans et al. (60) strongly recommend aggressive therapy of PP as soon as it is diagnosed. They found in their review of 57 reported infants with PP that the survival rate was better in those treated with pericardiocentesis than in those treated conservatively despite the fact that the former group was presumably sicker. Because PP frequently recurs, they further suggest that it be treated with an indwelling pericardiocentesis catheter connected to suction.

Air in the anterior mediastinum may simulate PP. A diagnosis of PP rests on demonstrating air around the entire circumference of the heart; air along the left, right, or inferior border of the heart (Figs. 6-7d, 6-9b, 6-13) does not constitute adequate evidence of pneumopericardium (64). Such collections that do not entirely circumscribe the heart are usually due to pneumomediastinum or an anteromedial pneumothorax. Lateral views may be extremely helpful in patients in whom sagittal views are not diagnostic (60). Air beneath the heart may occur with pneumomediastinum (66) and is most probably due to dissection of air into the potential space between the parietal pericardium and diaphragm (Fig. 6-13).

Air Embolism

A uniformly fatal complication of IPE is air embolism (AE). It has been described in infants with hyaline membrane disease (15,67,68), in acute asthma (69), and in skin divers (39,70). However, to our knowledge, it has not been described in adults as a complication of PPB. Schaefer et al. (39) found that in dogs, AE occurred only when the transpulmonary pressure gradient exceeded 65 cm water. Lenaghan et al. (46) found that the status of the lungs had a profound effect upon the susceptibility to AE. In normal dogs AE did not develop until peak ventilator pressures reached 65 cm water. However, dogs with ARDS (induced by acute hemorrhagic shock) developed AE at pressures as low as 35 cm H_2O. Fatal AE has

been reported in a human infant with peak pressures as low as 40 cm water (68).

The radiographic diagnosis of AE depends upon identifying air in the cardiac chambers, hepatic veins, pulmonary arteries, or systemic arteries (15,33,67,68) (Fig. 6-14). Fatal AE may be more common than is recognized. It is difficult to diagnose at autopsy (15), and unlike systemic venous AE, very small amounts of embolized air in the coronary and cerebral arteries may be fatal. AE apparently occurs from rupture of dissecting perivascular air into the pulmonary veins and lymphatics. Bowen et al. (67) observed air bubbles in the pulmonary veins at autopsy in an infant who died of ARDS and CPPB. During the postmortem examination, they injected barium gel into the bronchus and noted that it appeared in the pulmonary veins and lymphatics.

One would expect pulmonary venous AE to be limited to the left heart and systemic arteries, but air is invariably found in the right heart chambers, pulmonary arteries, and the hepatic veins as well (Fig. 6-14). Right-sided air could conceivably be due to passage of air through the entire systemic circulation and back to the hepatic veins and right heart (15). Rupture of air into the pulmonary lymphatics with transport to the systemic veins would be another possible mechanism for right-sided AE. Another is that proposed by Lenaghan et al. (46): at the time of PPB-induced alveolar wall rupture of the lungs in dogs, they observed that there was actually a temporary *reversal* of blood flow in the pulmonary arteries, with transient pulmonary and tricuspid insufficiency and retrograde flow of air bubbles from the pulmonary vasculature to the right ventricle, right atrium, and hepatic veins.

Extraperitoneal Air Dissection and Pneumoperitoneum

Joannides and Tsoulos (34) showed that mediastinal air moves downward through the loose periesophageal connective tissues and from there into the extraperitoneal fascial planes of the anterior, posterior, and lateral abdominal walls as well into the mesentery. The exact path that air takes to gain access to the peritoneal cavity in patients with pneumoperitoneum is uncertain, but there are at least three possible mechanisms: (a) bubbles form in the retroperitoneal tissues and, with in-

---

* Higgins et al. (65) reported that a radiographic decrease in cardiac size indicates hemodynamic compromise and tamponade.

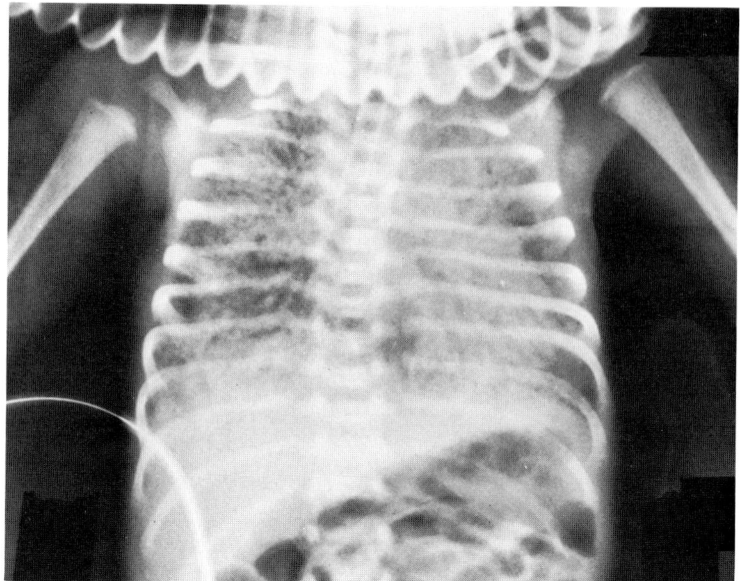

a

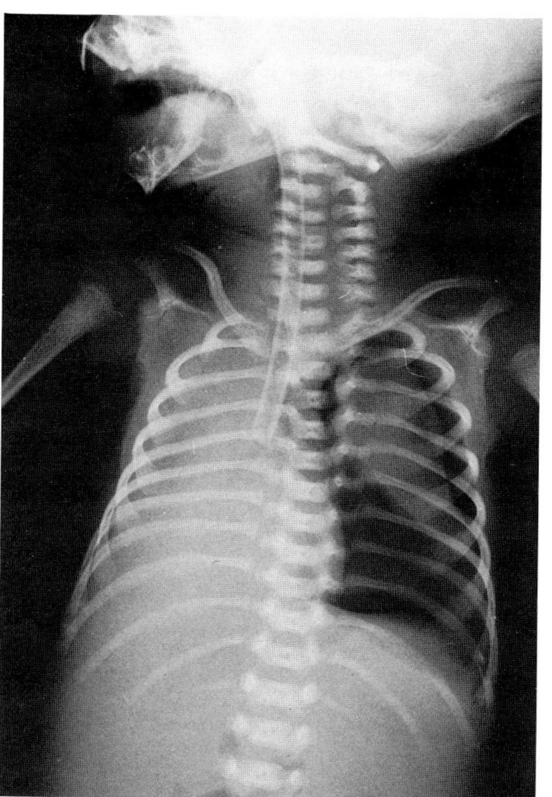

b

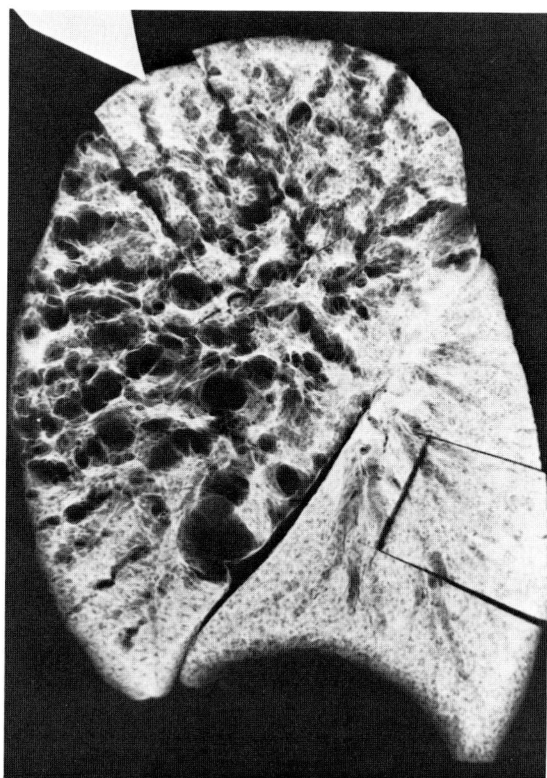

c

Fig. 6-11, a–d. **Fatal pneumothorax.** Premature infant with RDS receiving CPPB. **a** Chest x-ray on second day reveals extensive IPE. The infant subsequently became suddenly dyspneic, cyanotic, and died. **b** Postmortem radiograph reveals unsuspected left tension pneumothorax with displacement of the heart and compression of both lungs. **c** postmortem radiograph of section of fixed inflated left lung reveals extensive upper lobe IPE with cysts measuring up to 1 cm in diameter.

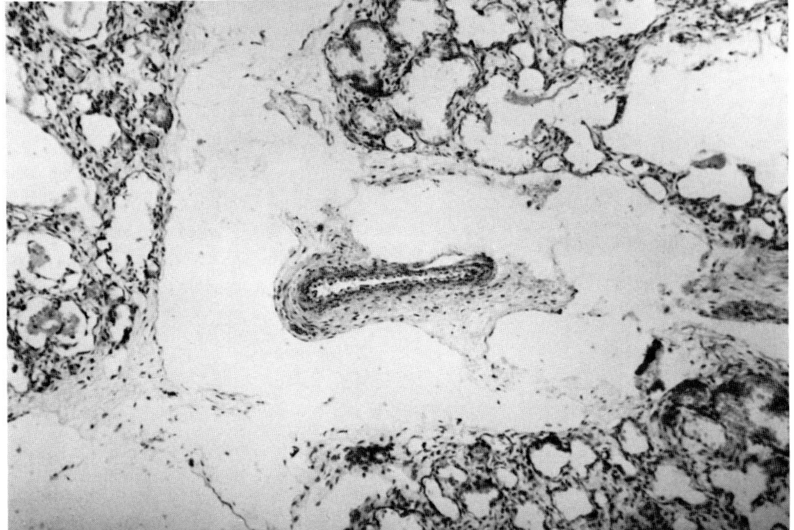

Fig. 6-11. (cont.) **d** Microscopic section of left upper lobe reveals total collapse of a vein secondary to extensive perivascular air in the interlobular septum. The air has completely torn away the perivascular connective tissues of the vein from the adjacent septum.

d

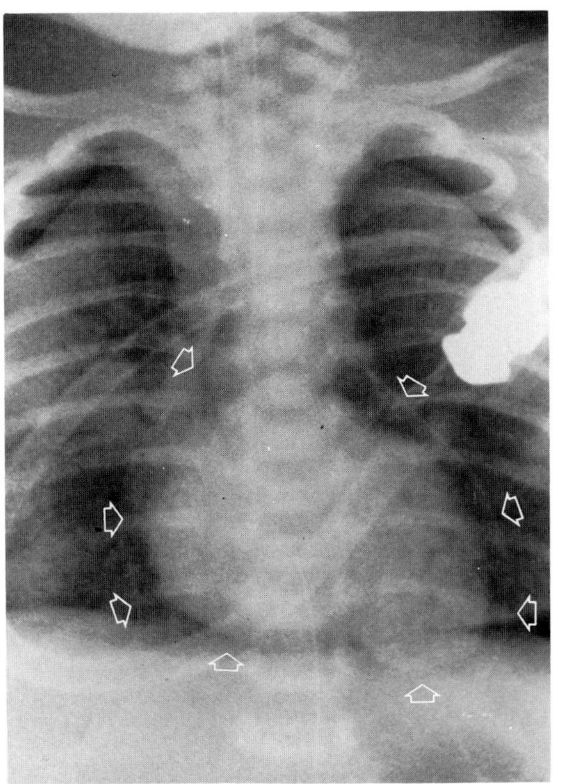

Fig. 6-12. Pneumopericardium. Premature infant with RDS treated with PEEP and O_2. Respiratory distress and cyanosis were increasing. Chest x-ray revealed bilateral pneumothorax and pneumopericardium (air seen about the entire circumference of the heart, *arrows*). The peak inspiratory pressures were reduced, and the pneumothoraces were treated with chest tubes. Repeat x-ray two hours later showed no pneumopericardium. The infant temporarily improved but died several days later of respiratory failure.

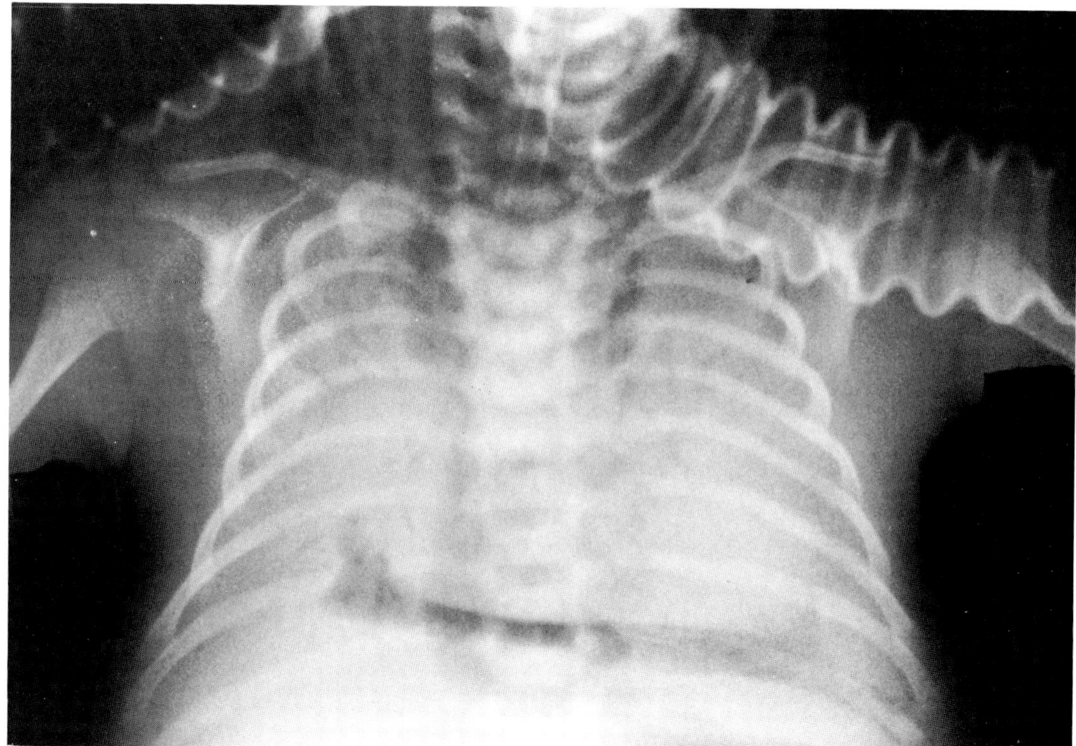

a

b

Fig. 6-13, a and **b. Tension pneumomediastinum simulating pneumopericardium.** Premature infant receiving CPPB for RDS. **a, b** Chest x-rays reveals large pockets of mediastinal air superior, anterior, posterior, and inferior to the heart. The inferior collection most probably represents dissection of air into the potential space between the parietal pericardium and diaphragm and should not be confused with pneumopericardium. The infant died of respiratory failure, and autopsy revealed immature lungs, diffuse pneumonia, edema, and IPE.

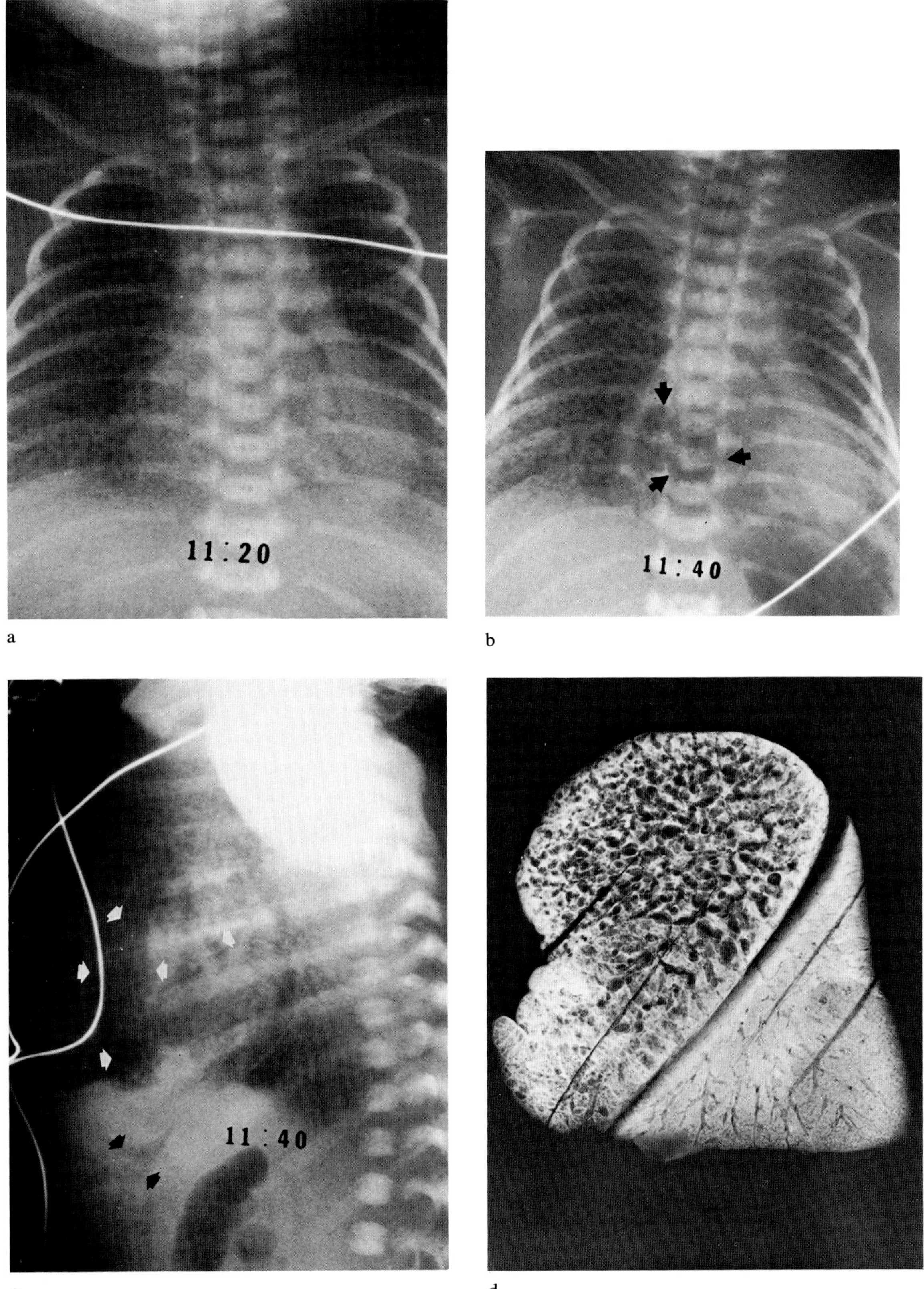

Fig. 6-14, a–d. Air embolism. A 1.5-kilogram premature infant with RDS treated with PEEP and up to 100% O_2. **a** An 11:20 AM chest x-ray revealed granular lungs with small mottled radiolucencies characteristic of IPE. **b, c** At 11:40 AM, 20 minutes later, there were increasing respiratory distress, cyanosis, and bradycardia. Repeat x-rays revealed extensive air in the right atrium, right ventricle, and hepatic veins (*arrows*). Death occurred within several hours, and autopsy confirmed the presence of air embolism in the right heart and systemic circulation. **d** Postmortem radiograph of fixed inflated section of left lung shows dense lungs with IPE; it is much more extensive in the upper lobes. Microscopic examination revealed immature lungs with hyaline membranes, IPE, and pulmonary hemorrhage.

creasing tension, may rupture directly into the peritoneal cavity; (b) air may enter the capillary beds of the retroperitoneum or mesentery and from there rupture into the peritoneal cavity; and (c) air in the pleural cavity may possibly pass into the peritoneal cavity through gaps in the diaphragm (33,71–74).

While pneumoperitoneum itself is not usually a serious complication, it creates diagnostic problems, since pneumoperitoneum from air dissection must be differentiated from a perforated viscus. In adult patients, if other signs of air leak (PM, PTX, IPE, etc.) are present, pneumoperitoneum can usually be assumed to be due to the air leak rather than a perforated viscus (48). However, in infants, the presence or absence of pneumomediastinum and other extraalveolar air collections does not allow a prediction of cause (75). Campbell et al. (72) stated that the presence of gaseous distention of the stomach and absence of intraabdominal fluid favors air dissection rather than a ruptured viscus as the cause of pneumoperitoneum. Obviously, air-fluid levels suggest a perforated viscus. Water-soluble contrast studies of the upper gastrointestinal tract may be extremely valuable in doubtful cases.

CPPB may occasionally be responsible for the development of a perforated viscus. Golden and Chandler (76) reported three patients with emphysema who developed marked colon dilatation and cecal perforation while receiving CPPB, and Leonidas et al. (75) described the same finding in infants receiving PPB.

Hemodynamic Effects

As the volume and relative tension of air in the perivascular connective tissues of the lung and mediastinum increase, the pulmonary vessels and mediastinal veins become progressively more collapsed (Figs. 6-4d, 6-5f–j, 6-11d). The preferential location of IPE in the larger interlobular septa, hilar regions, and mediastinum places it in an ideal position to cause compression of the major pulmonary vessels and systemic veins. In advanced cases, compression and obstruction of the pulmonary and mediastinal vessels may become extreme, resulting in tachycardia, falling cardiac output, and systemic hypotension (8,28,32,35–37,39,45) (Figs. 6-5, 6-7,

6-9, 6-10, 6-15). The patient may develop shock and cyanosis, and the pulses may become imperceptible. Acute dilatation of the right side of the heart has been shown at autopsy in both patients and experimental animals with extensive IPE and PM (27,28,32,36). The veins are usually more compressed than the arteries, presumably because their thinner walls and lesser distending pressure render them less resistant to compression. Since IPE causes relatively greater obstruction of the pulmonary veins than of the arteries, it should temporarily obstruct outflow from the lungs more than inflow and presumably result in the formation of acute pulmonary edema. When IPE and PM are extreme, a radiologic pattern may be observed suggesting that such a sequence does in fact occur. The peripheral portions of the lungs may become extremely radiopaque (Figs. 9c, 10a), resulting in a reversal of the more common pattern of pulmonary edema. If the acute "air block" is relieved, the peripheral edema clears rapidly (Figs. 6-9d, 6-10b). The hemodynamic situation usually improves rapidly if it is possible to decrease the driving pressures used during PPB or if there is a sudden release of air into the neck, pleural space, mediastinum, or abdomen (9,77).

Changes in Pulmonary Function

Since IPE occupies part of the total available intrathoracic volume, it will diminish functioning total lung capacity in direct proportion to the amount of interstitial air present. This effect is probably not important except in those cases in which pulmonary function is already severely compromised or when IPE is extensive (Fig. 6-16). Of far greater importance is the stiffening of the lungs that occurs because of the relatively unyielding, distended interstitial air pockets. Macklin and Macklin (38) observed that extensive IPE "splinted" the lung and increased resistance to both inspiration and expiration. Nennhaus et al. (44) believed that a rise in resistance to pulmonary inflation (decreased compliance) was the outstanding clinical feature of IPE and should suggest its presence. Other investigators (8,28,51) have reported a decrease in arterial oxygen saturation at the time that IPE was observed radiologically. We have observed several patients who developed both an increase in airway resistance and a lowered arterial oxygen saturation coinciding with the time that widespread IPE was observed radiologically (Figs. 6-5a, 6-7b, 6-11a, 6-15b). It appears that, in some cases, a vicious cycle is created in which IPE increases airway resistance, necessitating higher peak pressures, which in turn drive more air into the interstitial compartments of the lung, mediastinum, and soft tissues. The lungs become progressively stiffer and severely hyperexpanded (Figs. 6-15, 6-16). These severe changes are unlikely to develop unless the peak inspiratory pressures exceed 50 cm water.

Secondary Infection

While IPE and subpleural air cysts are known to follow various types of pneumonia, the reverse sequence may also occur. Subpleural air cysts secondary to PPB may become secondarily infected. Radiologically, thickening of the cyst wall or the presence of air-fluid levels may be observed if the cysts become infected. Persistence of a subpleural cyst for more than a few days also strongly suggests the presence of secondary infection (Figs. 6-6, 6-7, 6-16). IPE may also contribute to the spread of infection (31,39). IPE is frequently accompanied by the formation of interstitial edema and hemorrhage (Figs. 6-4a,b, 6-15c), and the proteinaceous fluid forms an ideal medium for bacterial growth. Boiset (31) states that the interstitial air dissection forms "air corridors" which facilitate the spread of infection in the interstitial and perivascular connective tissues. We examined several patients at autopsy with extensive IPE who also showed extensive acute inflammation of the perivascular and septal connective tissues; and frequently, acute interstitial inflammatory changes were observed in areas in which interstitial air was also present (Figs. 6-7f, 6-16d). Similar changes were also observed in pigs subjected to several hours of PPB (Fig. 6-4b).

Whether infection precedes IPE or follows it is not as important as the recognition that the combination of IPE and infection is an ominous and frequently lethal combination (Figs. 6-7, 6-16). The infection is often refractory to treatment, and such patients are especially likely to develop a blowout of an infected subpleural air cyst and tension pneumothorax.

IPE-Induced Changes in Pulmonary Morphology

Several histologic abnormalities are observed in patients with IPE; these include interstitial proteinaceous material containing fibrin, interstitial hemorrhage, fibroblastic proliferation, and patchy hyaline membrane formation within the alveoli. In patients who have been treated with PPB for ARF, it is impossible to tell whether these changes are due to the underlying pulmonary disease, secondary infection, the effects of supplemental oxygen, or the mechanical effects of PPB. Many investigators have shown that the pulmonary complications ascribed to PPB (inflammation, hemorrhage, capillary damage, edema, hyaline membranes, necrosis, and fibrosis) can be produced by high concentrations of inspired oxygen without the use of PPB (11,78–80). The role of PPB by itself as a cause of lung damage is unclear. In experimental animals, neither Morgan et al. (78) nor Nash et al. (79) were able to demonstrate pathologic effects in the lungs from PPB alone. However, Nash et al. used inspiratory pressures of only 13 cm water, and the peak pressures used by Morgan et al. were not stated.

Other studies, using higher inspiratory pressures, have demonstrated anatomic changes in the lungs associated with IPE. Arbulu et al. (28) described the presence of edema and hemorrhage in the interlobular septa and subpleural connective tissues in a patient with extensive IPE who had received positive pressure anesthesia. Ovenfors (25) observed hemorrhage in the lungs of dogs who had developed IPE using inspiratory pressures of 30 cm H_2O.

We have recently completed a study attempting to assess the effects of CPPB and IPE on the lungs of 15 pigs in the absence of supplemental oxygen (27). The pigs were maintained with CPPB with peak pressures ranging from 30 to 50 cm water for periods ranging from 17 to 136 hours. All the animals ventilated at pressures greater than 25 cm water uniformly developed marked IPE, and it was most marked in those ventilated at the highest pressures. Histologic examination of the lungs revealed interstitial edema and fibrin, focal hemorrhage, and fibroblastic proliferation (Fig. 6-4). These findings were not observed in the pigs ventilated at pressures of 20 cm water or less. In several

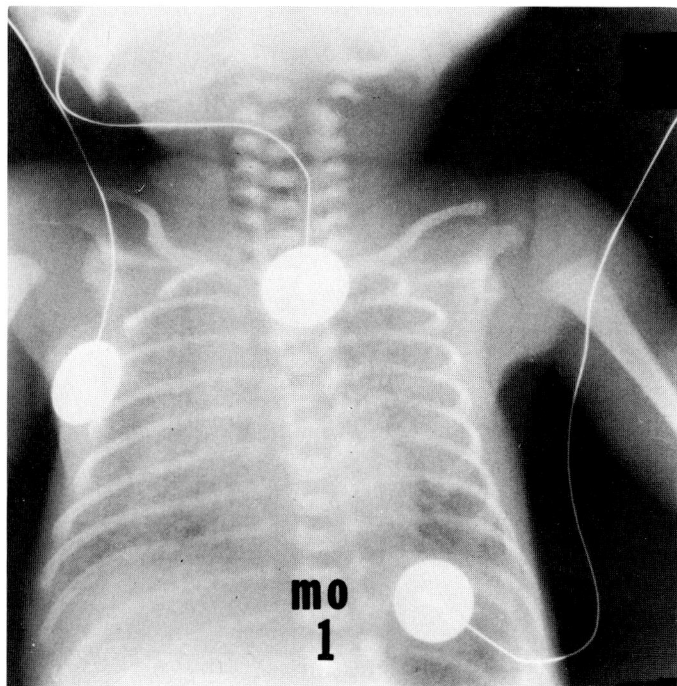

a

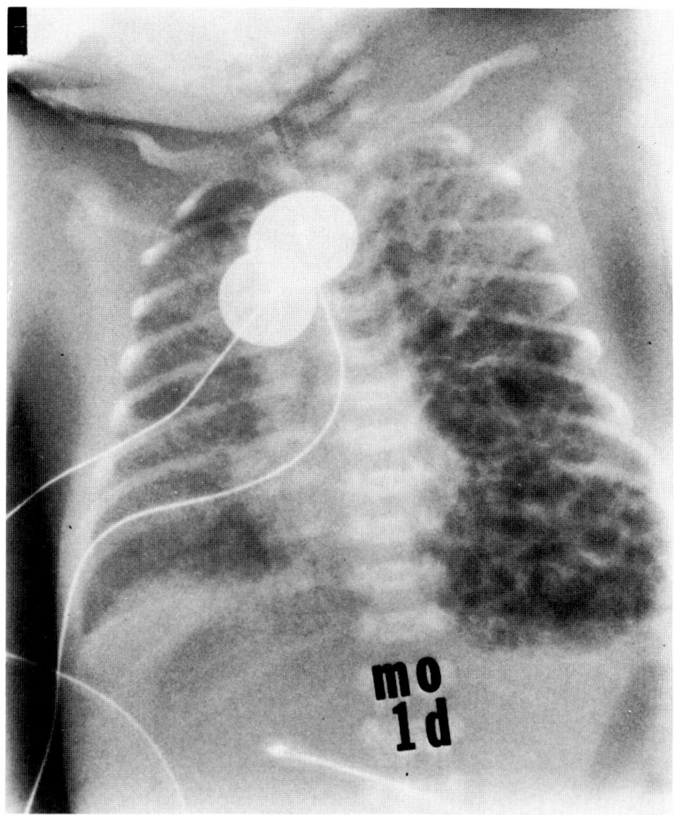

b

Fig. 6-15, a–d. Tension IPE in a premature infant with RDS. a Chest x-ray five hours after tracheal intubation revealed the endotracheal tube in the right intermediate bronchus with obstruction and atelectasis of the right upper lobe and entire left lung. The atelectasis completely resolved upon repositioning the tube in the trachea. **b** Chest x-ray at one day revealed a markedly hyperexpanded cystic-appearing left lung. The infant was severely dyspneic, cyanotic, hypotensive, and he died several hours later.

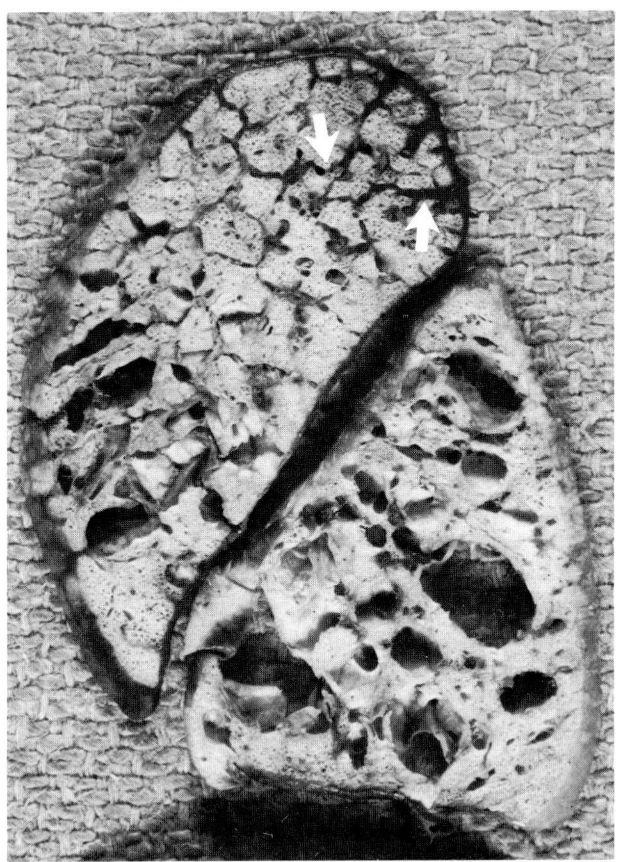

c

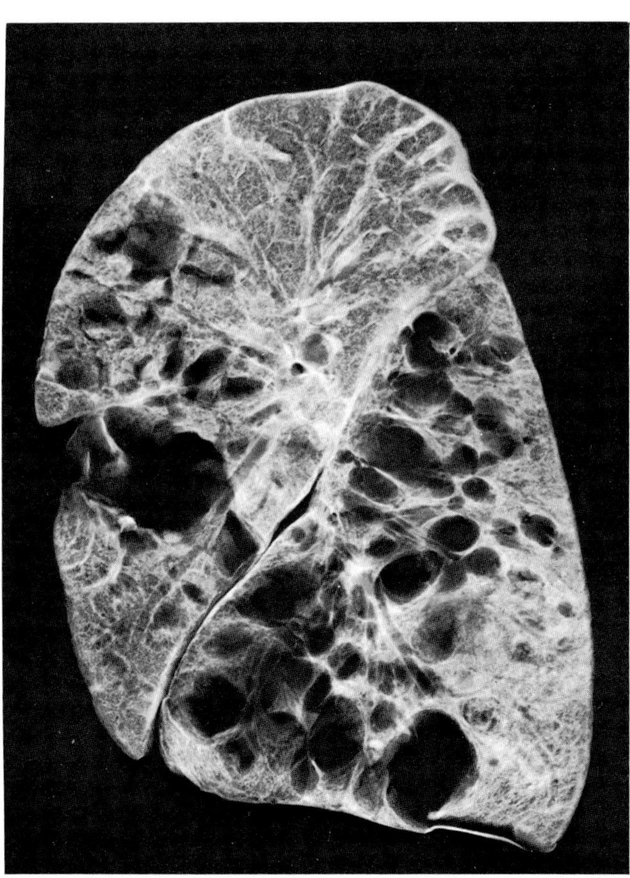

d

Fig 6-15 (cont.) **c** Postmortem section of fixed inflated left lung. At autopsy, the left lung was tense, hyperexpanded, and would not deflate. The fixative could not be introduced into the bronchus until the IPE was decompressed by needling one of the subpleural cysts. The cystic collections of IPE are visualized in the subpleural connective tissues and interlobular septa. There are also areas of septal hemorrhage, especially in the right upper lobe (*arrows*). Histologic examination confirmed the presence of extensive IPE with interstitial hemorrhage, edema, and inflammation. **d** Radiograph of another left lung section reveals extensive interstitial and subpleural emphysema.

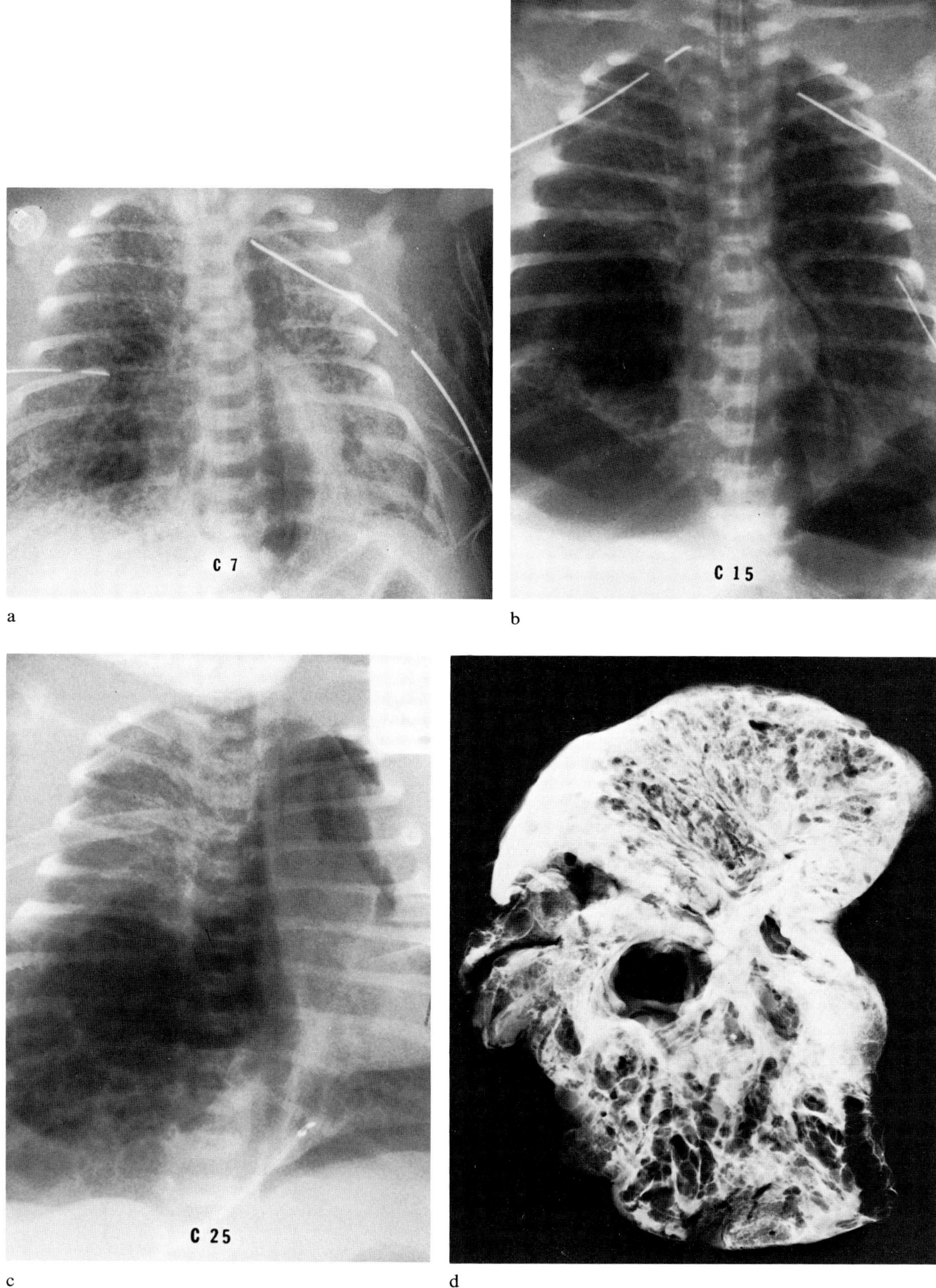

Fig. 6-16. Legend on page 107.

pigs ventilated at peak pressures of 30 cm water or more with room air, hyaline membranes were observed. This study does not deny the role of supplemental oxygen in producing lung damage, but it does suggest that CPPB alone can produce edema, hemorrhage, fibrosis, and hyaline membranes and that these changes may result from the mechanical damage produced by dissecting interstitial air.

Acknowledgment

Our thanks go to Christine M. Volzo for her continuing work in preparing this manuscript.

References

1. Ashbaugh DG, Petty TL, Bigelow DB, Harris TM: Continuous positive-pressure breathing (CPPB) in adult respiratory distress syndrome. J Thorac Cardiovasc Surg 57:31–41, 1969.
2. Kirby RR, Downs JB, Civetta JM, Medell JA, Dannemiller FJ, Klein EF, Hodges M: High level positive end expiratory pressure (PEEP) in acute respiratory insufficiency. Chest 67:156–163, 1975.
3. Pontoppidan H, Geffin B, Lowenstein E: Acute respiratory failure in the adult. N Engl J Med 287:690–698, 743–752, 799–806, 1972.
4. Sugerman HJ, Olofsson KB, Pollock TW, Agnew RF, Rogers RM, Miller LD: Continuous positive-end-expiratory pressure ventilation (PEEP) for the treatment of diffuse interstitial edema. J Trauma 12:263–274, 1972.
5. Uzawa T, Ashbaugh DG: Continuous positive-pressure breathing in acute hemorrhage pulmonary edema. J Appl Physiol 26:427–432, 1969.
6. Kirkpatrick BV, Felman AH, Eitzman DV: Complications of ventilator therapy in respiratory distress syndrome. Am J Dis Child 128:496–502, 1974.
7. Fleming WH, Bowen JC: Early complications of long-term respiratory support. J Thorac Cardiovasc Surg 64:729–738, 1972.
8. Leeming WA: Radiological aspects of the pulmonary complications resulting from intermittent positive pressure breathing. Aust Radiol 12:361–377, 1968.
9. Lightman DJ, Lincoln JC: Malignant pulmonary interstitial emphysema. Br J Anaesth 39:587–591, 1967.
10. MacPherson RI, Chernick V, Reed M: The complications of respirator therapy in the newborn. J Can Assoc Radiol 23:91–102, 1972.
11. Northway WH Jr, Rosan RC, Porter DY: Pulmonary disease following respirator therapy of hyaline-membrane disease. N Engl J Med 276–357, 1967.
12. Perna AM, Brawley RK, Bender HW, Gott VL: Fatal respiratory distress syndrome after prolonged mechanical ventilation: its pathogenesis and prevention. J Surg Res 11:584–589, 1974.
13. Relier JP: Mechanical complications of artificial ventilation in the newborn. Biol Neonate 16:122–132, 1970.
14. Sagel SS, Wimbush P, Goldberg D: Tension pneumopericardium following assisted ventilation in hyaline membrane disease. Radiology 106:175–178, 1973.
15. Vinstein AL, Gresham EL, Lim MO, Franken EA: Pulmonary venous air embolism in hyaline membrane disease. Radiology 106:627–630, 1972.
16. Baratz RA, Philbin DM, Patterson RW: Plasma antidiuretic hormone and urinary output during continuous positive pressure breathing in dogs. Anesthesiology 34:510–513, 1971.
17. Kumar A, Pontoppidan H, Baratz RA, Laver MB: Inappropriate response to increased plasma ADH during mechanical ventilation in acute respiratory failure. Anesthesiology 40:215–221, 1974.
18. Sladen A, Laver MB, Pontoppidan H: Pulmonary complications and water retention in prolonged mechanical ventilation. N Engl J Med 279:448–453, 1968.
19. White WA, Bergland RM: Experimental inappropriate ADH secretion caused by positive-pressure respirators. J Neurosurg 36:608–613, 1972.
20. Gett PM, Jones ES, Shepherd GF: Pulmonary oedema with sodium retention during ventilator treatment. Br J Anaesth 43:460–470, 1971.
21. Nicotra MB, Stevens PM, Viroslav J, Alvarez AA:

Fig. 6-16, a–d. Persisting interstitial pulmonary emphysema (PIPE). Full-term infant with meconium aspiration treated with PEEP and supplemental oxygen (FiO$_2$ 25–45%). **a** Day 7. There are diffuse bilateral IPE, marked hyperexpansion, bilateral pneumothorax (treated), and a large posterior collection of mediastinal air. **b** On day 15, large air cysts are developing in the lungs. There are soft-tissue air and persisting pneumothoraces. Heart size is markedly reduced, possibly reflecting a decrease in cardiac output. **c** Day 25. There has been progressive enlargement of the IPE cysts in the right lower lobe, resulting in displacement of the heart and compression of the right upper lobe and left lung. The infant was never weaned from the respirator, and death occurred on day 32. **d** Sagittal postmortem radiograph of a right lung section reveals diffuse consolidation (pneumonia), extensive IPE, and large cysts in the lower lobe. Microscopic examination confirmed the presence of pneumonia and extensive IPE with chronic inflammation of the interstitial air cysts.

Physiologic evaluation of positive and expiratory pressure ventilation. Chest 64:10–15, 1973.

22. Ashbaugh DG, Petty TL: Positive end-expiratory pressure: physiology, indications, and contraindications. J Thorac Cardiovasc Surg 65:165–170, 1973.

23. Colgan FJ, Marocco PP: The cardiorespiratory effects of constant and intermittent positive-pressure breathing. Anesthesiology 36:444–449, 1972.

24. Jardin F, Farcot J, Boisante L, Curien N, Margairaz A, Bourdarias J: Influence of positive end-expiratory pressure on left ventricular performance. N Engl J Med 304:387–392, 1981.

25. Ovenfors C: Pulmonary interstitial emphysema. Acta Radiol (Suppl 224), 1964.

26. Westcott JL, Cole SR: Interstitial pulmonary emphysema in children and adults: roentgenographic features. Radiology 111:367–378, 1974.

27. DeGraff AC, Cole SR, Horowitz SM, Davis JM, Sandals HE, Westcott JL: The long term effects of positive pressure breathing and interstitial pulmonary emphysema. (in press.)

28. Arbulu A, Belamaric J, Norton ML: Hyperinflation interstitial rupture of the lung. Ann Otol Rhinol Laryngol 81:825–31, 1972.

29. Fisher JH, Macklin CC: Pulmonic interstitial and mediastinal emphysema. Am J Dis Child 60:102–115, 1940.

30. Macklin CC: Pneumothorax with massive collapse from experimental local overinflation of the lung substance. Can Med Assoc J 36:414–420, 1937.

31. Boisset GF: Subpleural emphysema complicating staphylococcal and other pneumonias. Pediatrics 81:259–266, 1972.

32. Emery JL: Interstitial emphysema, pneumothorax, and "air-block" in the newborn. Lancet 1:405–409, 1956.

33. Gregory GA, Tooley WH: Gas embolism in hyaline membrane disease. N Engl J Med 282:1141–1142, 1970.

34. Joannides M, Tsoulos GD: The etiology of interstitial and mediastinal emphysema. Arch Surg 21:333–339, 1930.

35. Kelman SR: Experimental emphysema. Arch Intern Med 24:332–346, 1919.

36. Kirschner PA, Strauss L: Pulmonary interstitial emphysema in the newborn infant. Dis Chest 46:417–426, 1964.

37. Macklin CC: Transport of air along sheaths of pulmonic blood vessels from alveoli to mediastinum. Arch Intern Med 64:913–926, 1939.

38. Macklin MT, Macklin CC: Malignant interstitial emphysema of the lungs and mediastinum as an important occult complication in many respiratory diseases and other conditions. Medicine 23:281–358, 1944.

39. Schaefer KE, McNulty WP Jr, Carey C, Liebow AA: Mechanisms in development of interstitial emphysema and air embolism on decompression from depth. J Appl. Physiol 13:15–29, 1958.

40. Reid L: The connective tissue septa in the adult human lung. Thorax 14:138–145, 1959.

41. v Hayek H: Die menschliche Lung. Berlin: Springer-Verlag, 1953.

42. Bhatia JL, Thind GS: Interstitial and mediastinal emphysema complicating acute miliary tuberculosis. Indian J Chest Dis 12:76–79, 1970.

43. Torrey RG, Grosh LC: Acute pulmonary emphysema observed during the epidemic of influenzal pneumonia at Camp Hancock, Georgia. Am J Med Sci 157:170–181, 1919.

44. Nennhaus HP, Javid H, Julian OC: Alveolar and pleural rupture. Arch Surg 94:136–141, 1967.

45. Marcotte RJ, Phillips FJ, Adams WE, Livingstone H: Differential intrabronchial pressures and mediastinal emphysema. J Thorac Surg 9:346–355, 1940.

46. Lenaghan R, Silva YJ, Walt AJ: Hemodynamic alterations associated with expansion rupture of the lungs. Arch Surg 99:339–343, 1969.

47. Kumar AN, Falke KJ, Geffin B, Aldredge CF, Laver MB, Lowenstein E, Pontoppidan H: Continuous positive-pressure ventilation in acute respiratory failure. N Engl J Med 283:1430–1436, 1970.

48. Rohlfing B, Webb W, Schlobohm R: Ventilator-related extra-alveolar air in adults. Radiology 121:25–31, 1976.

49. Avery ME: The Lung and Its Disorders in the Newborn Infant. Philadelphia: WB Saunders Co, 1968, p 187.

50. Campbell RE: Intrapulmonary interstitial emphysema: a complication of hyaline membrane disease. AJR 110:449–456, 1970.

51. Fletcher BD, Outerbridge EW, Dunbar JS: Pulmonary interstitial emphysema in the newborn. J Can Assoc Radiol 21:273–279, 1970.

52. Herrnheiser G, Whitehead JP: Pulmonary interstitial emphysema. Br J Radiol 26:519–524, 1953.

53. Clarke TA, Edwards DK: Pulmonary pseudocysts in newborn infants with respiratory distress syndrome. AJR 133:417–421, 1979.

54. Bauer CR, Brennan MJ, Doyle C, Poole CA: Surgical resection for pulmonary interstitial emphysema in the newborn infant. J Pediatr 93:656–661, 1978.

55. Drew JH, Landau LI, Acton CM, Kent M, Campbell PE: Pulmonary interstitial emphysema requiring lobectomy. Am J Dis Child 53:424–426, 1978.

56. Fletcher BD, Outerbridge EW, Youssef S, Bolande RP: Pulmonary interstitial emphysema in a newborn infant treated by lobectomy. Pediatrics 54:808–810, 1974.

57. Stocker JT, Madewell JE: Persistent interstitial pulmonary emphysema: another complication of the respiratory distress syndrome. Pediatrics 59:847–857, 1977.

58. Watts JL, Arviagno RL, Brady JP: Chronic pulmonary disease in neonates after artificial ventilation: distribution of ventilation and pulmonary interstitial emphysema. Pediatrics 60:273–281, 1977.

59. Robbins JJ: Letter to the editor. Chest 59:469, 1971.

60. Brans YW, Pitts M, Cassady G: Neonatal pneumopericardium. Am J Dis Child 130:393–396, 1976.

61. Grosfeld JL, Kilman JW, Frye TR: Spontaneous pneumopericardium in the newborn infant. J Pediatr 76:614–616, 1970.

62. Pomerance JJ, Weller MH, Richardson CJ, Soule JA: Pneumopericardium complicating respiratory

63. Reppert SM, Ment LR, Todres ID: The treatment of pneumopericardium in the newborn infant. J Pediatr 90:115–117, 1977.

64. Varano LA, Maisels MJ: Pneumopericardium in the newborn: diagnosis and pathogenesis. Pediatrics 53:941–945, 1974.

65. Higgins CB, Broderick TW, Edwards DK, Shumaker A: The hemodynamic significance of massive pneumopericardium in preterm infant with respiratory distress syndrome. Radiology 133:363–368, 1979.

66. Levin B: The continuous diaphragm sign. A newly recognized sign of pneumomediastinum. Clin Radiol 24:337–338, 1973.

67. Bowen FW, Chandra R, Avery GB: Pulmonary interstitial emphysema with gas embolism in hyaline membrane disease. Am J Dis Child 126:117–118, 1973.

68. Mahmud F: Air embolism from mechanical ventilation in respiratory distress syndrome. South Med J 72:783–785, 1979.

69. Segal AJ, Wasserman M: Arterial air embolism: a cause of death in status asthmaticus. Radiology 99:271–272, 1971.

70. Polak B, Adams H: Traumatic air embolism in submarine escape training. US Naval Med Bull 30:165–177, 1932.

71. Aranda J, Stern L, Dunbar J: Pneumothorax with pneumoperitoneum in a newborn infant. Am J Dis Child 123:163–166, 1972.

72. Campbell R, Boggs T Jr, Kirkpatrick J: Early neonatal pneumoperitoneum from progressive massive tension penumomediastinum. Radiology 114:121–126, 1975.

73. Donahoe PK, Stewart DR, Osmond JD III: Pneumoperitoneum secondary to pulmonary air leak. J Pediatr 81:797–800, 1972.

74. Summers B: Pneumoperitoneum associated with artifical ventilation. Br Med J 1:1528–1530, 1979.

75. Leonidas J, Berdan W, Baker D: Perforation of the gastrointestinal tract and pneumoperitoneum in newborns treated with continuous lung distending pressures. Pediatr Radiol 2:241–246, 1974.

76. Golden GT, Chandler JG: Colonic ileus and cecal perforation in patients requiring mechanical ventilatory support. Chest 68:661–664, 1975.

77. Unger DL, Pifarre R: Tracheostomy for subcutaneous emphysema and pneumomediastinum complicating asthma. Chest 61:691–692, 1972.

78. Morgan WW, DeLemos R, Wolfsdorf J, Nachman R, Block J, Leiby G, Wilkonson HA, Allen T, Averym M, Haller JA: A quantitative assessment of lung injury from oxygen with and without assisted ventilation, and air with assisted ventilation in lambs. Surg Forum 19:265–267, 1968.

79. Nash G, Bowen JA, Langlinais PC: "Respirator lung": a misnomer. Arch Pathol 21:234–240, 1971.

80. Nash G, Blennerhassett JB, Pontoppidan H: Pulmonary lesions associated with oxygen therapy and artificial ventilation. N Engl J Med 276:368–374, 1967.

7 Radiographic Features of Thoracic Complications Occurring in Infants in the Intensive Care Nursery

G. B. Clifton Harris

The past two decades have witnessed outstanding progress in the rates of survival as well as in the subsequent quality of life of tiny, preterm infants and of neonates with respiratory disorders. These accomplishments can be attributed to the painstaking attention provided by attending physicians, nurses, and respiratory therapists based on an escalating understanding of perinatal physiologic and pathologic processes. Concomitant technologic advances in life-support devices and physiologic monitoring instruments, adapted and designed for use in extremely small infants, have played a significant complementary role.

Babies under 1500 grams pose the major management problems in the intensive care nursery, and increasing numbers of babies even under 750 grams are being admitted to such nurseries. These tiny infants are so frail and puny that all aspects of their care, even when performed by those with considerable experience, are fraught with perilous, potentially life-threatening mishaps.

The immediate care of these babies usually includes effective resuscitation and treatment to maintain adequate oxygenation. When gas exchange is severely impaired, therapy requires high oxygen concentration in the inspired air and the use of mechanical ventilation with intermittent positive pressure and with positive end-expiratory pressure. Intravascular catheters are required to monitor vital data as well as for nutritional purposes. Endotracheal intubation and suctioning are frequently essential, as is gastrointestinal intubation. While these invasive procedures have proved effective in dramatically improving survival, acute complications and harmful late sequelae of their use must be anticipated.

This chapter deals with the radiologic features of some of the thoracic complications that may occur during the care of these fragile occupants of the intensive care nursery. It is based largely on my own experience at the Children's Hospital Medical Center and the Lying-In Division of the Boston Hospital for Women.

Endotracheal Intubation

A common problem with endotracheal intubation is malposition of the tube. Ideally, the tube should be securely fixed in place such that the lower tip lies about 1 cm above the carina (1), which usually is at the level of the fourth thoracic vertebra. It should be a cardinal rule regarding endotracheal intubation that the procedure is not complete until a radiologic examination has shown that the tube is in appropriate location. Prompt recognition of an inappropriately placed tube is of vital importance. If too high, the tube may be dislodged from the trachea with a change in head position (Fig. 7-1). More often the tube is inserted too far, and the usual faulty placement causes the tube to extend down below the carina into the right main or right intermediate bronchus, where it often results in collapse of the right upper lobe as well as of the entire left lung (Fig. 7-2). Malposition can cause collapse or hyperaeration of various other lobes, depending on the depth of the abnormal insertion and on the location of the tube wall and its orifice in relation to the various bronchial openings (Fig. 7-3a, b).

Malposition of the endotracheal tube can cause

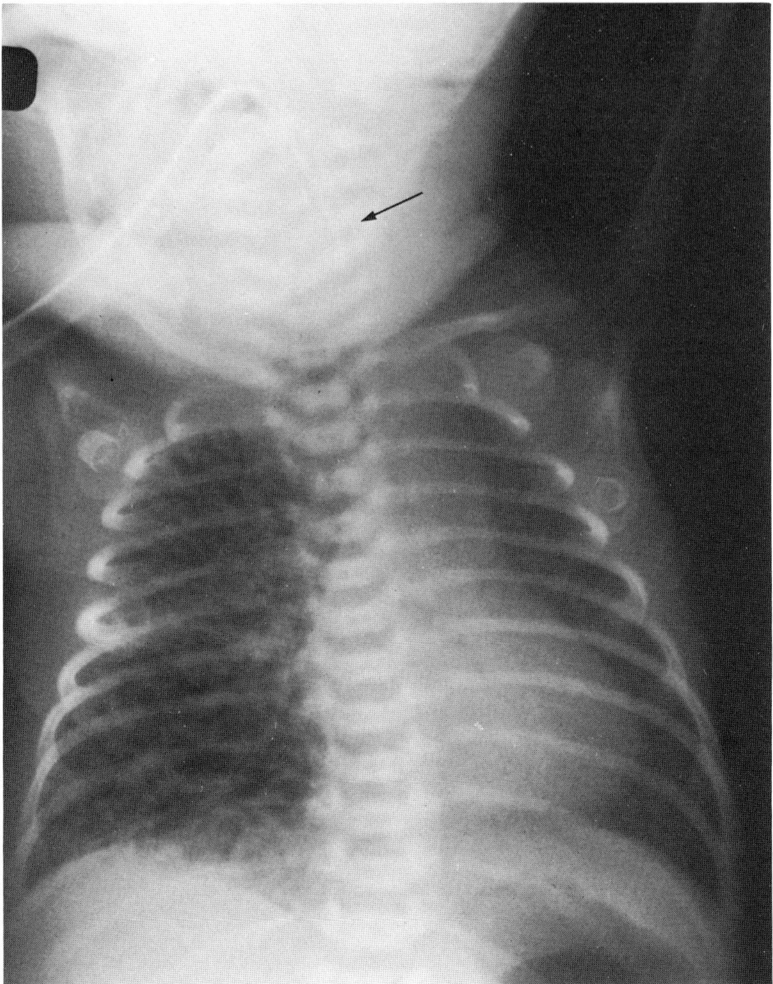

Fig. 7-1. High endotracheal tube (*arrow*). When the ET tube is this high, it might easily become entirely dislodged from the airway. The tip of the ET tube should be about 1 cm above the carina. Notice the extensive interstitial emphysema involving the right lung.

severe damage to bronchial mucosa, and ultimately this can lead to granulation tissue formation and scarring. These lesions may then result later in lobar collapse or obstructive emphysema (2,3). Polypoid granulations secondary to such trauma may be successfully treated by endoscopic excision if they seriously compromise the lumen of the airway (2). The presence of an endotracheal tube even in good position may impair mucociliary function and cause squamous metaplasia of the tracheobronchial mucosa (4,5), and lobar collapse may develop secondarily to this even after the baby has been successfully weaned from its artificial airway (6) (Fig. 7-4).

Superficial laryngeal and tracheal lesions are commonly associated with endotracheal intubation and seem to result in few serious acute or permanent problems (5,7–9). A small number of infants, however, may have narrowing of the subglottic airway and have hoarseness and stridor following extubation. More significant endotracheal lesions can be granulomas, mucosal cysts, or stenosis, which may become clinically manifest months after the tube has been removed (10) (Fig. 7-5).

On occasion, the endotracheal tube may inadvertently be placed in the esophagus. This may be recognized radiographically if the air column and tube are not appropriately superimposed (Fig. 7-6). It is possible, however, for the ET tube to be in the esophagus but be directly superimposed

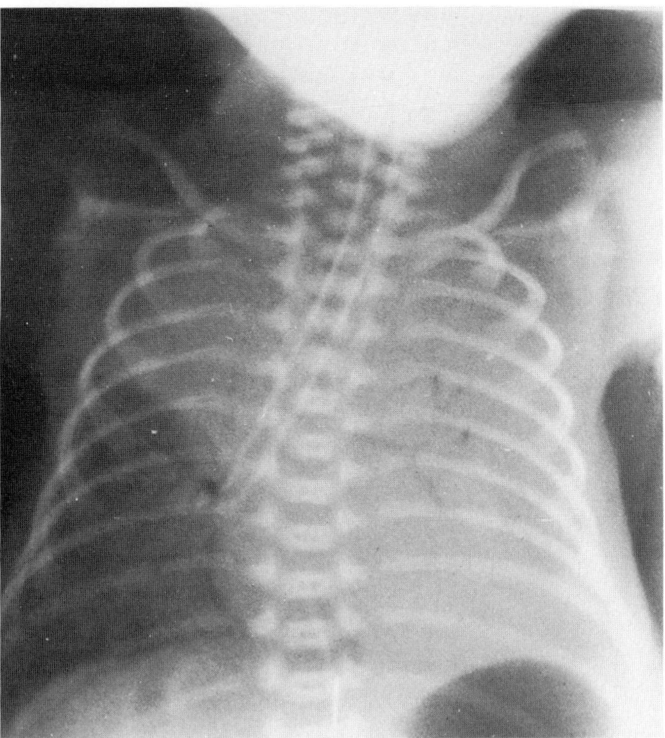

Fig. 7-2. Malpositioned endotracheal tube. The ET tube has been inserted too far and extends down into the right intermediate bronchus. This has caused collapse of the right upper lobe and of the entire left lung, presumably because the walls of the ET tube block the bronchial openings of those regions.

on the tracheal air column as seen on a frontal chest film. One can suspect the ET tube may be in the esophagus by noting distention of the esophagus with air and an excessive amount of air in the stomach and small bowel (Fig. 7-7).

Malposition of an ET tube usually causes some deterioration in the patient's clinical status or blood gases, and such changes are appropriate justification for prompt radiographic examination of the infant's chest.

Ventilator Therapy and Pulmonary Air Leaks

Pulmonary Interstitial Emphysema

Advances in techniques of mechanically assisted ventilation are responsible for much of the reduced mortality among small immature infants and newborns with respiratory disorders. The basic princi-ple of assisted ventilation is to maintain a pressure differential between the atmosphere and the alveoli to sustain expansion of alveoli, which would otherwise collapse. Even with skillful application and constant vigilance, mechanically assisted ventilation is obviously invasive, and the incidence of associated complications is high. Uneven ventilation of alveoli allows some alveoli to be subjected to transpleural forces that exceed normal and tear the connective tissue and permit alveolar air to enter the interstitial spaces of the lung. The immature lung appears to be especially susceptible to barotrauma. While pulmonary interstitial emphysema and its sequelae may occur spontaneously in infants with respiratory distress syndrome, the disorder appears to be aggravated by the use of positive pressure ventilators (11–13). Pulmonary interstitial emphysema (PIE) may be followed by pneumothorax, pneumomediastinum, pneumopericardium, loculated interstitial emphysema (pulmonary pseudocyst), pneumoperitoneum, and intravascular air embolism.

PIE may occur in as many as 40% of ventilated

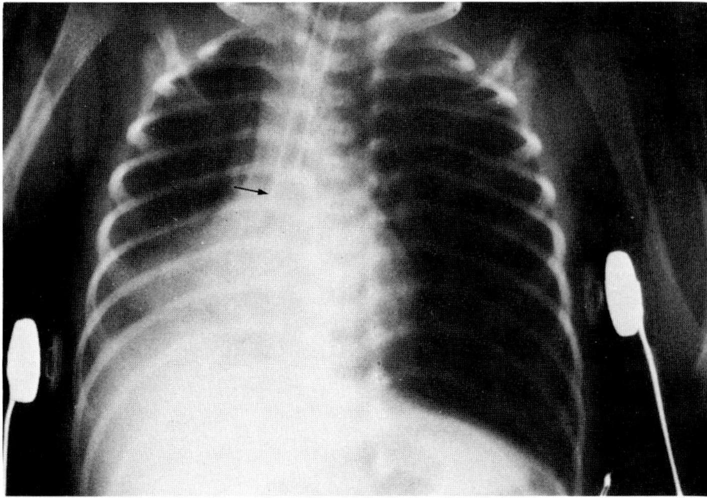

a

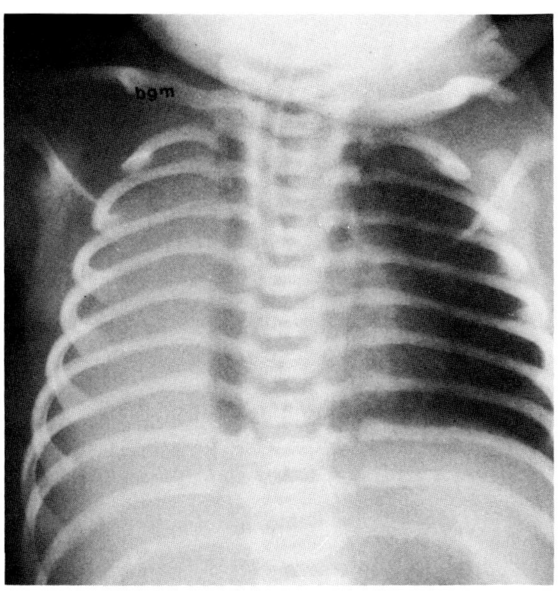

b

Fig. 7-3, a and b. Malpositioned endotracheal tube. a Endotracheal tube in right bronchus (*arrow*) has resulted in collapse of the right middle lobe and right lower lobe. **b** Endotracheal tube has been inserted into the left bronchus, resulting in collapse of the right lung.

infants, and major air leaks are associated with increased mortality especially in infants under 1.5 kg (11–14). The overall incidence of air leaks in infants with hyaline membrane disease at the Lying-In Division of the Boston Hospital for Women was 27% (11). Those in whom air leaks occurred were significantly more premature and had lower birth weights than those without air leaks.

Prompt early recognition and appropriate treatment of such air leaks may favorably influence survival rates. Transillumination of the chest has proved to be a useful technique for early recognition of large collections of air in the pleural, mediastinal, and pericardial spaces (15,16).

PIE may be recognized radiographically as small bubbles and streaks of air (Fig. 7-8) readily apparent if the lung otherwise is generally increased in density, as is likely to be the case in infants with hyaline membrane disease and pulmonary immaturity. PIE usually develops within the first week. It may persist unchanged for several days, worsen, spontaneously disappear, or go on to pneumothorax or some other complication. PIE may accumulate locally and expand to form large, loculated, cystlike collections (Fig. 7-9) within the lung (17–19). The masslike effect of such expanding pseudocysts or of extensive PIE can compress and further compromise adjacent lung. The pres-

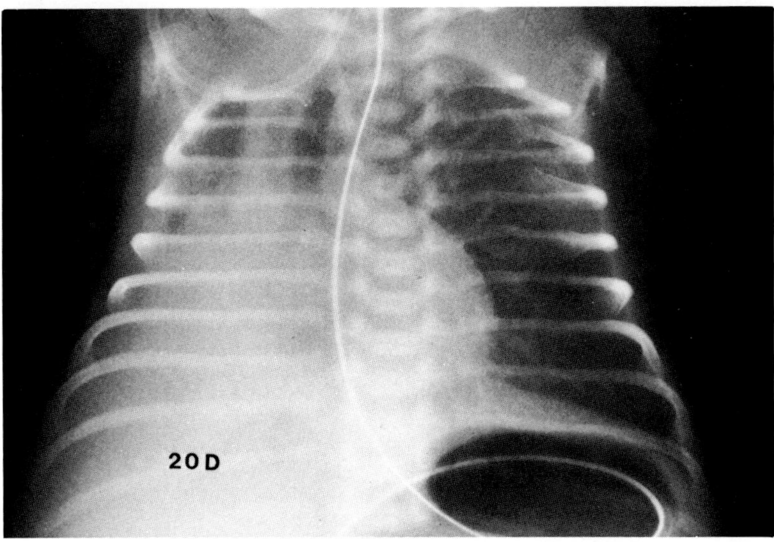

Fig. 7-4. Postextubation collapse. This baby had previously required endotracheal intubation. Transient collapse of the right lower and middle lobes occurred following extubation.

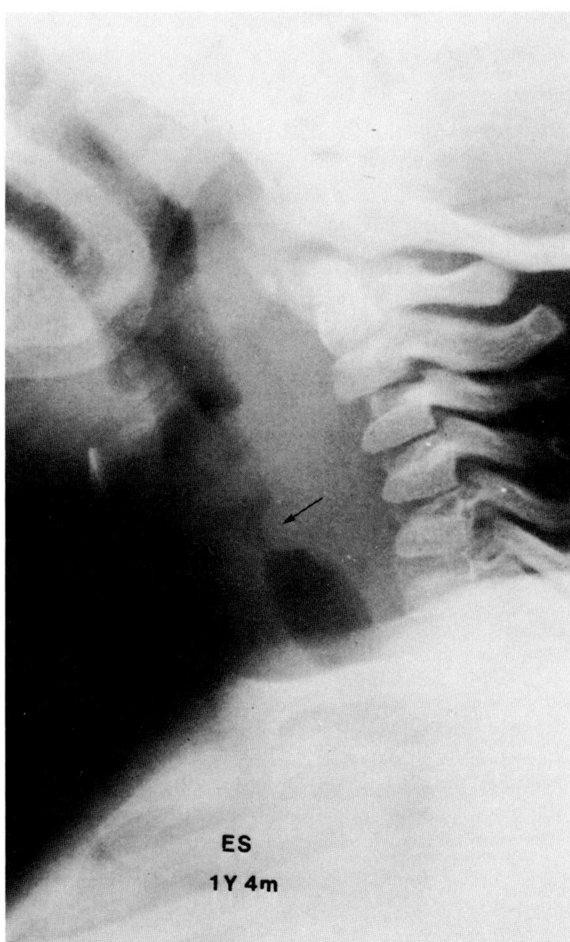

Fig. 7-5. Tracheal granuloma is evident as a subglottic mass narrowing the tracheal airway (Age 16 months). At birth this infant weighed 1200 grams and was intubated for 13 days for repeated apneic spells. Granuloma was excised by laser beam surgery. A similar appearance could be due to postintubation mucosal cysts or cicatricial stenosis.

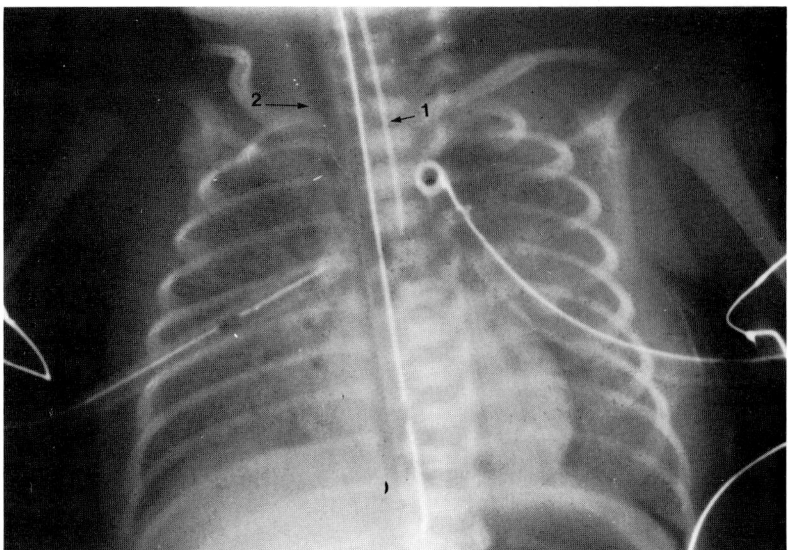

Fig. 7-6. Endotracheal tube in esophagus. Close inspection reveals that the endotracheal tube (*arrow #1*) is not in the trachea (*arrow #2*). A nasogastric catheter is also in the esophagus.

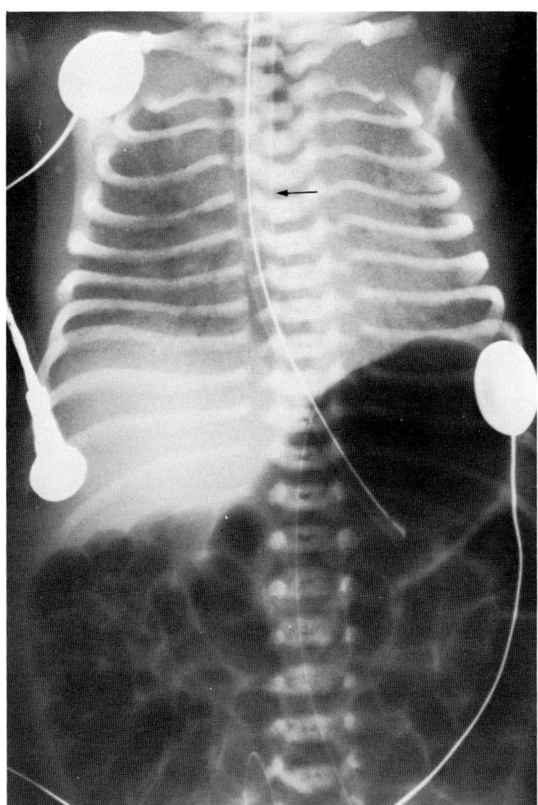

Fig. 7-7. ET tube in esophagus. The ET tube (*arrow*) could be in the trachea and too low in position. However, note the excessive amount of air in the gastrointestinal tract, strongly suggesting that the ET tube is probably in the esophagus.

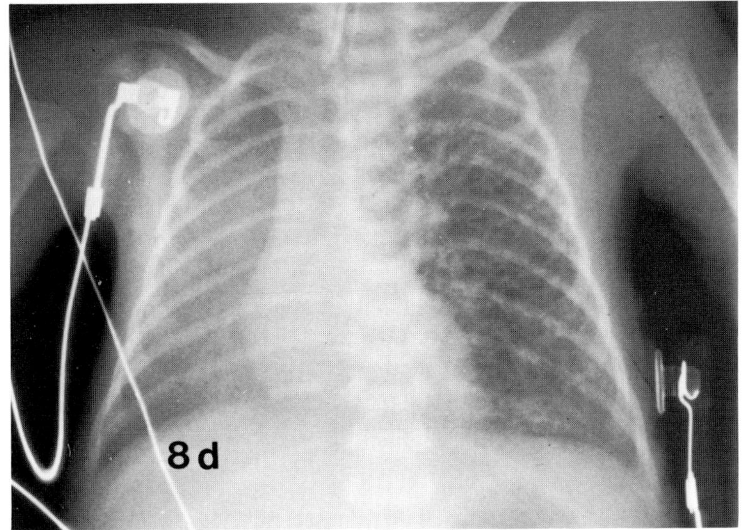

a

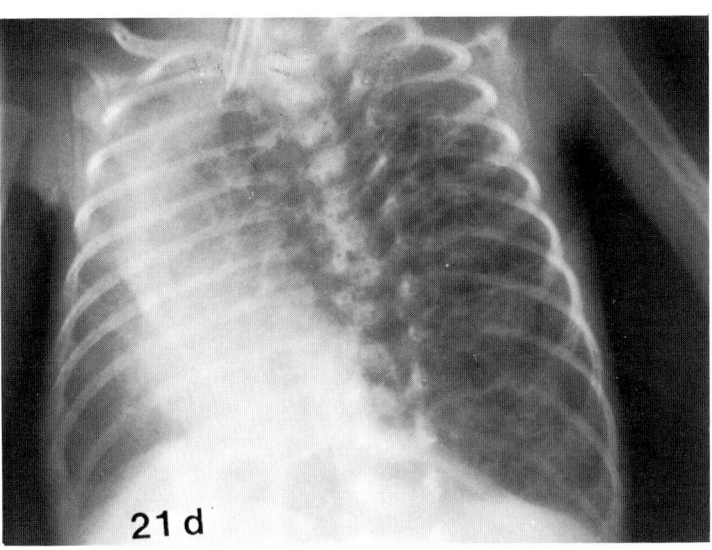

b

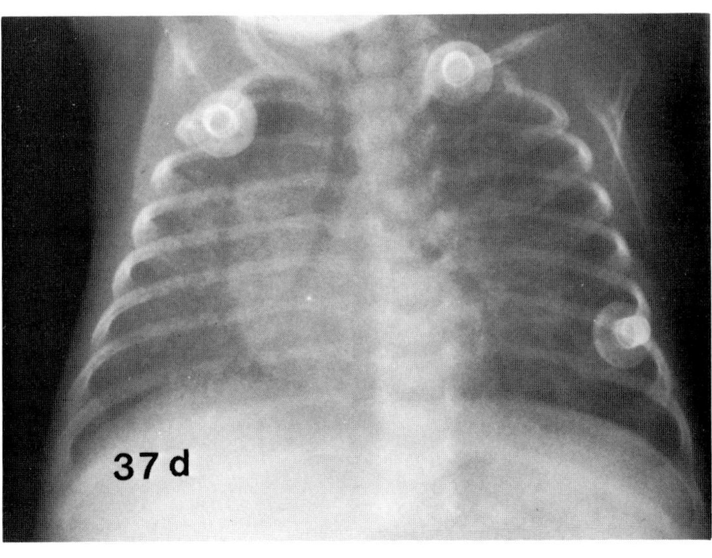

c

Fig. 7-8, a–c. Pulmonary interstitial emphysema—spontaneous resolution. a PIE is evident in left lung as tiny rounded and streaky lucencies scattered throughout the lung, which has increased in volume. Compare with the uniform gray appearance of the right lung. **b** Massive enlargement of the left lung due to progressive accumulation of PIE. The enlarging lung has displaced the heart and mediastinum to the right and compromised the right lung. **c** Spontaneous reabsorption of the interstitial emphysema has occurred, and the lung has returned toward normal.

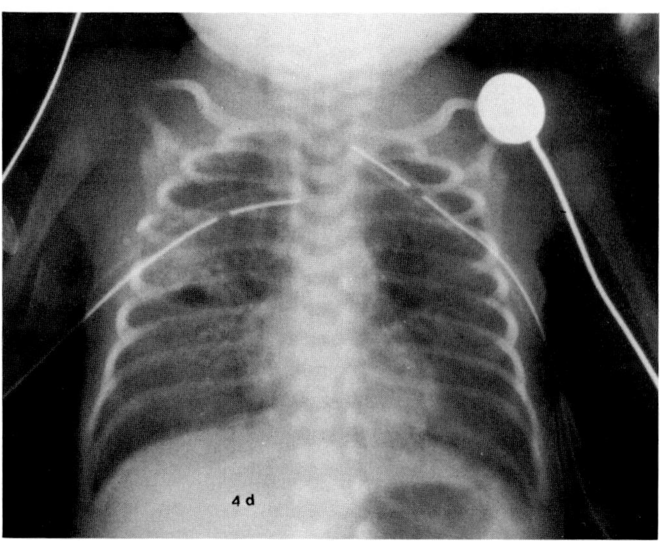

a

Fig. 7-9, a–c. Pulmonary interstitial emphysema—pseudocyst. a A small cystlike accumulation of air in the right midlung region is evident after satisfactory evacuation of bilateral pneumothoraces. Some perihilar PIE is also present bilaterally. **b** The loculated collection of PIE has shown considerable increase in size. Elsewhere the PIE has resorbed. **c** Persistent pseudocystic collection of PIE is still present at five months. The patient, however, was asymptomatic and growing well. No further follow-up films are available, but the patient is clinically well several years later.

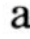

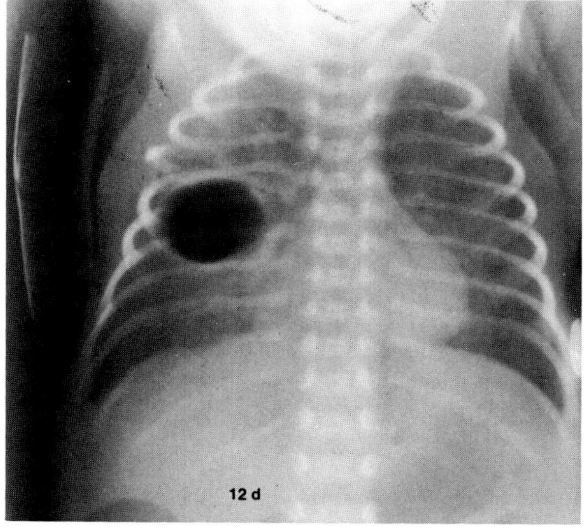

b

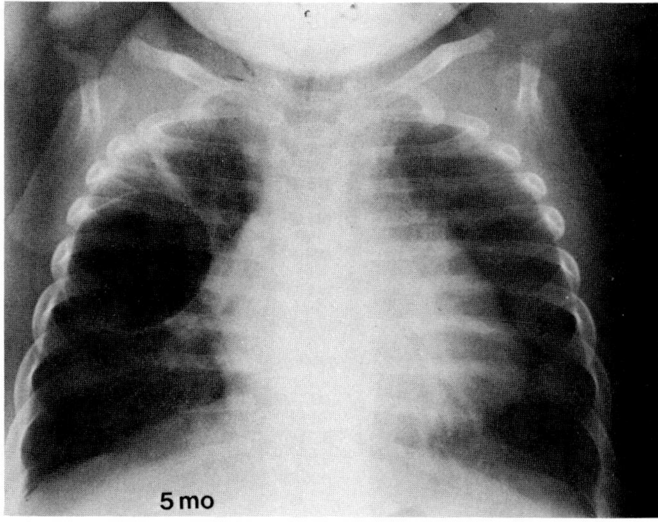

c

ence of PIE also causes a decrease in pulmonary blood flow through the areas of lung involved (13). PIE and pseudocysts generally undergo spontaneous absorption over a period of several days to a few weeks. Rarely, a pseudocyst may persist for many months, but surgical intervention is not required as long as the patient is clinically not deteriorating (21) (Fig. 7-9). In a few reported instances, progressive increase in the extent of PIE has contributed to the death of the infant or has required lobectomy (20).

In addition to surgery (20,22), a variety of techniques have been used to deal with the problem of very large localized or extensive and persistent PIE which appears to be compromising the patient's respiratory status. Selective intubation of the main bronchus on the side opposite the region of the PIE has occasionally been crowned with success (23), but in our experience (Fig. 7-10) it has often failed. More recently, high-frequency ventilators have been used in some infants with severe PIE under tension. High-frequency ventilation is characterized by very rapid rates up to 1800 per minute with low peak inspiratory and mean airway pressures. The exact mechanisms by which this technique supports ventilation are not completely known. Nevertheless, improved oxygenation and elimination of carbon dioxide does

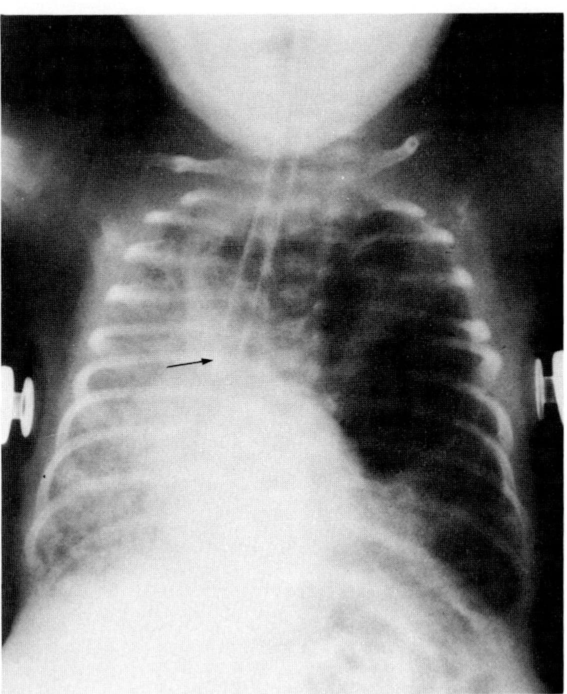

Fig. 7-10. PIE—selective intubation. Very extensive PIE has caused marked enlargement of the left lung, which in turn has compromised the right lung. An attempt was made to selectively ventilate the right lung by deliberately inserting the endotracheal tube into the right bronchus (*arrow*). Such attempts to treat unilateral PIE have not been very successful in our experience and failed in this particular baby. The PIE eventually disappeared spontaneously.

occur effectively. It has been used successfully to treat several infants with severe PIE (24) (Fig. 7-11).

Pneumothorax

Pneumothorax occurs more commonly in the newborn than in any other period of life. Spontaneous asymptomatic pneumothorax occurs in healthy newborns with an incidence of about 1% and needs no direct treatment other than vigilance. In infants requiring ventilatory assistance, as many as one-third develop pneumothorax (12,25).

The clinical signs of a pneumothorax are variable (12,25). Changes in respiratory rate, cyanosis, apnea, bradycardia, shift of heart sounds, reduction of breathsounds, distention of the involved side of the chest, and sudden deterioration of vital signs are some of the clinically apparent alterations.

Radiographically the diagnosis usually presents no difficulty (Fig. 7-12). One must be familiar, however, with the fact that in the supine infant the air may lie anterior and medial within the thorax, with the lung falling posteriorly (Fig. 7-13). The air may thus appear as a medial pneumothorax (26) and may mimic pneumomediastinum. Pleural air that lies predominantly anteriorly may be evident only as an apparent small difference in radiolucency between the two sides of the chest. An occasional useful clue to the presence of a pneumothorax is a sharp, clear demarcation of the edge of the heart on the side on which the pleural air is present. Since most of these infants have lung disease, the heart border, in the absence of a pneumothorax is usually ill-defined. A horizontal beam lateral view or a lateral decubitus view with the involved side uppermost can at times be useful to demonstrate the presence of a pneumothorax more definitely. If the accumulation of air is particularly large, there may be a marked shift of the mediastinum and inversion of the diaphragm. The air enters the pleural space presumably by rupturing from the interstitial tissues of the lung directly through the pleura. It has been assumed that the interstitial air tracked back to the mediastinum and then ruptured from the mediastinum out into the pleural space. In our clinical experience, however, there is a very low frequency of association of pneumomediastinum with pneumothorax, and it seems more likely that the interstitial air extends to the visceral pleural surface and ruptures out through it into the pleural space (12).

Pneumomediastinum

Following rupture of alveoli and development of PIE, the air may track along the perivascular and peribronchial tissue planes back to the mediastinum and cause an accumulation of air there (13). This usually has no great clinical consequences. Radiographically (Fig. 7-14) the air often insinuates itself between the thymus and pericardium, elevating one or both lobes of the thymus upward, anteriorly and laterally. It is important to recognize this phenomenon and not confuse the displaced shadows of the thymus for areas of pneumonia or collapse in the upper lobes. If the

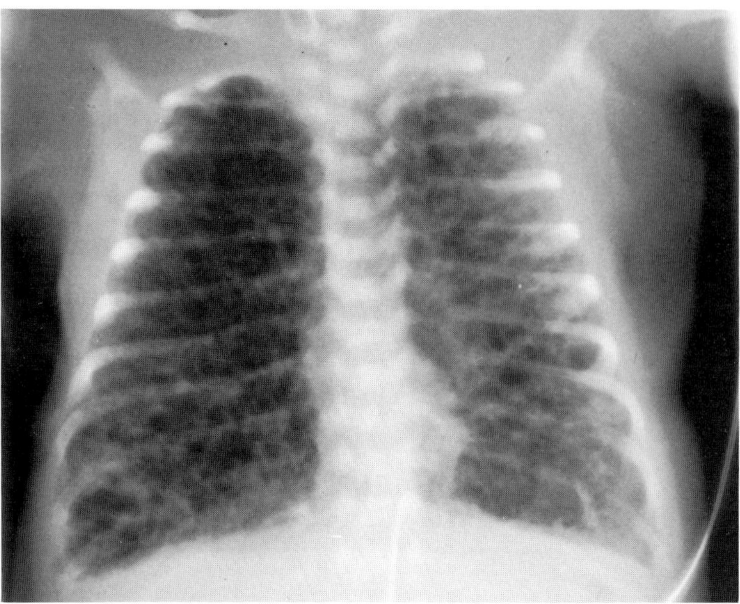

Fig. 7-11. PIE—high-frequency ventilator treatment. Very extensive and severe PIE, present throughout both lungs, has caused striking increase in the volume of both lungs. The diaphragm is depressed and the heart is very small, probably from interference with pulmonary artery circulation and systemic venous return due to the PIE. This baby was treated with high-frequency ventilation, and the PIE disappeared within 24 hours.

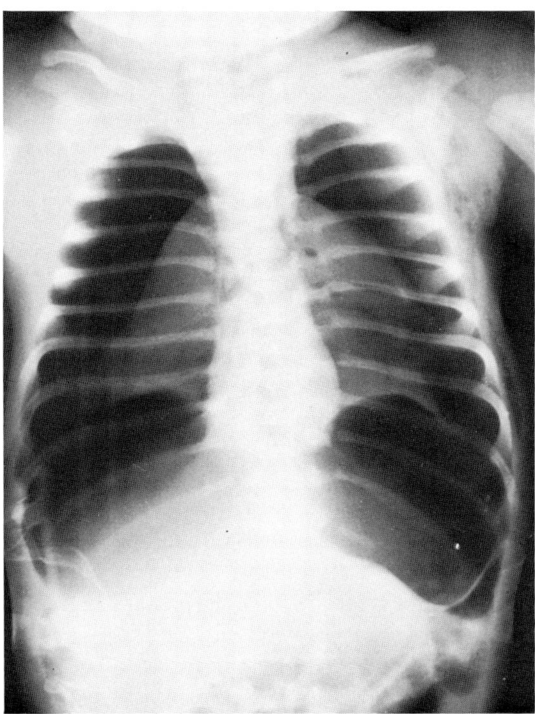

Fig. 7-12. Pneumothorax. Very large bilateral tension pneumothoraces developed during overly vigorous resuscitation of this infant. Diaphragm is inverted, lungs are collapsed, and the heart volume is very small.

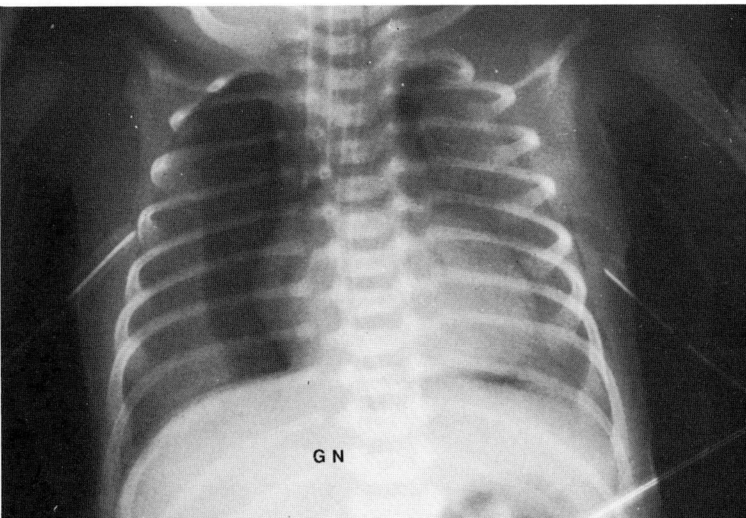

Fig. 7-13. Right medial pneumothorax. Medial and anterior accumulation of the air in the pleural space is a frequent manifestation of pneumothorax in infants. It is related to the supine position of the infant. The lung tends to fall posterior and lateral. Note that the right and left thoracostomy tubes were not properly secured and have fallen out of the pleural spaces.

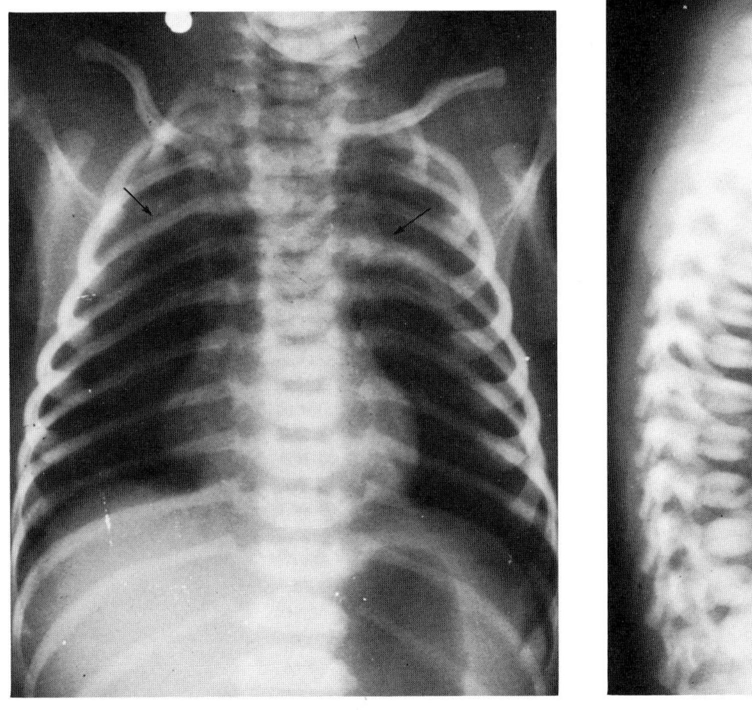

a

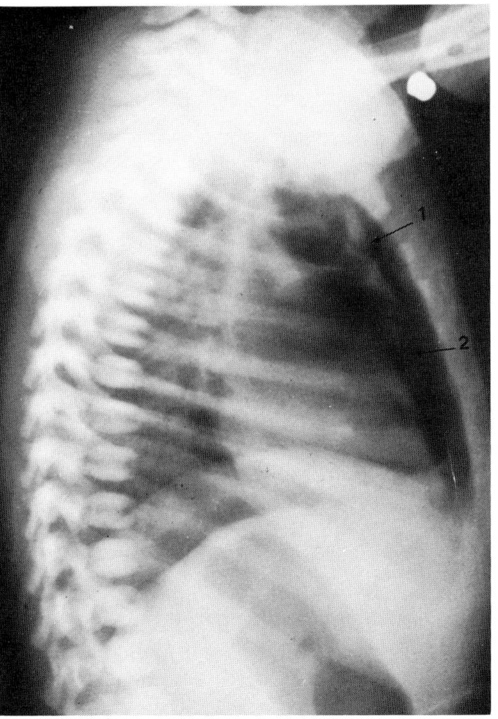

b

Fig. 7-14, a and b. Pneumomediastinum. Frontal (a) and lateral (b) views. The mediastinal air often displaces the lobes of the thymus laterally and superiorly (*arrows #1*). If not recognized as such, these shadows may be misconstrued as areas of lobular pneumonia or atelectasis. Arrow #2 shows a large collection of mediastinal air displacing the heart posteriorly.

accumulation of air in the mediastinum is large, the systemic and pulmonary venous return may be compromised.

Pneumopericardium

The exact method by which pulmonary interstitial air extends into the pericardial space is not known. It has been suggested that the air actually dissects initially into the mediastinum and then into the pericardial space at the reflection of the pericardium onto the aorta and pulmonary artery (27). It is possible that it also extends along the perivenous tissue planes and gains entrance into the pericardial space as the veins enter the left atrium.

The clinical signs depend on the volume that accumulates within the pericardial space. Small volumes may cause no particular change in the clinical status. Rapid and large collections result in severe cardiac tamponade, leading to death of the infant unless immediate pericardial decompression is performed. Signs of pneumopericardium are sudden onset of bradycardia, cyanosis, hypotension, and diminished heart sounds (27,28).

Transillumination of the chest with a high-intensity fiberoptic light source has been useful to demonstrate the pneumopericardium (16). If radiographs can be obtained promptly, the pneumopericardium is readily evident (Fig. 7-15) outlining the entire cardiac contour, being limited superiorly by the reflection of the pericardium on the great vessels. It may be difficult to differentiate from pneumomediastinum unless the air is visible entirely around the undersurface of the heart.

If signs of cardiac tamponade are present, immediate percutaneous pericardiocentesis provides relief. In some instances, indwelling pericardial catheters may be very helpful if the problem is recurrent (29). Prompt recognition and adequate therapy have permitted survival of many infants suffering this complication.

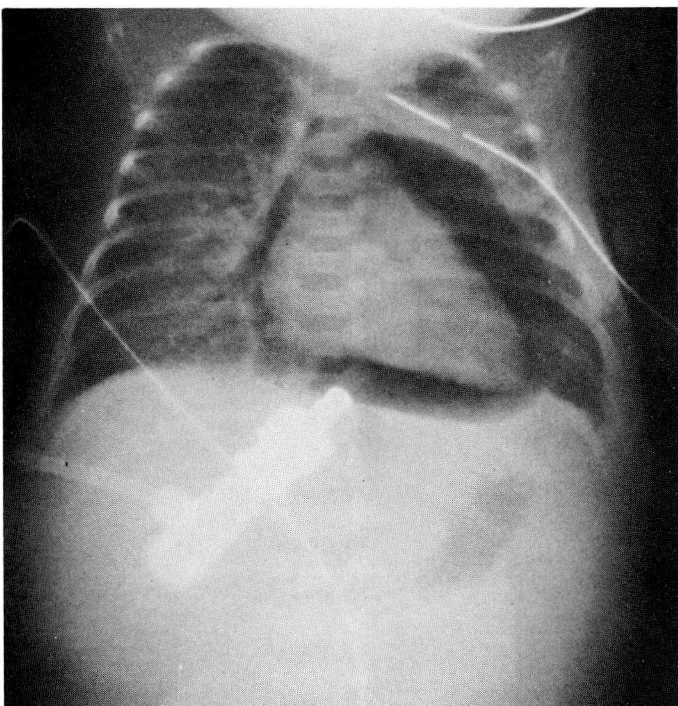

Fig. 7-15. Pneumopericardium. The accumulation of air within the pericardial sac completely outlines the cardiac shadow. The air is confined superiorly by the reflection of the pericardium at the level of the aorta and pulmonary artery. It can result in cardiac tamponade and requires immediate evacuation.

Pneumoperitoneum

Air that accumulates in the mediastinum may extend through the potential tissue planes that exist between the mediastinum and the retroperitoneal space and then extend from the retroperitoneal space into the peritoneal cavity (14,30). Mediastinal air can extend around the periaortic adventitial planes; or since the infant is usually in the supine position, the air can dissect along the anterior communications through the diaphragm.

A sudden appearance of gas in the peritoneal

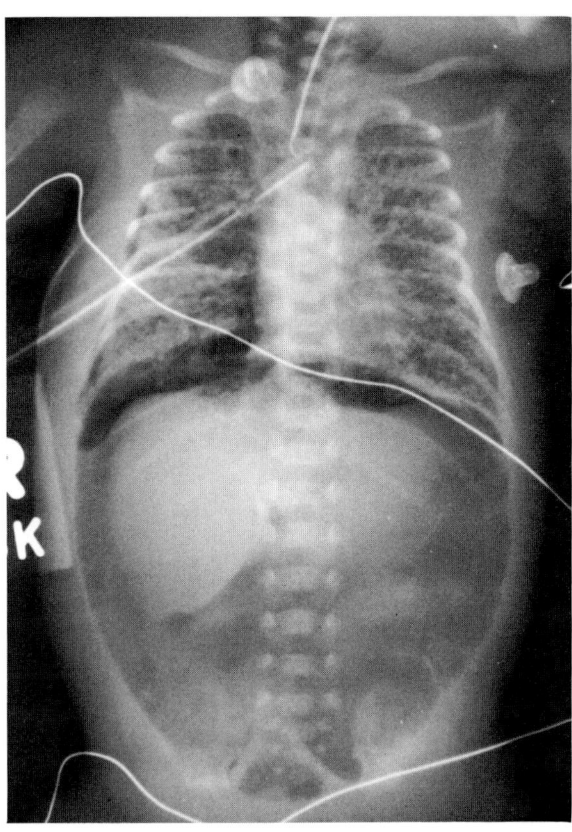

a

Fig. 7-16. **Pneumoperitoneum.** This pneumoperitoneum developed as a complication of pulmonary interstitial emphysema. The absence of fluid in the peritoneal space tends to exclude intestinal perforation as a cause of the pneumoperitoneum. Both lungs show extensive PIE, and some mediastinal emphysema has tracked up into the soft tissues of the neck as seen on the anteroposterior and lateral projections.

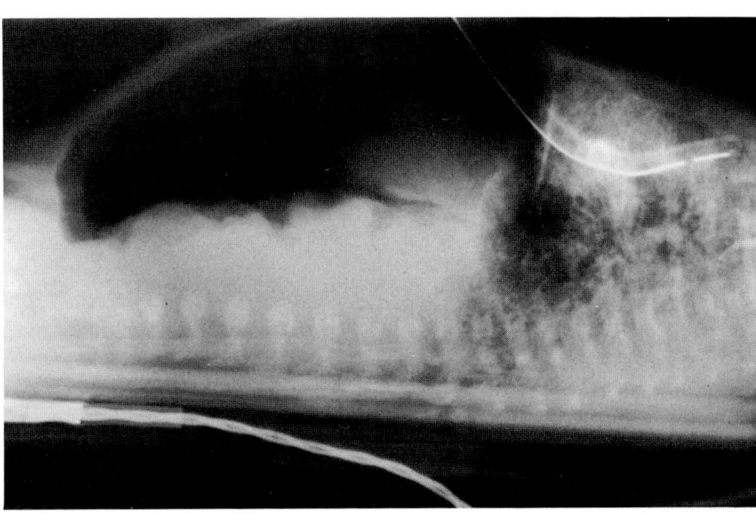

b

cavity naturally raises concern about the possibility of perforation of the bowel. Differentiation between such perforation (as the cause for peritoneal gas) and air that has dissected down from the mediastinum can be difficult. When the air has extended from the mediastinum into the peritoneal cavity there is usually no accompanying fluid or an insignificant amount (Fig. 7-16) in the peritoneal space, whereas if a perforation of the bowel has occurred, there is usually intestinal content as well as inflammatory exudate present. If one suspects that the air in the peritoneal cavity has developed secondary to pulmonary interstitial emphysema and pneumomediastinum, it is possible to remove some of the air from the peritoneal space and check its oxygen concentration and compare it with the oxygen concentration being used in the respirator (31). If gas is present in the peritoneal cavity secondary to rupture of the bowel, then the oxygen concentration, of course, would be quite low. Oral metrizamide may also be useful to exclude an intestinal perforation (32).

Intravascular Air Embolism

Air embolism complicating the evolution of pulmonary interstitial emphysema is fortunately rather rare, since it is almost always fatal (33,34). The mechanism by which air enters the vascular system is probably variable. It is possible that dissection of air within the connective tissue supporting structures of the lung allows air to enter the lymphatics of the lung, which in turn drain into the systemic venous system. Support for this hypothesis is provided in the fact that the intravascular air in many of these unfortunate instances is evident in the right side of the heart and in the hepatic veins and inferior vena cava (Fig. 7-17). It is also possible that rupture of air into the interstitial compartment of the lung and tearing of the connective tissue permits air to enter directly into the pulmonary venous system and thereby gain entrance into the left atrium and systemic circulation. The air that may be evident on the right side of the heart and in the vena cava and hepatic veins could occur from passage of air across the foramen ovale from the left atrium. No matter what the mechanism, this disastrous complication usually leads to death.

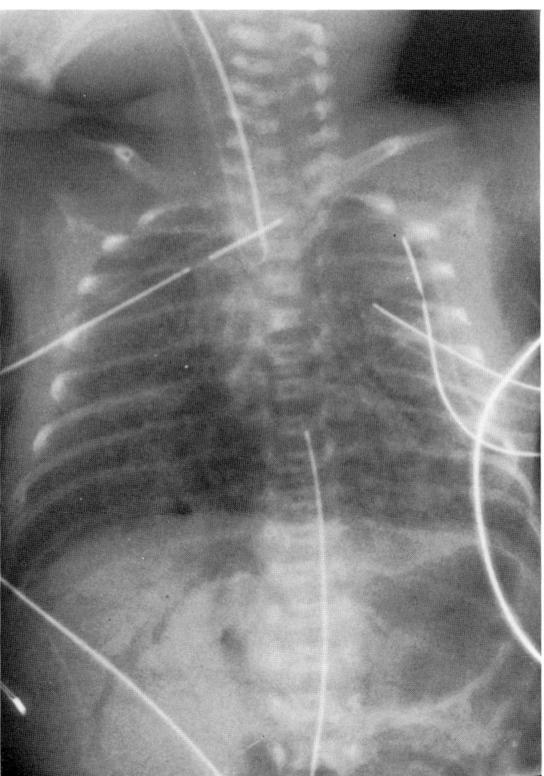

Fig. 7-17. Intravascular air is evident filling the chambers of the heart, the hepatic veins, the inferior vena cava, as well as vessels in the neck.

Thoracostomy Tubes

The most frequent complication of chest tube drainage of pneumothorax in the newborn is perforation of the lung. This is particularly likely to occur if a trocar is used to aid in the insertion of the catheter, but penetration of the lung by a chest tube may also occur even when the tube is inserted using blunt dissection (35,36). The immature lung, particularly when affected by hyaline membrane disease, pneumonia, or hemorrhage, does not have normal resiliency and is more likely to be damaged by a tube than is a normal lung. Pneumothorax is usually preceded by the development of pulmonary interstitial emphysema, and the presence of such interstitial emphysema adds to the stiffness of the lung. Penetration of the lung by a tube can be suspected clinically if a pneumothorax enlarges, persists, or recurs after the tube is placed.

Whenever chest tubes are inserted it is imperative to obtain frontal and lateral radiographs in order to reconstruct the spatial relationships of the chest tube. In this way not only is it usually possible to recognize that a chest tube is not in a satisfactory position to remove the pleural air, but also one can appreciate that a chest tube may be penetrating the parenchyma of the lung (Fig. 7-18). In infants with tension pneumothorax that has proven unresponsive to multiple chest tube insertions one must consider such an injury to the lung.

Perforation of the lung by a chest tube can have other detrimental effects on the respiratory management of the infant. Positive end-expiratory pressure may increase the air leak through the bronchopleural fistula, leading to a decreased utilization of oxygen. Most reports of such iatrogenic complications indicate that the mortality rate is high. Grosfeld et al. (37) report that emergency thoracotomy and suture closure of the bronchopleural fistula can be a lifesaving procedure.

Less frequent complications of thoracostomy tube use include pulmonary hemorrhage, hemothorax, and traumatic arteriovenous fistula between the chest wall and lung (38,39). Roentgenographic verification of chest tube position may show that the tube has failed to enter the pleural space—it may be in the soft tissues of the chest wall (Fig. 7-19) or may enter the abdomen (Fig. 7-20).

Feeding and Suction Catheters

The care of the premature infant with respiratory difficulties frequently requires the use of pharyngeal and endotracheal suction catheters, and the

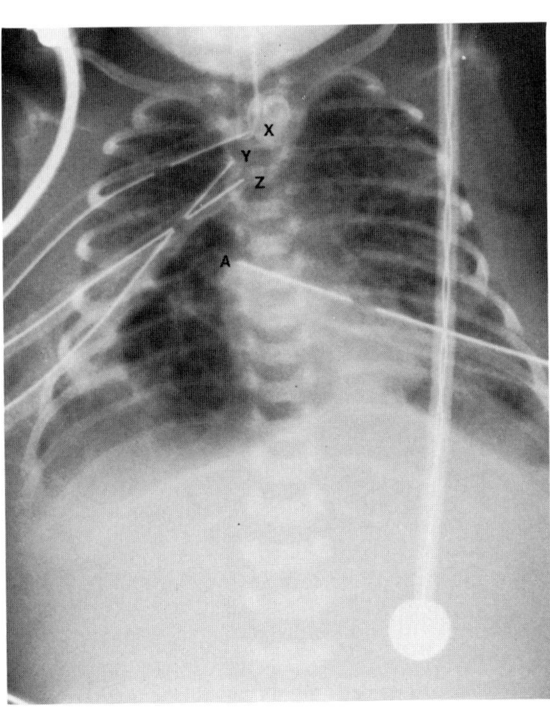

a

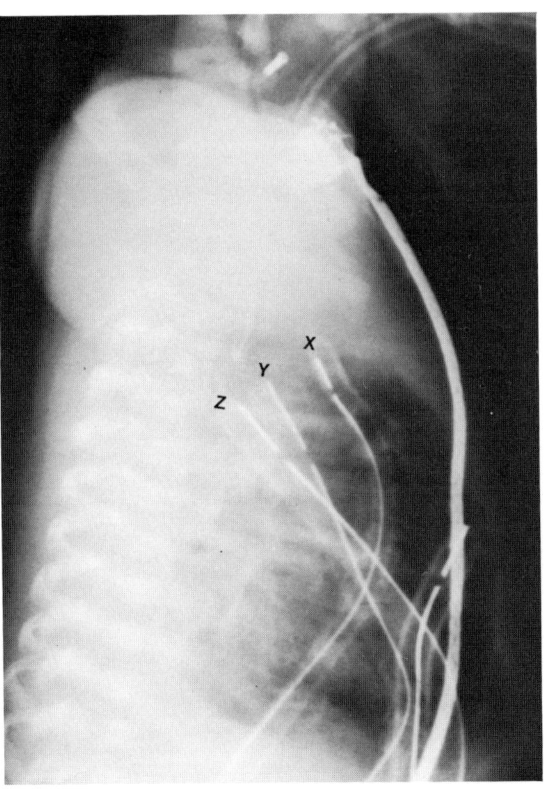

b

Fig. 7-18, a and b. Thoracostomy tube perforation of the lung can be identified by localizing the position of the tubes on the frontal (**a**) and lateral (**b**) films. The tips of X, Y, and Z must have penetrated the right lung. Both lungs are compromised by the presence of extensive PIE. The multiple thoracostomy tubes had been placed for recurrent pneumothoraces. At autopsy there was evidence of perforation of the right lung by the tubes.

                                                                                  G. B. C. Harris

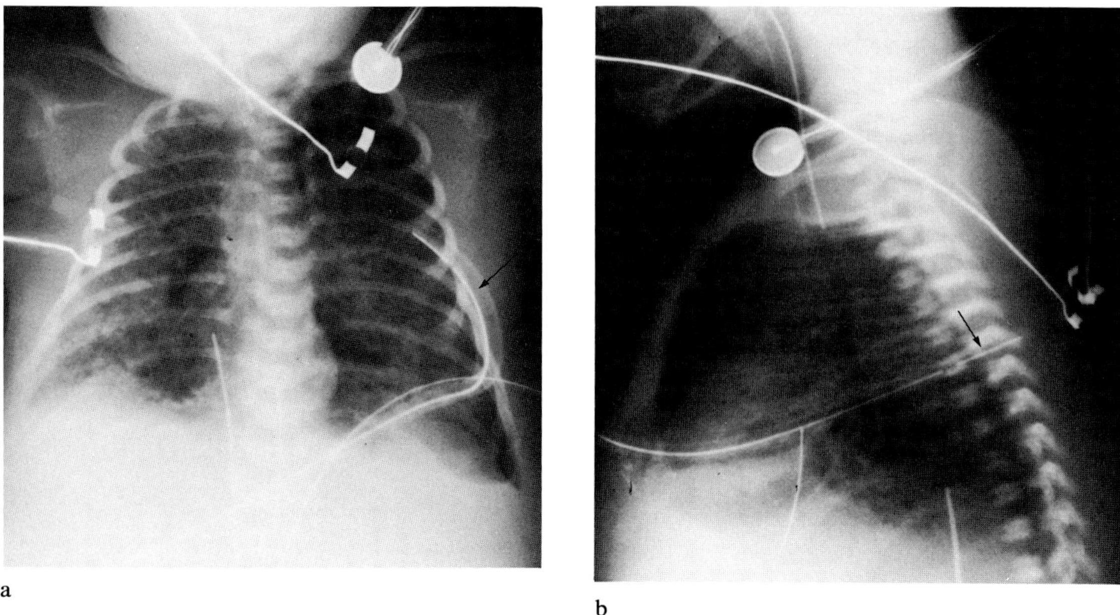

a

b

Fig. 7-19, a and **b. Misplaced thoracostomy tube.** AP **(a)** and lateral **(b)** views show that the thoracostomy tube has failed to enter the pleural space (*arrow*). It lies subcutaneously. An umbilical vein catheter has its tip in the right atrium, and the end of the umbilical artery line lies at the level of T10.

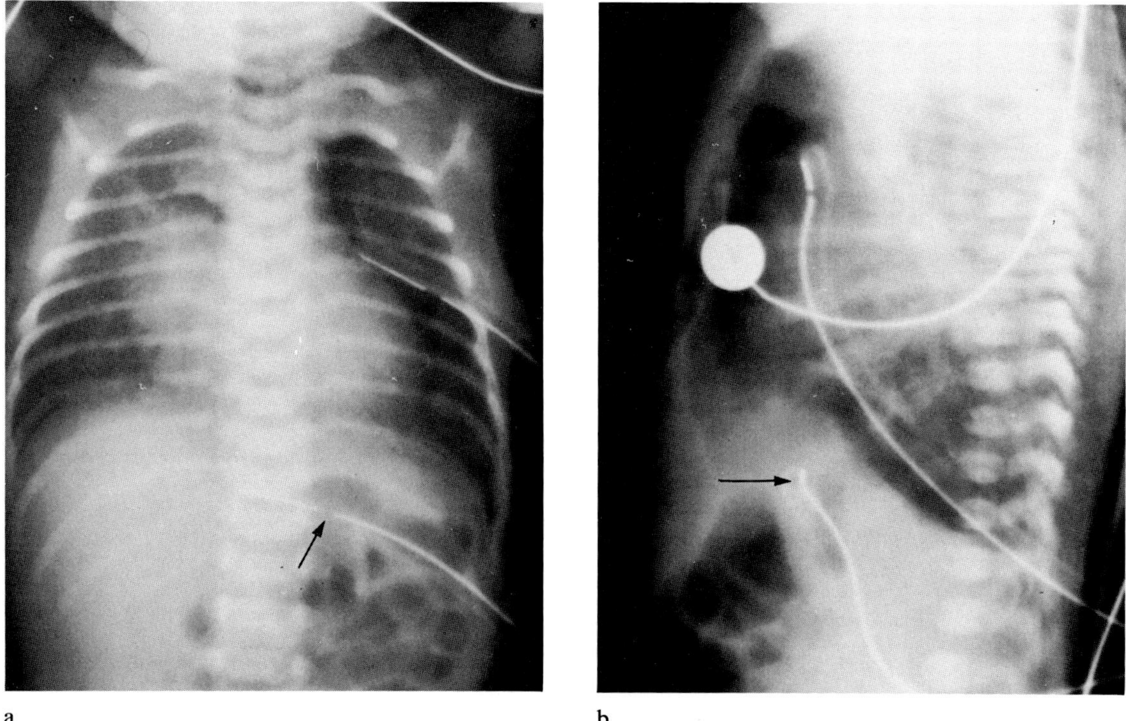

a   b

Fig. 7-20. Misplaced thoracostomy tube. The films show that the tube (*arrow*) lies inferior to the level of the left diaphragm. The tube had been inserted in an effort to remove pleural air that appeared to be loculated in the lower chest.

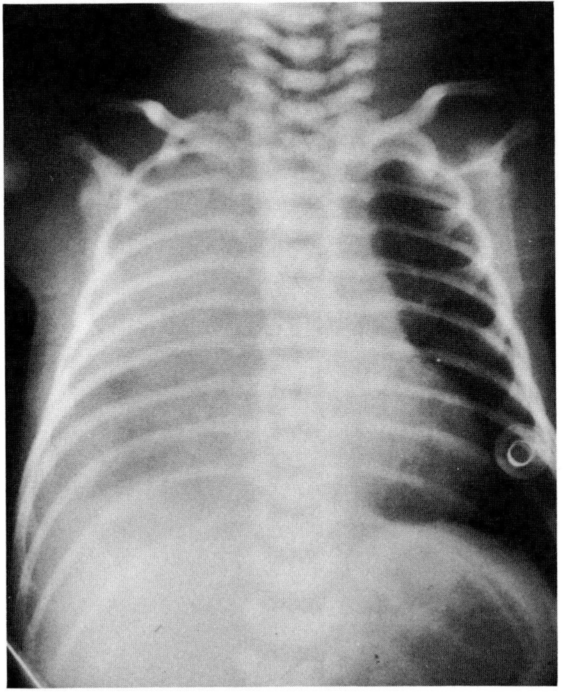

a

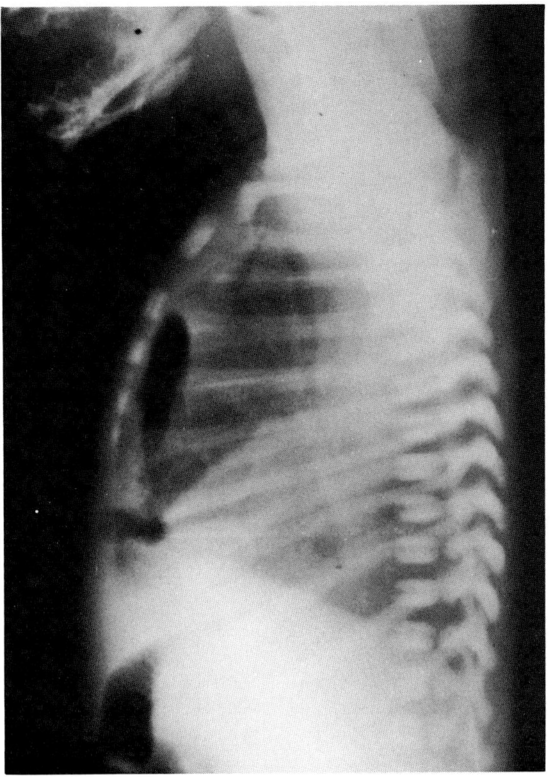

b

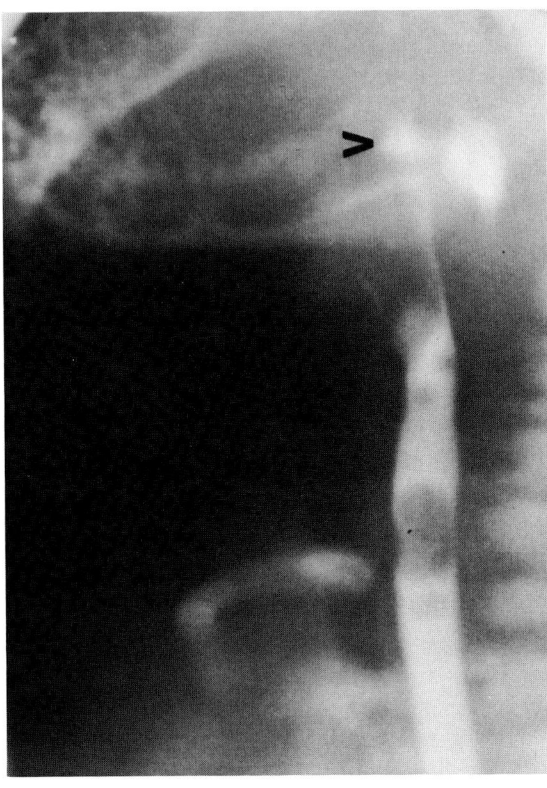

c

Fig. 7-21, a–c. Perforation of posterior pharynx by a feeding tube resulting in a fistulous tract extending from the pharynx to the right pleural space. Clinically this complication had not been recognized, and the baby was believed to have pneumonia and empyema. Chest films **(a,b)** show evidence of pleural fluid and air in the right chest. The contrast study of the esophagus **(c)** shows the site of perforation of the posterior pharynx. The baby was treated conservatively and recovered.

common way of feeding low-birth-weight infants who may be unable to suck or swallow is with nasogastric or orogastric intubation. The insertion of these tubes can lead inadvertently to traumatic perforation of the pharynx and of the esophagus (40–42). This is an infrequent but very serious hazard of the use of these catheters. Traumatic perforation of the pharynx or esophagus during the insertion of these devices produces a mediastinal sinus tract which may extend, to varying degrees, into the mediastinum or may perforate out into a pleural space (43,44). Smaller traumatic sinus tracts in the posterior pharyngeal wall have probably been mistakenly diagnosed as congenital diverticula (45,46). If the sinus tract extends into the pleural space, it results in a pneumothorax, and feeding through such a misplaced nasogastric catheter can mimic empyema (Fig. 7-21) and may, of course, ultimately lead to superimposed infection.

The diagnosis is easy to make roentgenographically if the catheter is in place and can be seen in the chest. However, nasogastric tubes are often inserted temporarily for a gavage feeding and then promptly removed. Suctioning of the pharynx and trachea also is done intermittently, and the possibility of trauma secondary to such catheters may not be so readily apparent. One may suspect the possibility of perforation of the pharynx radiographically by recognizing the presence of air in the posterior pharyngeal wall. Fluoroscopic evaluation of the pharynx and esophagus with aqueous contrast material provides the diagnosis. Metrizamide is useful for this examination.

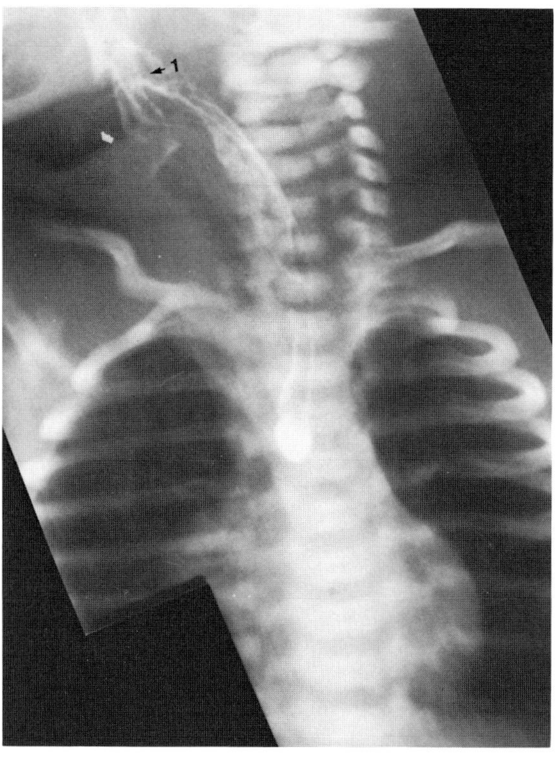

a

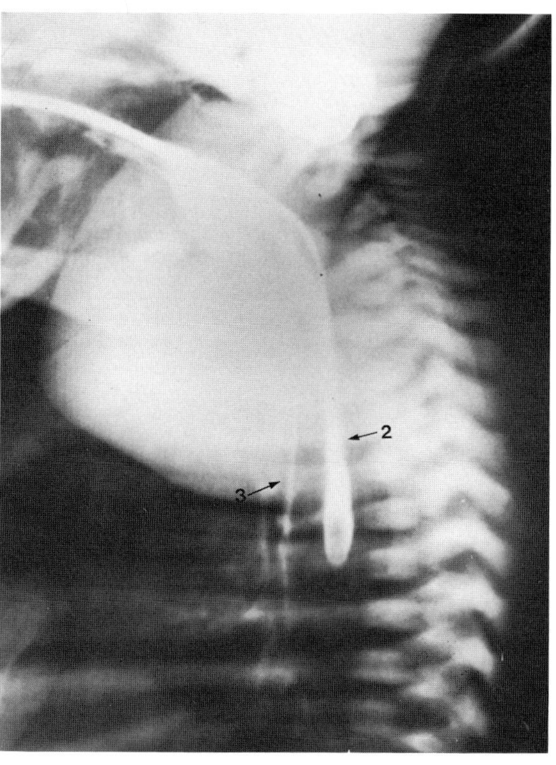

b

Fig. 7-22, a and b. Perforation of posterior pharynx by nasogastric tube simulating esophageal atresia. When a nasogastric catheter was placed, it could not be passed into the stomach, and the clinical suspicion of an esophageal atresia was raised. Contrast material was then inserted through the catheter, and an incorrect diagnosis of esophageal atresia was made before the infant was transferred for surgery. Arrow #1 (in **a**) shows the site of perforation of the posterior pharyngeal wall. Arrow #2 (in **b**) demonstrates contrast material in the mediastinal sinus tract, which was mistaken for esophageal atresia. Arrow #3 (in **b**) indicates the trachea outlined by aspirated contrast material. The true diagnosis can be made by observing the site of perforation, the increased distance between the trachea and the sinus tract, and the unusual size and shape of the sinus tract. These findings should alert one that this is not congenital esophageal atresia.

In some infants, traumatic perforation of the posterior pharynx has led to a mistaken diagnosis of congenital esophageal atresia (47). The episode is associated with failure to pass a nasogastric tube into the stomach, and this raises clinical concern about a possible esophageal atresia. These infants may also have excessive accumulation of secretions in the pharynx. Roentgen studies following instillations of a small amount of contrast material show a collection in the sinus tract that may lead the unwary into a mistaken diagnosis of congenital esophageal atresia (Fig. 7-22). There are usually important clues that one is not dealing with a congenital esophageal atresia but rather with a traumatic perforation of the pharynx. The catheter and the contrast material lie several millimeters posterior to the trachea, whereas the upper esophageal pouch in true congenital esophageal atresia is in immediate direct contact with the posterior wall of the trachea. The sinus tract tends to be irregular in outline and usually narrower than the pouch of congenital esophageal atresia.

Once recognized, conservative management appears to be successful, and spontaneous closure usually results without serious clinical sequelae. If empyema ensues, it may require treatment by closed tube thoracostomy. An exploratory thoracotomy with resection and ligation of the pseudo-diverticulum has been carried out in a few infants, but conservative management appears to be the treatment of choice in view of the experience that spontaneous closure is likely to occur. Total or partial parenteral nutrition may be necessary while awaiting such spontaneous closure.

Feeding tubes are often passed without the use of roentgen evaluation of position, and occasionally the tube may inadvertently pass into the airway (Fig. 7-23).

Vascular Catheters

Access to the arterial system is essential for monitoring blood gases, pH, and blood pressure. Frequent measurements of various biochemical and hematologic factors, as well as parenteral administration of fluids and drugs, are essential parts of the care of very-low-birth-weight infants. The umbilical artery is a commonly used route because of its accessibility. When the umbilical artery is

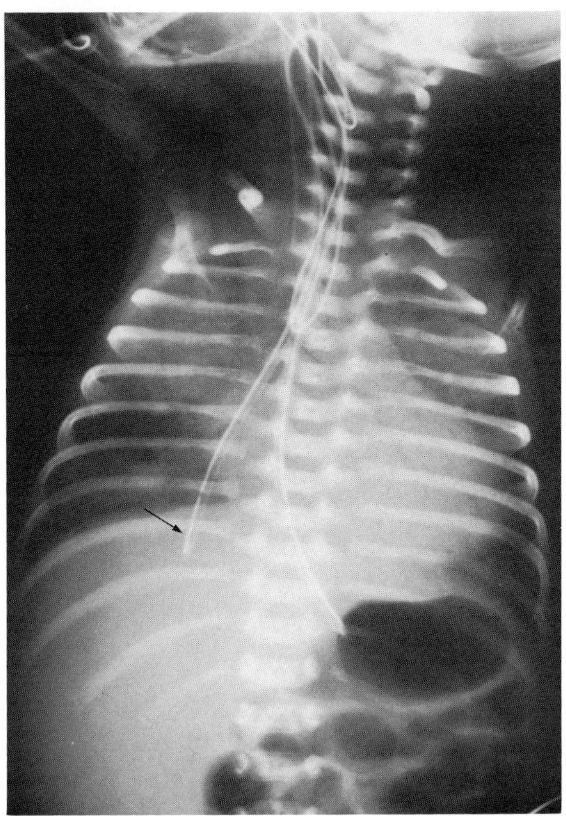

Fig. 7-23. Nasogastric catheter inadvertently placed in the trachea. It extends down to the right lower lobe bronchus (*arrow*).

catheterized, the catheter is advanced so that the tip lies in the aorta. The "ideal" level for the position of the tip of the catheter is the subject of some dispute. There are two approaches: those who advocate "high" and those who prefer "low" positions. The "high" school prefer to have the catheter tip between T6 and T10, and the "low" school keep the catheter tip at the L3–L4 level (48–50). The agreed upon area to avoid is the aortic region which gives rise to the celiac, renal, and mesenteric arteries.

The most common complication associated with indwelling aortic catheters is thrombus formation about the catheter (51,52). This has been reported as occurring in 95% of patients if the catheter is in place for more than 24 hours. Clinically recognizable complications of umbilical artery catheters, however, are quite infrequent and include embolism, vasospasm, blanching of an extremity, hemorrhage, necrotizing enterocolitis, infection, perforation, mycotic aneurysm, hypertension, and paraplegia (53,54). Roentgenographic recognition

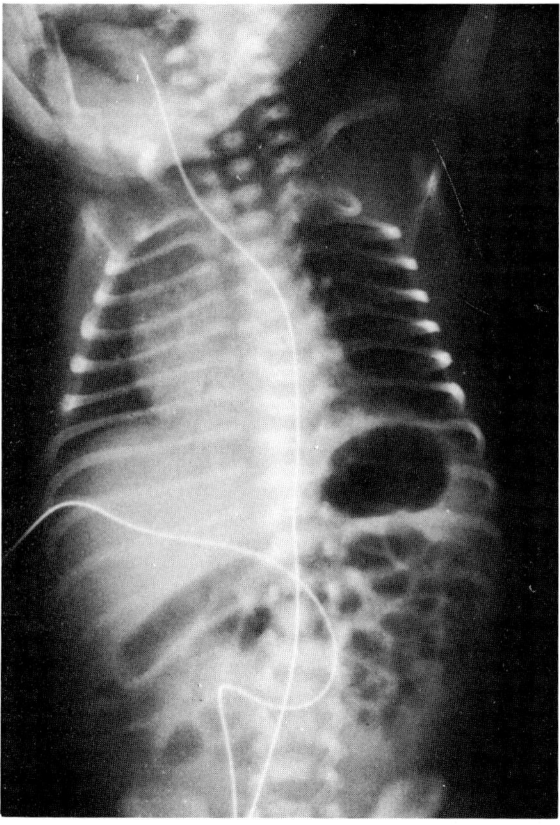

Fig. 7-24. Malpositioned umbilical artery catheter. It has been inserted too far and probably is in the right internal carotid artery.

of thoracic complications from the use of umbilical artery catheters is very difficult. Confirmation of the position of the catheter radiographically is essential following its placement. The tip may be too high, extending into one of the arteries arising from the aortic arch (Fig. 7-24). It may be at the level of the ductus arteriosus or pass through it into the pulmonary artery (Fig. 7-25) and give rise to misleading blood gases.

Catheter placement in the umbilical vein is occasionally used for drawing blood or as an access for fluid infusions. Ideally the tip of the catheter should be in the inferior vena cava just below its entrance into the right atrium, having passed from the umbilical vein through the portal vein and ductus venosus. Complications mostly affect the liver and gastrointestinal tract. If the tip of the catheter lies within the cardiac chambers, it may lead to arrhythmias, pulmonary embolism and infarction, nonbacterial endocarditis, hydrothorax, atrial perforation, and pericardial effusion (55–57). If the catheter is inserted too far, it may pass through the right atrium and extend up into the superior vena cava and into a neck vein (Fig. 7-26). It may also pass across the foramen ovale into the left atrium and out into a pulmonary vein. If the tip is in the left atrium, it may be a source for arterial embolism. In a pulmonary vein, the catheter can obstruct the vein and lead to pulmonary infarction (Fig. 7-27) and to pleural effusion. Late complications associated with prior insertion of umbilical vein catheters are splenic vein thrombosis, portal hypertension, and esophageal varices (58).

The location of an umbilical artery or umbilical vein catheter should always be studied roentgenographically immediately after it is inserted or its position changed (Fig. 7-28). A central venous

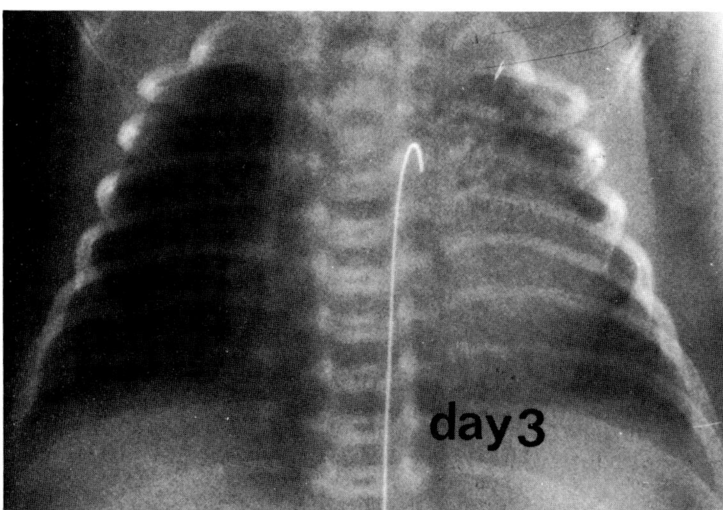

Fig. 7-25. Malpositioned umbilical artery catheter. The catheter is in too far. The tip has passed from the aorta through the ductus arteriosus. Note the presence of PIE in the left upper lobe.

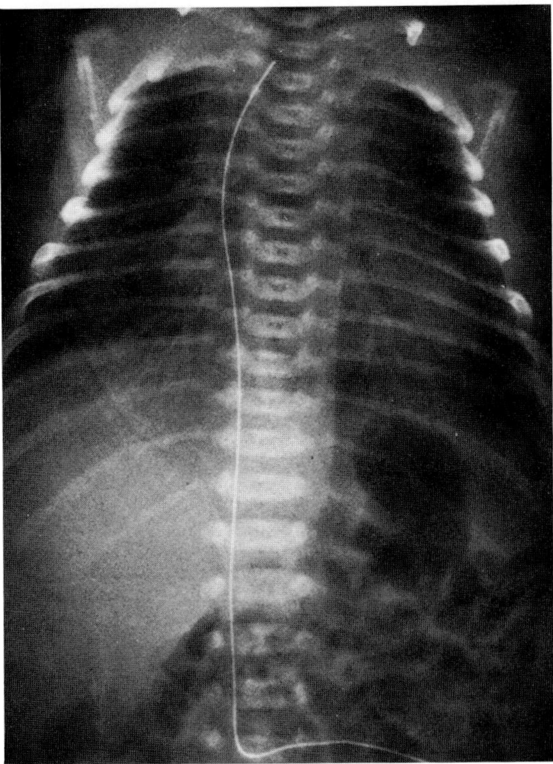

Fig. 7-26. Misplaced umbilical vein catheter. The catheter has been inserted too far and lies in a neck vessel. The tip should be at the junction of the inferior vena cava and right atrium.

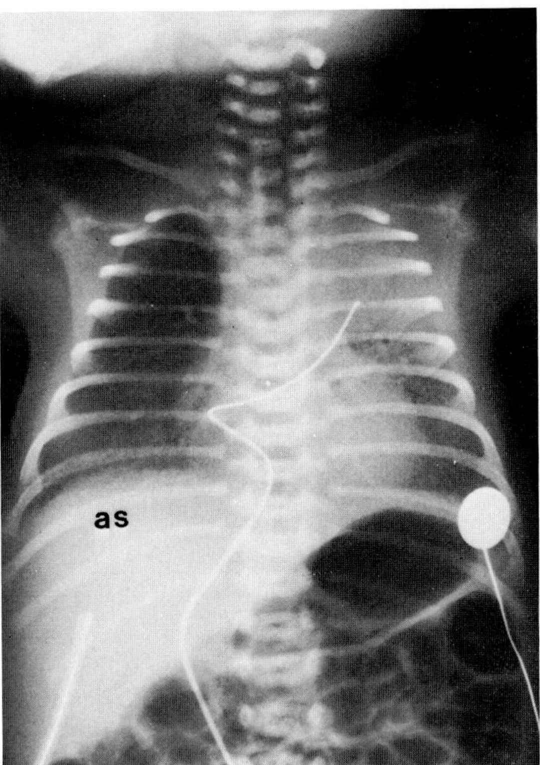

Fig. 7-27. Misplaced umbilical vein catheter. The catheter has been inserted too far. It extends from the right atrium across the foramen ovale into the left atrium and then out into a pulmonary vein. It caused obstruction of venous return from this lung segment, resulting in pulmonary hemorrhage, which is evident as an area of increased opacification in the left lung.

catheter inserted from an arm vein may perforate the superior vena cava and lead to hemothorax (Fig. 7-29).

Miscellaneous

Bronchopulmonary Dysplasia (BPD)

BPD is a form of chronic lung disease that develops in some newborn babies who have required intensive care for respiratory distress. In spite of numerous clinical, radiologic, and pathologic descriptions, the precise cause and pathophysiology are not entirely agreed upon (59). Such factors as high inspired oxygen concentration, high ventilating pressure, endotracheal intubation, mechanically assisted ventilation, severity of primary disease, immaturity of the lung, and patent ductus arteriosus have been incriminated.

Clinically the disorder is suspected in infants with severe respiratory distress who fail to improve in an expected fashion, who require high inspired oxygen concentrations, usually with mechanical ventilation, and who retain carbon dioxide. BPD may become the baby's primary problem. Radiographically the condition can be considered if the lungs fail to show progressive improvement in aeration and, instead, develop an increasing opacification and grossly disturbed aeration, with intermingled areas of patchy density, focal emphysema, and increased lung volumes (Fig. 7-30a–c). In infants who ultimately survive, the radiographic appearance gradually improves, but abnormal strandlike densities and small areas of uneven aeration may be evident for many months or even a few years (Fig. 7-31). Although the radiographic appearances of the lungs usually return to normal over a period of a few years, functional distur-

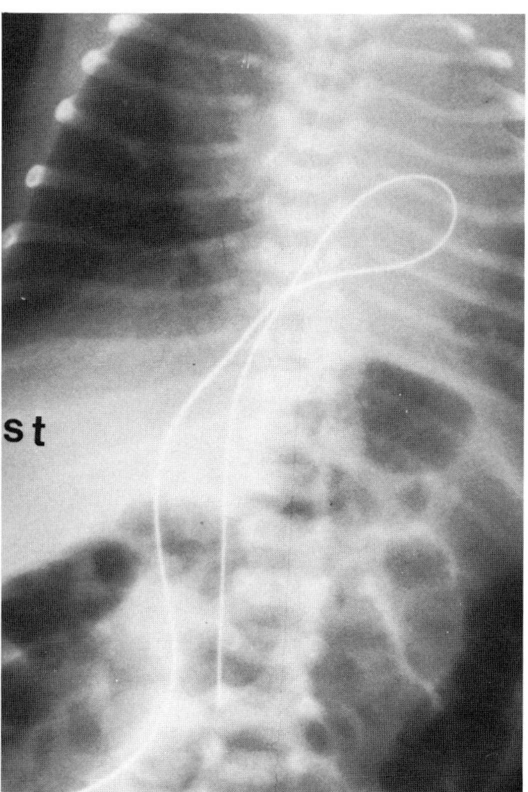

Fig. 7-28. Misplaced umbilical vein catheter. The catheter has extended up through the portal vein, ductus venosus, right atrium, through the foramen ovale, into the left atrium then back through the foramen ovale, right atrium, and down the inferior vena cava. Incidentally the ET tube has been badly positioned into the right intermediate bronchus.

bances persist and may provide a background for pulmonary disease in later years.

Pathologically BPD shows damage and repair of the bronchiolar and alveolar epithelium with interstitial fibrosis, squamous metaplasia of bronchial and bronchiolar epithelium, fibroproliferative bronchiolitis, bronchiectasis, atelectasis, and emphysema (60).

Infants who develop the condition require prolonged respiratory support with intubation, supplemental oxygen, and ventilation. Those who cannot be successfully weaned develop progressive pulmonary fibrosis, secondary infection, and cor pulmonale; and up to 40% of infants with severe BPD succumb, often around three to six months of age. Among those who survive there appears to be an increased risk for bronchiolitis and severe lower respiratory infections during their first year or two of life (61–63).

Patent Ductus Arteriosus (PDA)

The tiny premature baby has an increased risk of developing a PDA (64,65). The ductus is also likely to remain open in infants with hyaline membrane disease. The clinical diagnosis of a PDA may be difficult, as a murmur may not be present and it may be heralded only by deterioration in the clinical status of the infant. If a significant left-to-right shunt develops, the infant has increasing respiratory distress and seems to be at greater risk for developing bronchopulmonary dysplasia and necrotizing enterocolitis. Chest films (Fig. 7-32) occasionally may be helpful by showing progressive enlargement of the heart and an increase in pulmonary vascularity. The diagnosis can be substantiated by the use of ultrasound and radionuclide angiocardiography. Closure of a large PDA may improve lung compliance and thereby allow use of lower airway pressures. If medical management of the heart failure is unsuccessful, prompt closure of the ductus is imperative (66,67).

Pancuronium Bromide (Pavulon)

If the infant on a ventilator has asynchronous ventilation, i.e., "bucks" the ventilator, the patient's spontaneous respiratory efforts can be abolished with the muscle relaxant pancuronium bromide (Pavulon). This allows the full flexibility of the ventilator to be used to the patient's benefit, with reduction of peak inspiratory pressure. It results in an improving arterial-alveolar gradient, and the infants suffer fewer pneumothoraces (68–70). Radiographically the drug produces two interesting side effects (Fig. 7-33). It abolishes the swallowing of air, and the abdomen rather quickly becomes "gasless." Its use in some babies also results in development of conspicuous edema of the soft tissues of the thorax and abdomen. It is postulated that skeletal muscle activity and tissue motion are required to maintain lymph flow. Paralysis of muscles of the chest wall impairs the lymphatic drainage of the normal intercellular transudate, leading to excessive accumulation of fluid in the soft tissues.

Paralysis of the Diaphragm

Damage to the brachial plexus during delivery may be associated with forceps extraction or breech

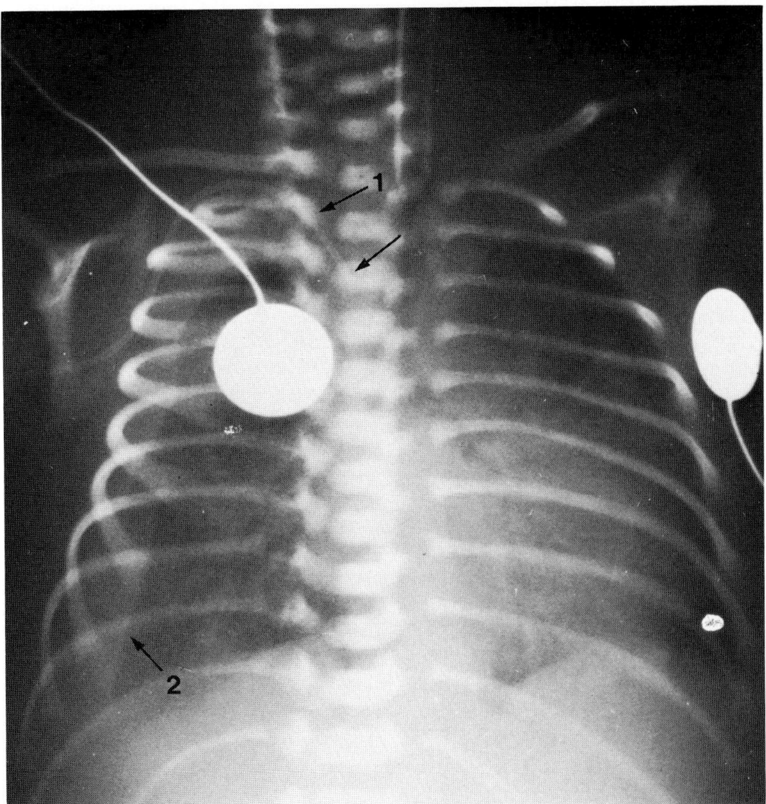

Fig. 7-29. Perforation of superior vena cava by a catheter (*arrow #1*). The catheter had been inserted from the right arm. At postmortem, it was found to have perforated the superior vena cava, causing bleeding into the right pleural space (*arrow #2*).

deliveries. This may result in paralysis of the diaphragm, usually unilateral, which can be a cause of respiratory distress (71). Radiographically (Fig. 7-34) the diaphragm on the affected side is higher than normal, and fluoroscopy will demonstrate the presence of paradoxical movements, which differentiate it from eventration of the diaphragm. About one-half of the babies will show complete recovery over a period of two or three months. In rare instances, the paralysis may result in severe respiratory distress, with the added problems of superimposed pneumonia and atelectasis. Plication of the diaphragm is essential in such babies.

Conclusion

For the very-low-birth-weight (VLBW—under 1000 grams) babies, the likelihood of survival continues to show remarkable improvement as expertise in their care has developed (72–77). According to the British Perinatal Mortality Survey, in 1958, only 7% of babies under 1000 grams survived and of these the majority suffered a major handicap. By 1970, the percent of survivors under 1000 grams had risen to 12% (78). In major intensive care units today, the survival rate for the smallest infant has now risen to 50% to 65%. During 1980, 116 babies under 1000 grams were cared for in the intensive care nurseries in the Children's Hospital Medical Center and in the Boston Hospital for Women. Of these, 71 survived (61%). It is difficult to evaluate the percent of survivors who are handicapped, because the definitions of major and minor handicaps vary. A major handicap generally includes definite cerebral palsy, an IQ below 70, severe deafness, or loss of vision. Major handicaps for VLBW infants range between 10% and 30%. These ameliorations in the care of extremely immature babies have been accompanied by much

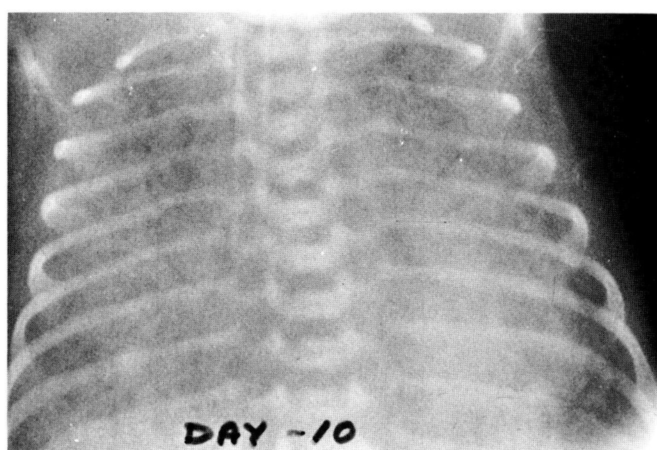

a

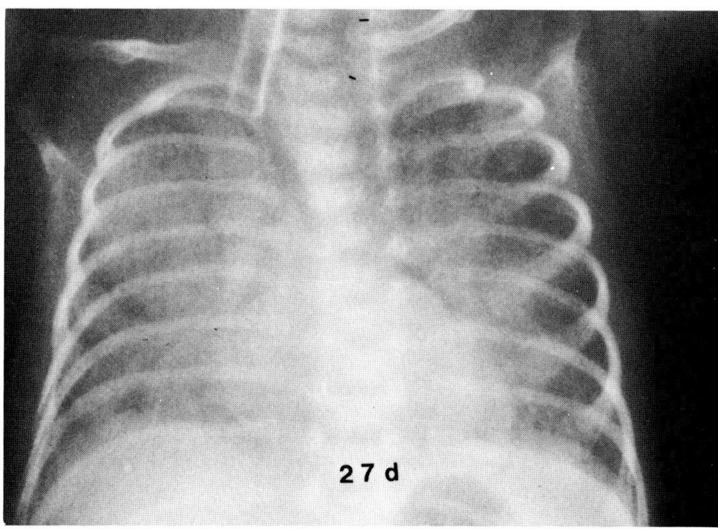

b

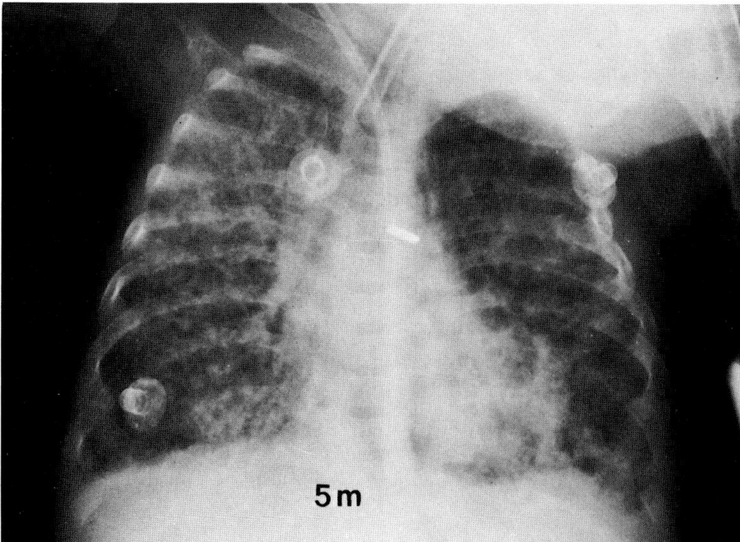

c

Fig. 7-30, a–c. Bronchopulmonary dysplasia. a and **b** Films of two patients, one at 10 days and one at 27 days, show almost complete opacification of both lungs, which are also somewhat increased in volume. **c** An infant at 5 months shows very irregularly aerated and voluminous lungs with confluent patchy and streaky densities and intermingled regions of focal emphysema. The patient still required intubation, had a PDA closed, and has a ventriculoperitoneal shunt in place for hydrocephalus.

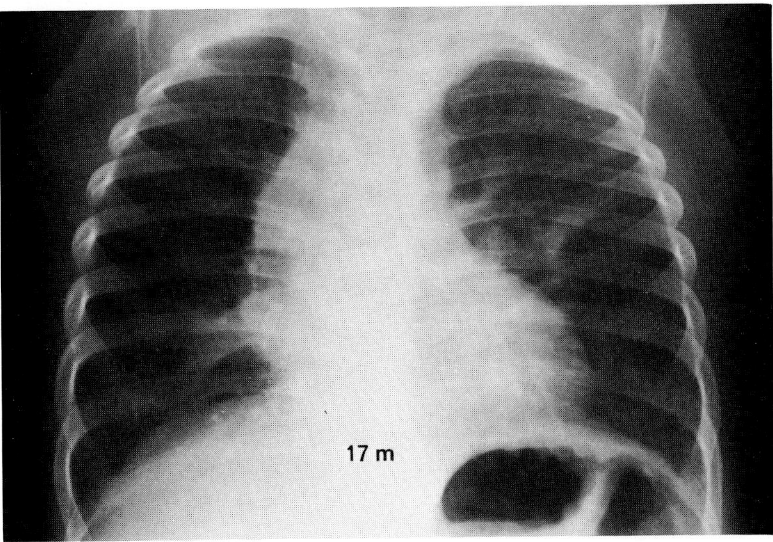

Fig. 7-31. Bronchopulmonary dysplasia. Changes persist in both lungs at the age of 17 months. Some improvement had occurred over the previous months, but aeration remains quite irregular and there are areas that appear locally emphysematous as well as having patchy and streaky shadows, which very likely represent areas of chronic lobular atelectasis and possibly some fibrosis.

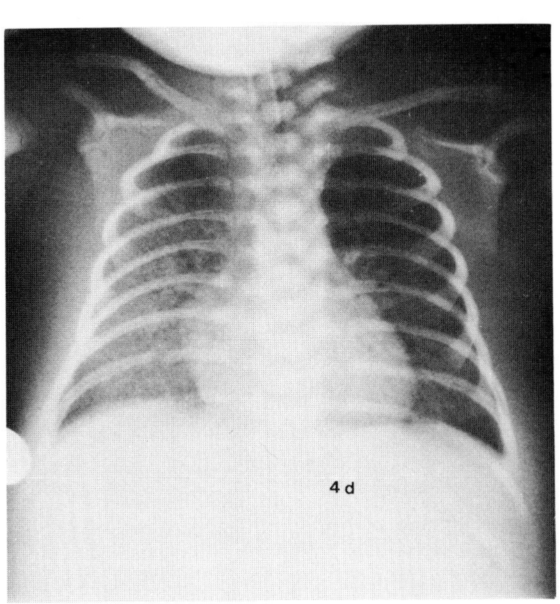

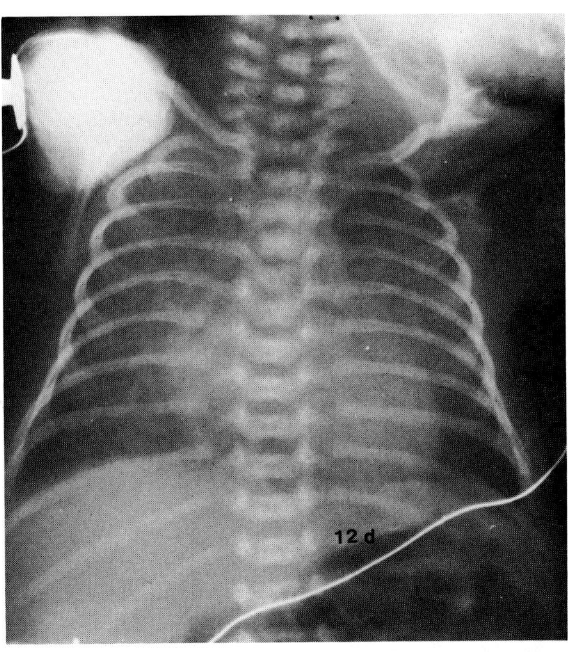

a   b

Fig. 7-32, a and **b. Patent ductus arteriosus.** At 4 days **(a)** the heart is normal in size. Both lungs do show some diffuse increase in density but actually had shown improved aeration with partial clearing of the changes of hyaline membrane disease. At 12 days **(b)** the heart is now considerably enlarged. There has been further increase in density of both lungs consistent with passive congestion and edema, and some of the perihilar vessels are larger than normal, although poorly seen because of the edema.

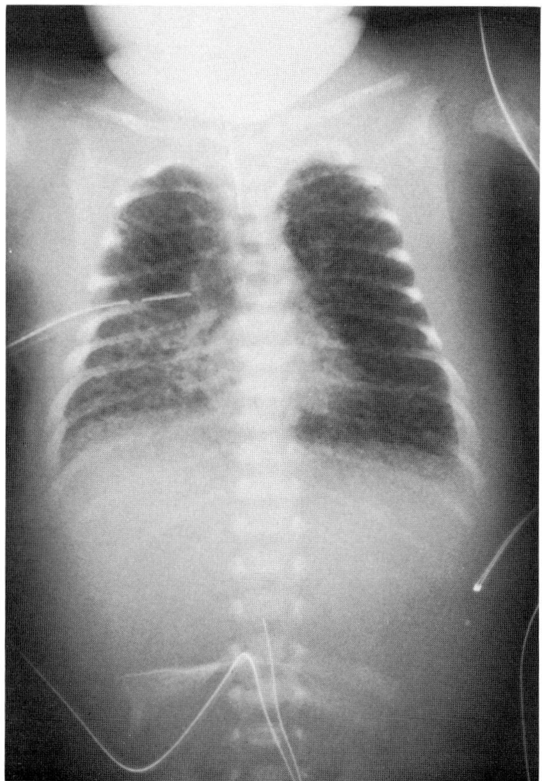

Fig. 7-33. Pancuronium bromide (Pavulon). Use of this paralytic agent often results in edema of the soft tissues of the chest and abdomen as well as an absence of air in the intestinal tract.

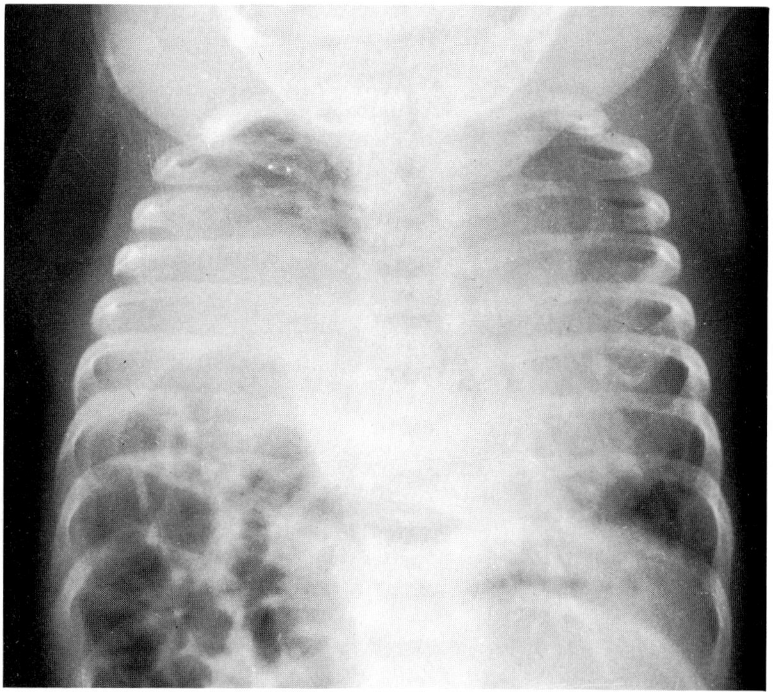

Fig. 7-34. Paralyzed diaphragm. Phrenic nerve paralysis may result from birth trauma. The right diaphragm is strikingly elevated, and expansion of the right lung is severely compromised. Paradoxical motion of the diaphragm was present at fluoroscopy. The baby suffered from recurrent pneumonias and responded to surgical plication of the diaphragm.

improved benefits accruing to the even larger population of higher-birth-weight infants who previously would have suffered significant neurologic sequelae and chronic lung disease.

An optimistic attitude for the immediate and long-term survival of the VLBW infants is justified. Continued vigilance, however, is essential. Complications associated with the treatment and investigation of these very tiny babies seem inevitable in spite of the diligent care of everyone involved in their management. Radiology is particularly important in helping to recognize and at times prevent many of these potentially life-threatening mishaps.

Acknowledgment

I am very grateful to Andrea Kelton for typing the manuscript.

References

1. Tochen ML: Orotracheal intubation in the newborn infant: a method for determining depth of tube insertion. J Pediatr 95:1050, 1979.
2. Nagaraj HS, Shott R, Fellow R, et al: Recurrent lobar atelectasis due to acquired bronchial stenosis in neonates. J. Pediatr Surg 15:411, 1980.
3. Miller KE, Edwards BK, Hilton S, et al: Acquired lobar emphysema in premature infants with bronchopulmonary dysplasia: an iatrogenic disease? Radiology 138:589, 1981.
4. Symchych PS, Cadotte M: Squamous metaplasia and necrosis of the trachea complicating prolonged nasotracheal intubation of small newborn infants. J Pediatr 71:534, 1967.
5. Joshi VV, Mandavia SG, Stern L, et al: Acute lesions induced by endotracheal intubation. Am J Dis Child 124:64, 1972.
6. Finer NN, Moriarty RR, Boyd J, et al: Post extubation atelectasis: a retrospective review and a prospective controlled study. J Pediatr 94:110, 1979.
7. Striker TW, Stool S, Downes JJ: Prolonged nasotracheal intubation in infants and children. Arch Otolaryngol 85:210, 1967.
8. Stewart AR, Finer NN, Moriarty RR, et al: Neonatal nasotracheal intubation: an evaluation. Laryngoscope 90:826, 1980.
9. Gregory G, Willis M: Complications of prolonged endotracheal intubation. Pediatr Res 12:561, 1976.
10. Papsidero MJ, Pashley NR: Acquired stenosis of the upper airway in the neonate: an increasing problem. Ann Otol Rhinol Laryngol 89:512, 1980.
11. Madansky DL, Lawson EE, Chernick V, et al: Pneumothorax and other forms of pulmonary air leaks in the newborn. Am Rev Respir Dis 120:729, 1979.
12. Monin P, Vert P: Pneumothorax. Clin Perinatol 5:335, 1978.
13. Plenat F, Vert P, Didier F, et al: Pulmonary interstitial emphysema. Clin Perinatol 5:351, 1978.
14. Stavis RL, Krauss AN: Complications of neonatal intensive care. Clin Perinatol 7:107, 1980.
15. Kuhns L, Bednarek F, Wyman M, et al: Diagnosis of pneumothorax or pneumomediastinum in the neonate by transillumination. Pediatrics 56:355, 1975.
16. Krowchuk D, Seashore JH: Thoracic transillumination: aid in the diagnosis and treatment of pneumopericardium. Pediatrics 64:958, 1979.
17. Leonidas JC, Bhan I, McCauley RCK: Persistent localized pulmonary interstitial emphysema and lymphangiectasis: a causal relationship? Pediatrics 64:165, 1979.
18. Clarke TA, Edwards DK: Pulmonary pseudocyst in newborn infants with respiratory distress syndrome. AJR 133:417, 1979.
19. Stocker JJ, Madewell JE: Persistent interstitial pulmonary emphysema: another complication of the respiratory distress syndrome. Pediatrics 59:847, 1977.
20. Reyes HM, et al: Pulmonary interstitial emphysema—surgical management. Report of 3 cases. J Pediatr Surg 15:266, 1980.
21. Leonidas JG, Hall RT, Rhodes PG: Conservative management of unilateral pulmonary interstitial emphysema under tension. J Pediatr 87:776, 1975.
22. Malginer AD, Capitanio MA, Wertheimer J, et al: Persistent localized pulmonary interstitial emphysema: an observation in 3 infants. Radiology 111:379, 1974.
23. Brooks JG, Bustamante SA, Koops SA, et al: Selective bronchial intubation for the treatment of severe localized pulmonary interstitial emphysema in newborn infants. J Pediatr 91:648, 1977.
24. Frantz ID, Stark AR, Dorkin HC: Ventilation of infants at frequencies up to 1800 per minute. Pediatr Res 14:642, 1980.
25. Ogata ES, Gregory GA, Kitterman JA, et al: Pneumothorax in the respiratory distress syndrome. Incidence and effect on vital signs, blood gases and pH. Pediatrics 58:177, 1976.
26. Moskowitz PS, Griscom NT: The medial pneumothorax. Radiology 120:143, 1976.
27. Lawson EE, Gould JD, Taeusch HW: Neonatal pneumopericardium: current management. J Pediatr Surg 15:181, 1980.
28. Higgins CD, Broderick TW, Edwards DK, et al: The hemodynamic significance of massive pneumopericardium in pre-term infants with respiratory distress syndrome. Radiology 133:363, 1979.
29. Emery RW, Lindsay WG, Nicoloff DN: Placement of pericardial drainage tube for the treatment of pneumopericardium in the neonate. Ann Thorac Surg 26:84, 1978.

30. Leonidas JC, Hall RT, Rhodes PG, et al: Pneumoperitoneum in the ventilated newborn. Am J Dis Child 128:677, 1974.
31. Chang JH, Hernandez J: Ventilator induced pneumoperitoneum—a rapid diagnosis. Pediatrics 66:135, 1980.
32. Cohen MD, Schreiner R, Lemons J: Neonatal pneumoperitoneum without adventitious pulmonary air: use of metrizamide to rule out perforation of the bowel. Pediatrics 69:587–589, 1982.
33. Oppermann HC, Wille L, Obladen M, et al: Systemic air embolism in the respiratory distress syndrome of the newborn. Pediatr Radiol 8:139, 1979.
34. Kogutt NS: Systemic air embolism secondary to respirator therapy in the neonate: 6 cases including one survivor. AJR 131:425, 1978.
35. Banagale RC, Outerbridge EW, Aranda JV: Lung perforation: a complication of chest tube insertion in neonatal pneumothorax. J Pediatr 94:973, 1979.
36. Moessinger AC, Driscoll JM, Wigger HJ: High incidence of lung perforation by chest tube in neonatal pneumothorax. J Pediatr 92:635, 1978.
37. Grosfeld JL, Lemons JJ, Ballantine TVM, et al: Emergency thoracotomy for acquired bronchopleural fistual in the premature infant with respiratory distress. J Pediatr Surg 15:416, 1980.
38. Oppermann H C, Wille L: Hemothorax in the newborn. Pediatr Radiol 9:129, 1980.
39. Jung AL, Minton SD, Roan Y: Pulmonary hemorrhage secondary to chest tube placement for pneumothorax in neonates. Clin Pediatr 19:624, 1980.
40. Touloukian RJ, Beardsley GP, Ablow RD, et al: Traumatic perforation of the pharynx in the newborn. Pediatrics 59:1019, 1977.
41. Nagaraj HS, Mullen P, Groff DB, et al: Iatrogenic perforation of the esophagus in premature infants. Surgery 86:583, 1979.
42. Clark TA, Coen RW, Feldman B, et al: Esophageal perforation in premature infants and comments on the diagnosis. Am J Dis Child 134:367, 1980.
43. Vaughn RS, Menke JA, Giacoia GP: Pneumothorax: a complication of endotracheal tube suctioning. J Pediatr 92:633, 1978.
44. Felming PJ: Esophageal perforation into the right pleural cavity in the neonate. J Pediatr Surg 15:335, 1980.
45. Urrutia J, Antonnattei S, Cordero L: Pseudodiverticulum of the esophagus in the newborn infant. Am J Dis Child 134:417, 1980.
46. Lucaya J, Herrera M, Salcedo S: Traumatic pharyngeal pseudodiverticulum in neonates and infants. Pediatr Radiol 8:65, 1979.
47. Heller RM, Kirchner SC, O'Neill JA: Perforation of the pharynx in the newborn: a near look-alike for esophageal atresia. AJR 129:335, 1977.
48. Mokrohisky ST, Levine RL, Blumhagen JL, et al: Low positioning of umbilical artery catheters increases associated complications in newborn infants. N Engl J Med 299:561, 1978.
49. Henriksson P, Wesstrom G, Hedner U: Umbilical artery catheterization in newborns. I. Thrombosis in relation to catheter type and position. Acta Paediatr Scand 68:575, 1977.
50. Harris MS, Little GA: Umbilical artery catheter: high, low or no. J Perinat Med 6:15, 1978.
51. Goetzman VW, Stadalnik RC, Bogren HC, et al: Thrombotic complications of umbilical artery catheters: a clinical and radiographic study. Pediatrics 56:374, 1975.
52. Henriksson P, Wesstrom G, Hedner U: Umbilical artery catheterization in newborns. III. Thrombosis—a study of some predisposing factors. Acta Paediatr Scand 68:719, 1979.
53. Marsh JL, King W, Barrett C, et al: Serious complications after umbilical artery catheterization for neonatal monitoring. Arch Surg 110:1203, 1975.
54. Spangler TG, Kleinberg F, Gulton RE, et al: False aneurysm of the descending aorta. Am J Dis Child 131:1258, 1977.
55. Symchych PS, Krauss AN, Winchester P: Endocarditis following intracardiac placement of umbilical venous catheters in neonates. J Pediatr 90:287, 1977.
56. Purohit DM, Levkoff AH: Pericardial effusion complicating umbilical venous catheterization. Arch Dis Child 52:520, 1977.
57. Kulkarni PB, Dorand RD: Hydrothorax: a complication of intracardiac placement of umbilical venous catheters. J Pediatr 94:813, 1979.
58. Vos LJM, Potocky V, Broker FHL, et al: Splenic vein thrombosis with esophageal varices: a late complication of umbilical vein catheterization. Ann Surg 180:152, 1974
59. Northway WH (Chairman): Workshop on bronchopulmonary dysplasia. J Pediatr 95:815, 1979.
60. Oppermann HC, Wille L, Bleyl U, et al: Bronchopulmonary dysplasia in premature infants. A radiological and pathological correlation. Pediatr Radiol 5:137, 1977.
61. Milner AD: Bronchopulmonary dysplasia. Arch Dis Child 55:661, 1980.
62. Edwards DK, Dyer WM, Northway WH: 12 years experience with bronchopulmonary dysplasia. Pediatrics 59:839, 1977.
63. Editorial: Bronchopulmonary dysplasia. The cost of survival for some pre-term infants? Lancet 1(8170):690, 1980.
64. Siassi B, Blanco C, Cabal LA, et al: Incidence and clinical features of patent ductus arteriosus in low birth weight infants. Pediatrics 57:347, 1976.
65. Friedman WF, Fitzpatrick KM, Merritt TA, et al: Patent ductus arteriosus. Clin Perinatol 5:411, 1978.
66. Obeyeseker HI, Pankhurst S, Yu VY: Pharmacological closure of ductus arteriosus in pre-term infants using indomethacin. Arch Dis Child 55:271, 1980.
67. Salomon NW, Anderson RM, Copeland JG, et al: A rational approach to ligation of patent ductus arteriosus in the neonate. Chest 75:671, 1979.
68. Krauss AN: Assisted ventilation: a critical review. Clin Perinatol 7:61, 1980.
69. Crone RK, Favorito JD, Todres ID: Muscle relaxation in treatment of critically ill infants with hyaline membrane disease. Crit Care Med 8:237, 1980.

70. Stark AR, Bascomb R, Frantz ID: Muscle relaxation in mechanically ventilated infants. J Pediatr 94:439, 1979.
71. Curran JA: Birth associated injury. Clin Perinatol 8:111, 1981.
72. Rothberg AD, Naisels MJ, Bagnato S, et al: Outlook for survivors of mechanical ventilation weighing less than 1250 grams at birth. J Pediatr 98:106, 1981.
73. Shannon DC, Crone RK, Todres ID, et al: Survival, cost of hospitalization, and prognosis in infants critically ill with respiratory distress syndrome requiring mechanical ventilation. Crit Care Med 9:94, 1981.
74. Schreiner RL, Kisling JA, Evans GM, et al: Improved survival of ventilated neonates with modern intensive care. Pediatrics 66:95, 1980.
75. Yu VY: Improving prognosis for infants weighing 1000 grams or less at birth. Arch Dis Child 55:422, 1980.
76. Brown ER, Taeusch HW: Intensive care and the very low birth weight infant. Lancet 2:362, 1979.
77. Hack M, Fanaroff AA, Merkatz IR: The low birth weight infant: evolution of a changing outlook. N Engl J Med 300:1162, 1979.
78. Editorial: The fate of the baby under 1500 grams at birth. Lancet 1(8168):461, 1980.

8 Thoracic Radiotherapy Changes

Herman I. Libshitz

Radiotherapy is frequently used in the treatment of malignancies in the thorax, on the thoracic wall, and near the thorax. Radiographic changes secondary to the radiotherapy will occur not only in the lesion being irradiated but also in adjacent normal structures that are included in the treatment fields. Many of these changes are an anticipated result of radiotherapy and cannot truly be considered complications. Other effects extend beyond this anticipated range and are more pronounced than those usually seen. Some are unexpected. The latter two groups of changes are considered complications.

Radiation effects may be seen in the lungs, pleurae, heart, esophagus, other mediastinal structures, and the bones of the thoracic wall. These various tissues and organs demonstrate different responses to irradiation and at varying times from the completion of radiotherapy. For example, pulmonary changes become apparent much more quickly than those in bones.

A variety of factors will influence the radiographic appearance of these changes. These include volume of tissue irradiated, shape of the portal, dose of irradiation, length of time from completion of therapy, and effects of other therapy. Both the expected and unexpected sequelae of radiotherapy to the thorax will be considered with these factors serving as a framework.

Lung

By the early 1920s it was realized that radiation therapy caused adverse effects in the lungs and pleurae (1–3). In 1925 Evans and Leucutia (4) recognized early and late radiotherapy effects. The former manifested by "infiltration," the latter by fibrosis. Desjardins (5) in 1926 suggested that the term *radiation fibrosis* was indicated only when tissue changes were permanent. Both of these ideas are still useful.

Pathologic Changes

The diagnosis of acute radiation pneumonitis is made from a combination of pathologic changes rather than from a pathognomonic feature (6,7). The findings include fibrin-rich membranes lining the alveoli (8); thickening of the alveolar septa, due to edema and mononuclear cell infiltration, which may either regress or progress to fibrosis (6–8); hyperplasia and prominence of alveolar lining cells with desquamation of cells into the alveolar lumen (6,7). Vascular lesions are also present, manifested by engorgement and thrombosis of capillaries (9,10) as well as edema, intimal proliferation, and medial changes. The vessels may become fibrosed (6,7,10).

This combination of pathologic findings explains the radiographic appearance of radiation pneumonitis. Should these changes not resolve, as is most often the case at therapeutic levels of irradiation, fibrosis ensues.

Factors Influencing the Radiographic Appearance

Volume

The likelihood of a patient developing significant clinical and radiographic changes is proportional to the volume of lung irradiated. Irradiation of all of both lungs to 3000 rad will most likely produce a fatal radiation pneumonitis. Irradiating approximately the equivalent of 25% to 33% of one lung to 3000 rad at standard fractionations is usually asymptomatic and rarely causes radiographic change. In the treatment of lung cancer, breast cancer, lymphoma, and the other malignancies usually treated, the volume of lung involved is usually sufficiently small so that it is not a limiting factor. The volume of lung irradiated occasionally becomes a serious consideration in therapy planning in patients with very large tumors or with compromised pulmonary function.

Field Size and Shape

While standard portals for various diseases are generally similar, institutional variations occur. It is important to be familiar with the portals used at one's institution and to have communication between diagnostic and therapeutic radiologists so that alterations in the usual portals or markedly unusual portals are recognized.

All change due to radiation pneumonitis should be within the irradiated volume. The borders of a well-established radiation pneumonitis conform to those of the field irradiated rather than to anatomic boundaries.

Most reports of radiation change outside of the irradiated fields (6,11–14) can be ascribed to dosimetric or technical errors. The clinical and radiographic features of some viral pneumonias and some chemotherapeutic effects in the lung may mimic radiation changes closely and account for some cases (15).

Radiation Dose

Radiation dose cannot be thought of as a given number of "rads." The number of fractions into which the dose was divided and the time period in which it was given are also important. It is obvious that the effects of a single treatment of 3000 rad will be appreciably different from the same total dose given in 15 fractions over a three-week period.

Most of our experience has been with ^{60}Co given 200 rad daily, five days a week; and unless otherwise specified, dosage figures will refer to this treatment schedule.

Radiographic evidence of pulmonary reaction is rarely seen under 3000 rad. It may be seen between 3000 and 3500 rad. It is usually seen between 3500 and 4000 rad and is almost always apparent at doses above 4000 rad. It is impossible, however, to predict which patient will develop radiation pneumonitis (6). Human variability is an unmeasurable factor.

Timing

Radiation pneumonitis is generally radiographically evident eight weeks after completion of therapy of a course of 3500–4000 rad or more (Fig. 8-1). It is usually well established at this time, indicating it was present one to two weeks earlier (16–20). Roentgenographic evidence of radiation pneumonitis is anticipated one week sooner for each 1000-rad increment above 4000 rad (19,20).

In most patients evidence of radiation fibrosis or retraction due to fibrosis will follow radiation pneumonitis (Fig. 8-2). Radiation fibrosis usually becomes stable by 9–12 months following completion of therapy (18–21).

Other Therapy

Various other therapies affect the severity and timing of radiation changes in the lung. A second course of radiation therapy is more likely to produce acute radiation pneumonitis than the first (22,23). Reactivation of the effects of radiation pneumonitis has been noted with actinomycin D and adriamycin administration (24–27) and also with steroid withdrawal (28,29).

The effects of chemotherapeutic agents given in conjunction with radiotherapy have not been completely worked out and will vary for different dosage schedules of both the medications and the radiotherapy. Radiotherapy given in conjunction with a chemotherapeutic agent that causes pulmonary parenchymal changes will generally cause at least additive changes (Fig. 8-3). Some agents, particularly actinomycin D and adriamycin, will cause synergistic changes (27,30,31).

Radiographic Appearance

The appearance of radiation pneumonitis may vary from minimal indistinctness of pulmonary vessels to marked consolidation. Minimal loss of sharpness of pulmonary vessels is often the first sign

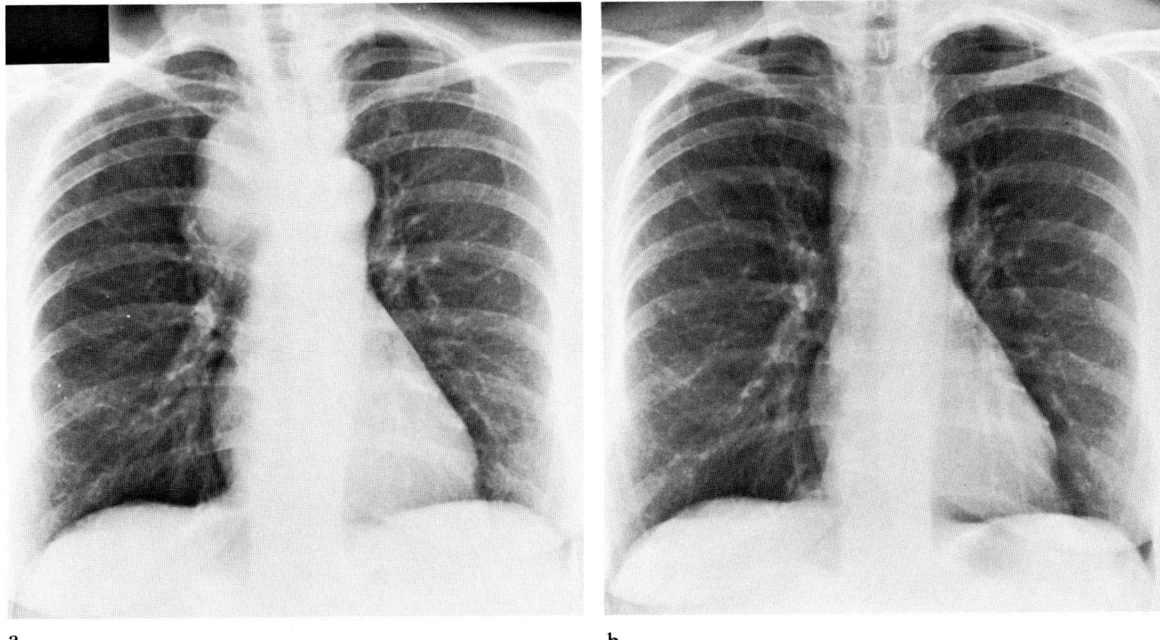

Fig. 8-1, a–d. Usual progression of radiation pneumonitis and fibrosis. A 61-year-old white female with poorly differentiated lymphocytic lymphoma treated with ^{60}Co irradiation; 4000 rad to the mediastinum and supraclavicular areas over four-week period. **a** Pretreatment radiograph showing right paratracheal and tracheobronchial adenopathy. **b** Three weeks following completion of therapy there is disappearance of enlarged nodes and no evidence of radiation pneumonitis. **c** Nine weeks following completion of radiotherapy, well-established radiation pneumonitis is present in both paramediastinal areas and in the apices. **d** At nine months following radiotherapy, radiation fibrosis is present. This was the final appearance in the patient. The minor fissure is elevated and pleural thickening is present in both apices.

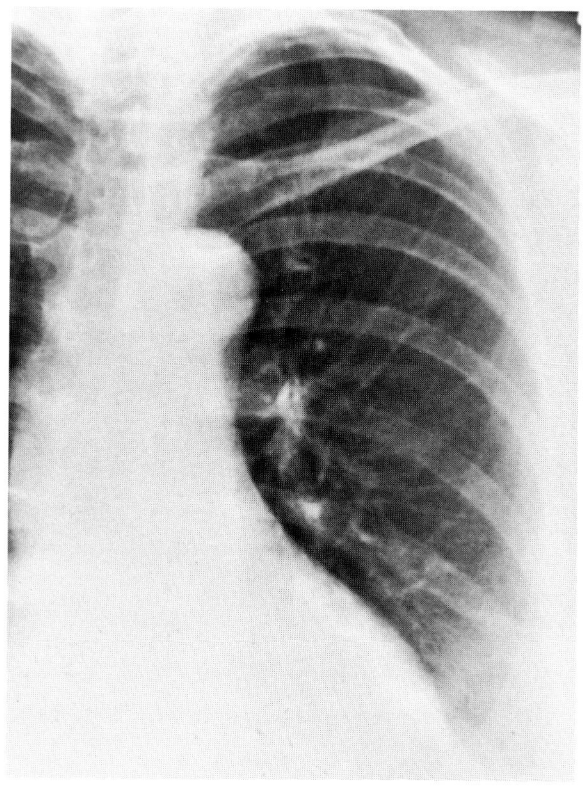

a

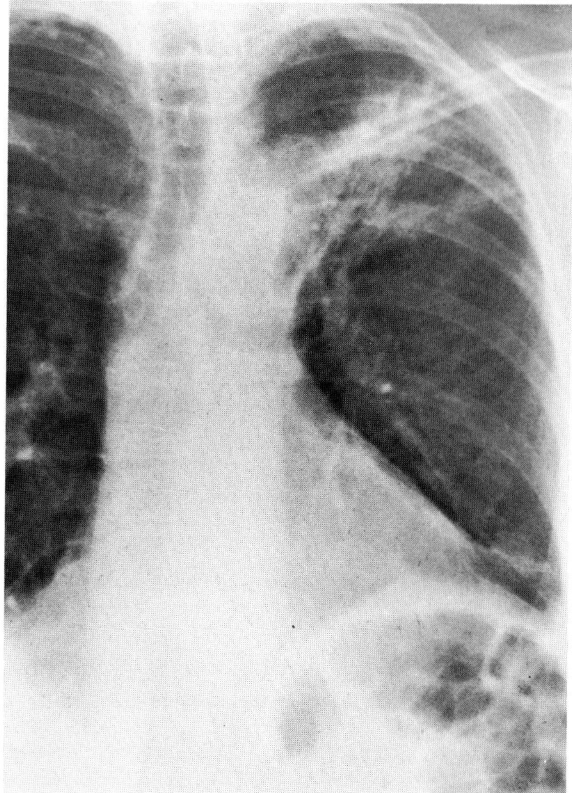

b

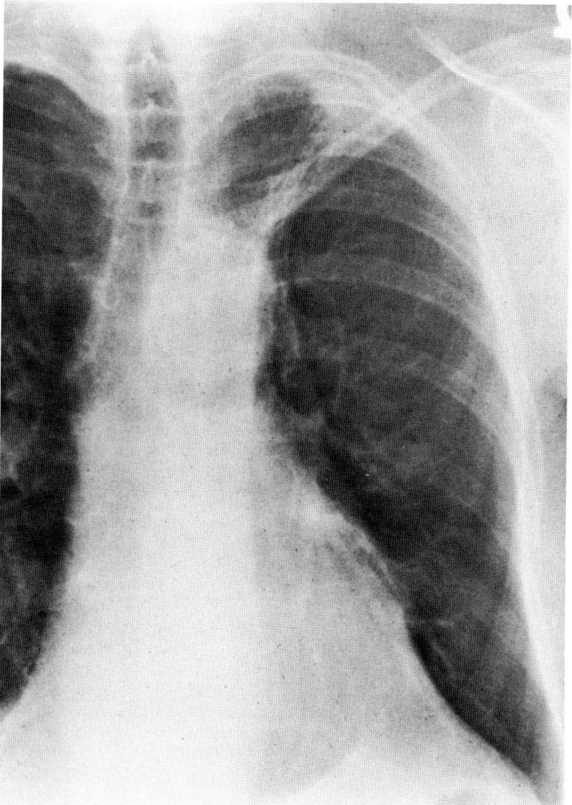

c

Fig. 8-2, a–c. Typical sequence of changes following postoperative radiotherapy for carcinoma of the breast. A 57 year-old-white female treated with postoperative radiotherapy following a modified radical mastectomy. Radiotherapy was given over a six-week period, 5000 rads to the internal mammary nodes, left supraclavicular area, and chest wall. **a** Pretreatment chest radiograph. **b** Eleven weeks following radiotherapy, typical radiation pneumonitis is present. **c** Radiation fibrosis is present 11 months after treatment, with contracture of the areas of prior radiation pneumonitis, apical thickening, and slight tenting of the left hemidiaphragm.

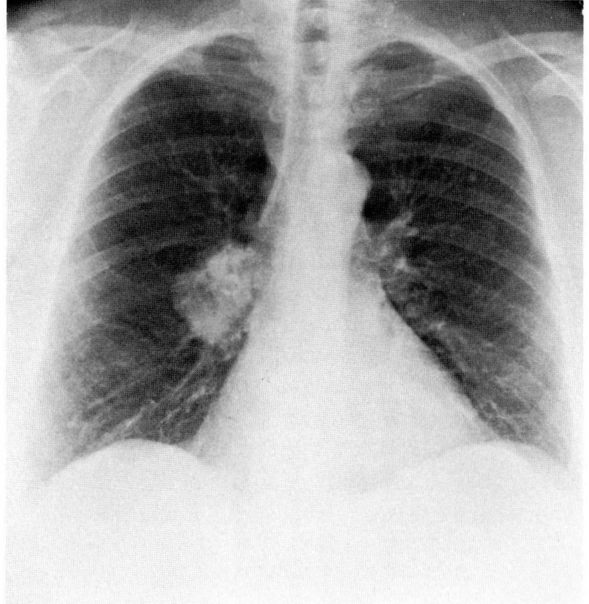

a

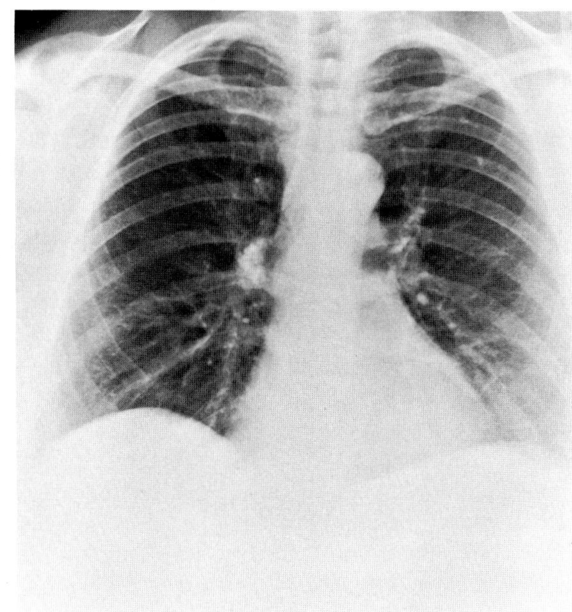

b

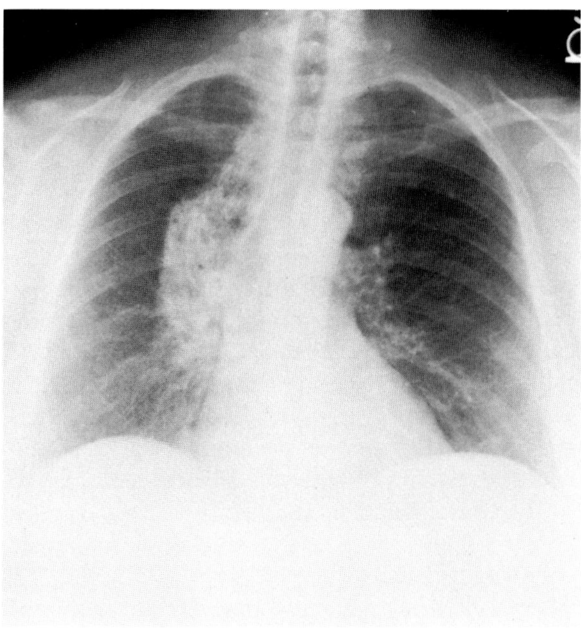

c

Fig. 8-3, a–c. Earlier-than-usual radiation pneumonitis. A 57-year-old white female with oat cell carcinoma of the lung. The patient had received several courses of chemotherapy (including adriamycin, cyclophosphamide, and vincristine) prior to radiotherapy. The patient received 3000 rads of radiotherapy in two weeks, 300 rads per day. The earlier-than-usual appearance of the changes is due to the chemotherapy and more rapid delivery of the radiotherapy. **a** Pretreatment radiograph showing large hilar mass of oat cell carcinoma. **b** Four weeks after completion of radiotherapy, mass is no longer present. Minimal indistinctness of the pulmonary vasculature is present in the suprahilar areas. The slightly earlier-than-usual appearance of radiation pneumonitis is related to chemotherapy and the rapidity with which radiotherapy was given. **c** Even more pronounced change is seen at seven weeks following completion of radiotherapy.

of radiation pneumonitis (Fig. 8-3b) and in some cases the only manifestation. Without pretreatment radiographs for comparison, this can easily be overlooked. Familiarity with the irradiation fields facilitates its identification. Importantly, as previously noted, the radiation change should be confined only to the irradiated portion of lung. More marked radiation pneumonitis is relatively easy to identify. The consolidation, frequently contains air bronchograms, has geometric boundaries (most often linear) and crosses normal tissue boundaries (Fig. 8-4). This combination of findings would be quite unusual in any other pulmonary inflammatory process.

When followed over short intervals, more pronounced consolidation may develop. The peak reaction usually occurs approximately 3–4 months following completion of therapy. From this point radiation fibrosis begins to develop with gradual retraction of the involved areas. this retraction continues to approxmately 9–12 months after therapy, when it becomes stable.

As expected, more extensive radiation pneu-

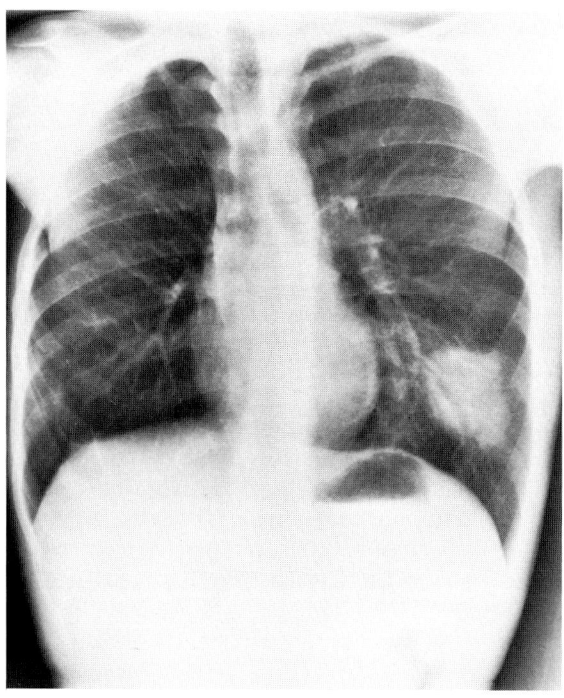

Fig. 8-4. Unusual portal. A square area of radiation pneumonitis is seen nine weeks following 3000 rad. A 5 cm × 5 cm portal was used to treat recurrent pulmonary parenchymal Hodgkin's disease. The patient had received multiple courses of combined chemotherapy prior to irradiation.

monitis usually results in a more severe radiation fibrosis. While complete resolution of radiation pneumonitis has been described, our experience has been that radiation fibrosis or evidence of contraction secondary to fibrosis can be identified in nearly all patients.

Radiation fibrosis is often identified in patients in whom there has been no prior evidence of radiation pneumonitis. This occurs most often when interval radiographs have not been obtained. There are, however, some patients in whom radiation pneumonitis is so minimal that it cannot be identified with certainty, if at all.

The findings of radiation fibrosis, while usually obvious, can be subtle. Minimal pleural thickening in the apex or elsewhere, slight elevation of a hilus or the minor fissure, minimal elevation of hemidiaphragm, or mild blunting of a cardiophrenic angle may be the only evidence of radiation fibrosis (20,32). Such changes are often identifiable only if pretreatment radiographs are available. The more obvious evidence of radiation fibrosis is strandlike densities in the irradiated lung. The patterns of fibrosis are consistent so that familiarity with the portals used makes less obvious sequelae easier to identify. Bronchiectatic and/or cystic changes may develop in the portions of lung involved in radiation fibrosis (33).

Less common complications include hyperlucency of an irradiated lung (34–36) and spontaneous pneumothorax (15,37,38). Pleural effusions secondary to radiotherapy can occur (16,39). These are extremely difficult if not impossible to distinguish from malignant effusions radiographically. Bachman and Macken (39) have offered the following diagnostic criteria for radiation pleuritis: effusion within six months of completion of therapy, coexistent radiation pneumonitis, and spontaneous resolution of the effusion. Reaccumulation of the effusion after thoracentesis or rapid increase in the amount of effusion suggests a malignant causation. Because cytologic examination of pleural fluid is frequently negative in neoplasia, prolonged observation may be the only way to distinguish radiation-induced from malignant effusions.

Occasionally, the effects of cardiac decompensation are superimposed on the pulmonary findings due to radiation pericarditis and/or myocarditis. The changes in the heart will be considered later.

Calcification of lymph nodes involved with lymphoma (most frequently Hodgkin's disease) can

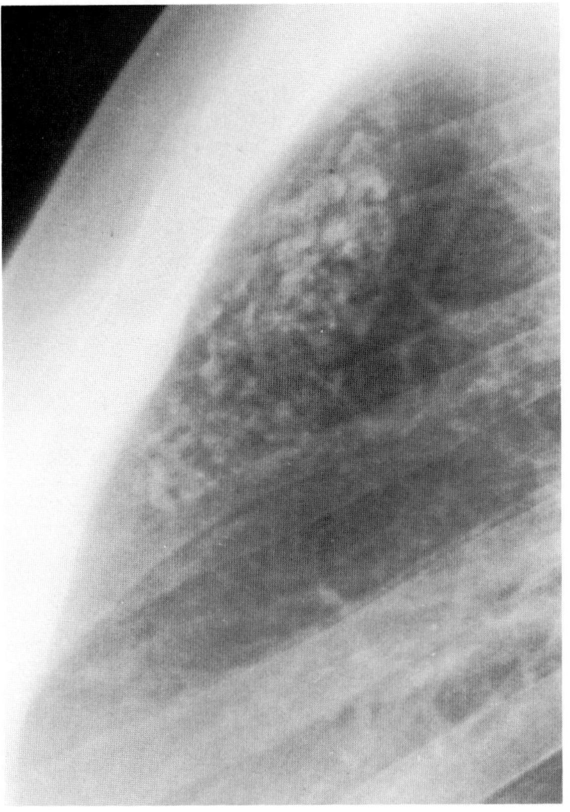

Fig. 8-5. Calcified node following radiotherapy. Lateral view of the anterior mediastinum showing calcification in a previously irradiated lymph node (Hodgkin's disease). The calcification became evident three and a half years postradiotherapy.

occur following radiotherapy (40,41) (Fig. 8-5). Recognizing this change is important so that a benign granulomatous etiology is not considered. The timing of the calcification varies from one to several years and may get denser with time. No definite dose dependency has been noted. It would appear that it is a favorable local response to treatment (40).

Differential Diagnosis

The differential diagnosis of radiotherapy changes includes infection, local recurrence of tumor (or occasionally development of a second primary), and lymphangitic spread. These can generally be distinguished based on awareness of the usual findings and their timing. Because the temporal relationships are so helpful in evaluating radiotherapy sequelae, we recommend that radiographs be ob-

tained at completion of therapy and at bimonthly intervals until the appearance of the chest has stabilized. As noted, fibrosis is generally stabilized by 12 months following completion of therapy. Routine follow-up suffices thereafter.

Lymphangitic spread is the easiest to exclude. Lymphangitic metastases are usually more prominent at the bases, and septal lines are usually obvious. That these changes are outside of the portals is also usually obvious. There is frequently a significant disparity between clinical and radiographic findings early in lymphangitic spread, with the clinical findings more pronounced than the radiographic findings suggest.

Recurrent tumor or the development of a second primary is usually identifiable by alteration in the contour of the stable appearance of radiation fibrosis (Figs. 8-6 and 8-7). Approximately three to four months after completion of therapy, the areas of radiation pneumonitis should start to contract. Any enlargement, particularly focally, should alert one to the possibility of recurrent tumor. Once a stable appearance has been reached, any alteration in that appearance is suspect and deserves evaluation.

Infection can often be excluded by knowledge of the field size and shape. Consolidation outside of the treated fields speaks for an infectious cause of the changes. Awareness of the timing of radiation pneumonitis also often affords the means of distinguishing a pneumonia from radiation reaction (Fig. 8-8). Unfortunately, it is often difficult, if not impossible, to exclude a superimposed pneumonia in areas of radiation pneumonitis. Appropriate clinical and bacteriologic studies may help. Occasionally, follow-up is the only way to make the distinction. While radiographic criteria have been suggested to distinguish infection, particularly tuberculosis, from radiation pneumonitis, we have not found any criteria particularly useful. A superimposed infection may cause increased lucency in areas of radiation fibrosis due to tissue destruction.

Clinical Correlation

None of the clinical manifestations of radiation pneumonitis are specific. Nor have we been able to correlate radiographic findings with symptoms. Many patients with extensive radiographic evidence of postradiotherapy change will be asympto-

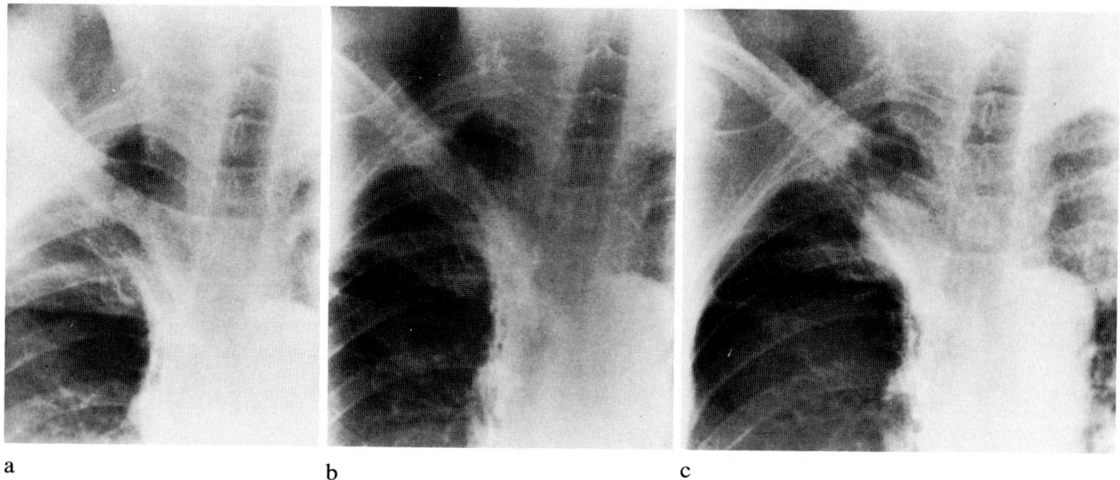

a   b   c

Fig. 8-6. Metastases developing in an irradiated area. This 66-year-old woman received 45000 rad to the internal mammary nodes (15 MeV electron beam) 13 months prior to the left radiograph. **a** This should be the stable appearance. **b** Seven months later, an increased soft-tissue density is seen just under the medial aspect of the left clavicle (middle radiograph). **c** Six months later (26 months postradiotherapy), an obvious mass is present (right radiograph) in this area representing metastatic breast cancer. There should be no alteration in stable radiation fibrosis.

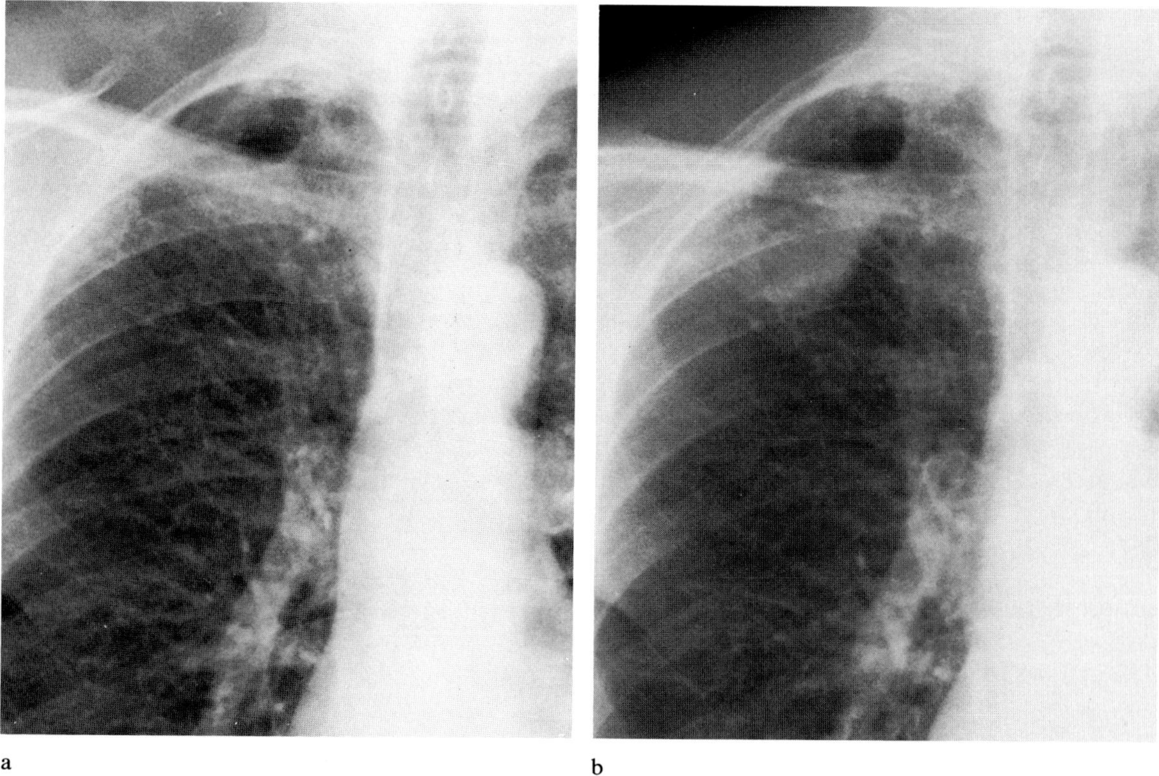

a   b

Fig. 8-7, a and b. Carcinoma developing in an irradiated area. A 59-year-old female who was irradiated following a right mastectomy seven years ago. **a** Chest radiograph showing stable postradiation changes four years after completion of radiotherapy. **b** An oat cell carcinoma has developed in the right upper lobe seven years postradiotherapy.

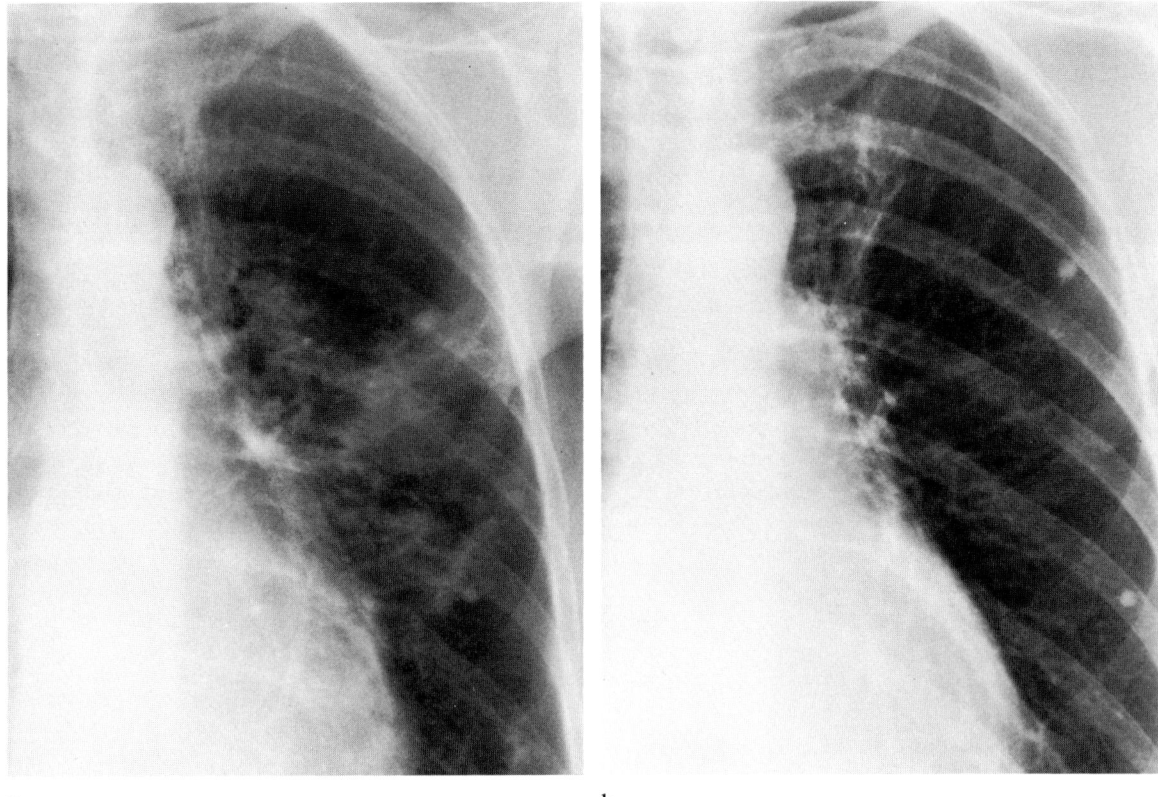

a   b

Fig. 8-8, a and b. Pneumonia outside of irradiated field. a A 68-year-old female who completed postoperative radiotherapy 20 weeks previous to the chest radiograph. Organized radiation pneumonitis is present in the left paramediastinal area. **b** Four months later a pneumonia has developed in the left lung. There is further contraction of radiation changes previously seen. The pneumonia is outside of the portals, and no evidence of radiation pneumonitis was previoulsy seen in this region.

matic or nearly so, whereas others with only minimal changes may be profoundly symptomatic. It is apparent that when a large volume of lung is irradiated in a patient with compromised pulmonary function, significant respiratory distress can occur. It is likely that pulmonary function tests are more sensitive than roentgen appearance in anticipating clinically significant radiation effects (15).

There is incomplete correlation between pulmonary function tests and the roentgenographic appearance of radiotherapy changes. A decrease in vital capacity and forced expiratory volume that is transient has been described in patients receiving mantle-field irradiation for Hodgkin's disease (42). This change begins at two to three months after the onset of therapy, reaches a maximum at four to six months, and returns to normal by almost eight months, in keeping with the timing of radiographic findings. Unfortunately, earlier reports of

changes in pulmonary function following radiotherapy do not give a clear picture of the physiologic disturbances.

Addendum

The computed tomographic appearance of acute and chronic radiation change in the thorax were recently described. Acute radiation pneumonitis demonstrates patchy, confluent regions of increased pulmonary attentuation. Chronic changes include soft tissue density fibrotic changes that blend smoothly with the pleural surfaces and adjacent mediastinal structures. Also seen are bronchiectatic changes and distortion of normal intrathoracic anatomic relationships. Both the acute and chronic changes usually make linear lateral margins with adjacent aerated lung. Development of a discrete mass or focal cavitation after the radiation changes have become stable is suspect for recurrent tumor or infection (43).

Heart

The clinical significance of radiation-induced heart disease has been appreciated only in the past 10 to 15 years. Prior to that time, radiation changes in the heart had been considered an incidental finding. Cardiac changes have been observed following radiotherapy for breast cancer, Hodgkin's disease and other lymphomas, lung cancer, thymic tumors, and other mediastinal tumors (1–17).

Pathologic Changes

Radiation injury to the heart may present as exudative pericarditis, constrictive pericarditis, myocardial fibrosis, and/or coronary artery disease (13,18–21). The basic lesion is injury of the capillary endothelial cell with decrease in the microcirculation (19,20). The posibility of direct cellular injury is also possible, because fibrosis does not always corresond to areas of vascular injury (2). Functionally, the changes prevent normal cardiac action as a result of impaired contractiblity and/or inability of the heart to handle normal volumes of blood (12,16). Mitral insufficiency secondary to myocardial fibrosis has been noted (4).

Factors Influencing the Radiographic Appearance

About 5% of patients receiving 4000 rad mean total dose in four weeks will have recognizable heart disease. Another 5% of patients will have asymptomatic alterations in the cardiac silhouette. The effects are dose-related. When the dose to the heart reaches 6000 rad, approximately 40% of patients will have recognizable changes (13,22). The incidence of radiation-induced heart disease has been related to the nominal standard dose received (23). There is a gradual rise up to 1500 ret, (radiation equivalent therapy) a steeper rise to 1600 ret, and a very steep rise thereafter. As in the lung, individual variation in sensitivity is unpredictable.

The volume of the heart irradiated is also a factor. There is an increased incidence of cardiac damage when larger volumes of the heart are irradiated (23).

The timing of radiation changes is variable. About 60% of injuries will be detected within one year, about 80% by two years, and the remaining 20% thereafter (20). Acute pericarditis may present during, or a few months after, treatment (24).

Chemotherapeutic agents given with radiotherapy may cause additional or synergistic effects. Adriamycin, particularly, has been identified as causing synergistic effects, and there are more profound changes seen in patients who have received radiotherapy and adriamycin. Changes can occur at lower radiation doses or be worse at usual doses in patients who have received both (25,26).

Radiographic Findings

Radiation pericarditis is the most common radiation injury. It presents as any other pericarditis (Fig. 8-9). The cardiac silhouette is enlarged, and diminished pulsations are evident at fluoroscopy (33,35). The effusion may be transitory and asymptomatic (24). An asymmetric configuration of the pericardial effusion may result (Fig. 8-10) if the effusion occurs after pericardial adhesions develop (27). Echocardiography is usually the best way of identifying the effusion.

As in any other type of cardiomyopathy or pericarditis, evidence of congestive heart failure and/or pulmonary edema may be present.

Differential Diagnosis

The most difficult differential diagnosis—and one that is often impossible—is the distinction between a radiation-induced pericardial effusion and an effusion from malignancy. The only positive evidence of a malignant causation is the presence of malignant cells in the effusion (28). The diagnosis of concomitant radiation pericarditis and myocarditis is also extremely difficult and at times is made only at autopsy.

Radiation-induced coronary artery disease may also be present and be the cause of cardiac decompensation. This possibility should be evaluated in the same manner as coronary artery disease of other causes (18,19). The presence of coronary

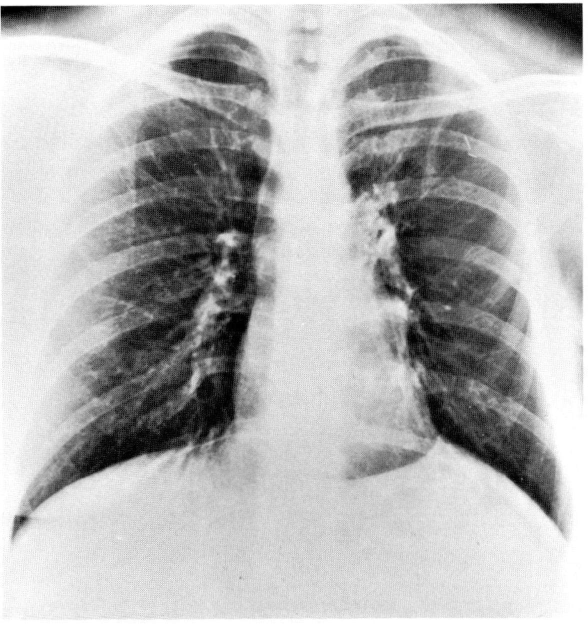

a

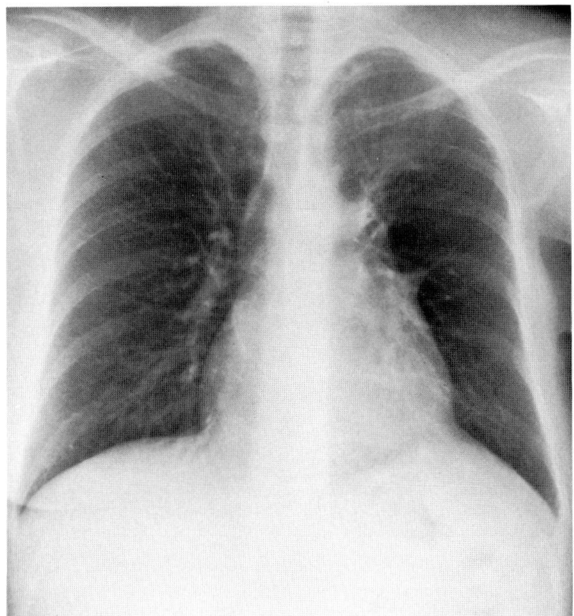

b

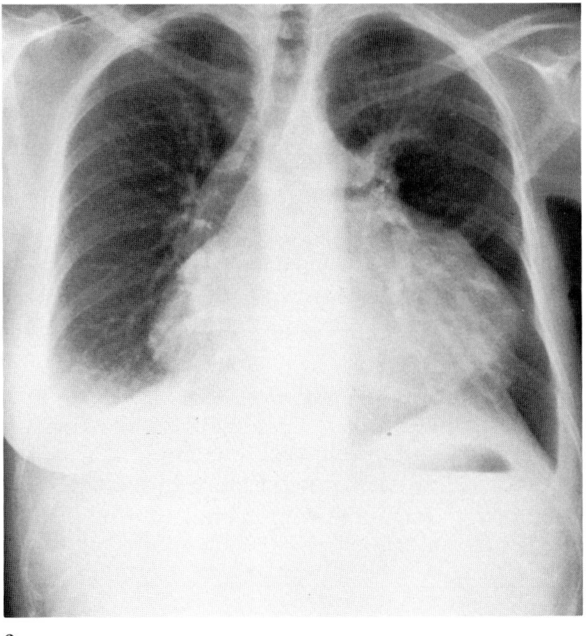

c

Fig. 8-9, a–c. Pericardial effusion following radiotherapy and chemotherapy. A 36-year-old white female who had a radical mastectomy and postoperative radiation therapy (5000 rad internal mammary nodes, 15 MeV electron beam). She also received eight courses of combination chemotherapy (5-fluorocytosine, adriamycin, and cyclophosphamide). a Five months following radiotherapy, well-established postradiotherapy changes are present in the left upper lobe. Some tenting of the diaphragm is also seen. b A pericardial effusion is present 15 months after completion of radiotherapy. The effusion was documented at echocardiography. c The pericardial effusion worsened despite medical therapy. At 22 months following completion of therapy a markedly larger pericardial effusion is seen, as well as bilateral pleural effusions. No evidence of tumor was found at surgery when a pericardial window was made.

artery disease at an earlier-than-usual age in a patient who has had cardiac irradiation points strongly to irradiation as the causative factor.

Clinical Correlation

The presentation of radiation-induced heart disease is variable (13,20,21). The changes may be asymptomatic and identified only by an increase in "cardiac" size. There may be tamponade, with mechanical constriction due to fibrosis, myocardial damage, or coronary artery damage (13,18–21,29). The clinical findings reflect these changes and include increased venous pressure, hepatomegaly, peripheral edema, pulsus paradoxus, friction rub, hypotension, and gallop rhythm (16). It is not always possible to sort out the relative effects of

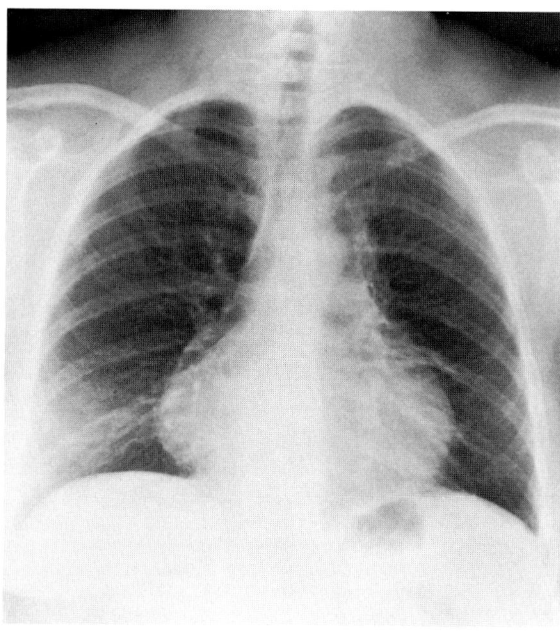

Fig. 8-10. Slightly asymmetric pericardial effusion. A 35-year-old white female who received 4500 rad (15 MeV electron beam) to the internal mammary nodes following left radical mastectomy. Prior to radiotherapy, she received six courses of combination chemotherapy (5-fluorocytosine, adriamycin, and cyclophosphamide). Eight months after completion of radiotherapy this somewhat eccentric pericardial effusion developed. Organizing radiation pneumonitis is present in the left paramediastinal area.

the various possible injuries (24). Treatment may include antiinflammatory drugs and/or pericardiocentesis. Pericardiectomy may be necessary in some patients (12) (Fig. 8-9c). Evaluation and treatment for radiation-induced coronary artery disease are as for any other causation (18,19,30).

Esophagus

Radiation reaction in the esophagus is frequently a limiting factor in the treatment of intrathoracic malignancies. While the esophagus is almost always included in mediastinal radiotherapy fields, few reports concerning the radiographic appearance of radiation esophagitis are available.

Pathologic Changes

Little information is available concerning the acute changes of radiotherapy in the esophageal mucosa

of humans. It is felt, however, the human changes are similar to those found in experimental animals. Acute changes in the opossum esophagus include erythema, patchy white exudates, areas of mucosal ulceration, and sloughing (1). These findings are dose-related and generally similar to those found in the rat and mouse (2,3).

Following epithelial damage and subsequent repair, which may be incomplete, chronic damage may develop, including marked thickening of the submucosal and muscular layers due to edema and fibrosis (4). Vascular damage is thought to be less prominent than the direct radiation effect upon the submucosal layers (5).

Factors Influencing the Radiographic Appearance

The effects of the various factors described relating to the heart and lungs are less clearly worked out for the esophagus. As in other organs, the effects are expected only in the treated portions of the esophagus. The dosage range causing change has generally been 4500–6000 rad in six to eight weeks (4,6). Far fewer changes have been identified in patients who have received under 4000 rad. Reports in the past few years (7–11) indicate that adriamycin and radiotherapy act synergistically in causing esophagitis; radiation changes, both acute and chronic, can be seen at doses under 2000 rad when patients receive both.

The timing of acute changes is not certain, though we have seen acute radiation changes as early as three weeks into therapy. The dose to the esophagus at that time is approximately 3000 rad. More chronic changes, including stenosis and stricture, have been noted from approximately two months onward following completion of therapy (6).

Radiographic Appearance

The majority of patients who present with dysphagia following mediastinal irradiation have no morphologic abnormality of the esophagus. Abnormal esophageal motility (Fig. 8.11) is the most common radiographic manifestation of radiation damage in the esophagus (4). This abnormal motility is most frequently characterized by interruption of the primary peristaltic wave. This interruption generally

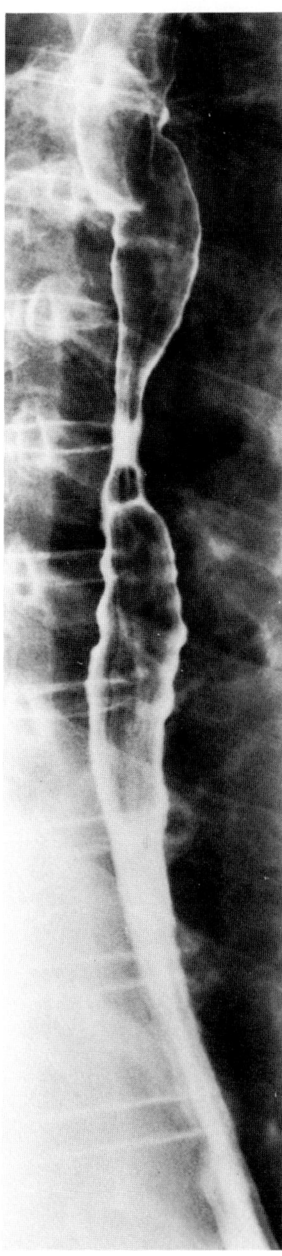

Fig. 8-11. Disordered esophageal motility. Disordered motor function seen on double-contrast esophagogram six months following 5000 rad of radiotherapy to the mediastinum for carcinoma of the lung.

occurs at the upper margin of the irradiated portion of the esophagus. Contractions similar to those seen in tertiary peristalsis are common. Failure of relaxation of the distal esophageal sphincter may occur in both man and experimental animals (1,6). Dilatation of the esophagus usually does not occur in the absence of stricture formation.

In Seaman's series approximately 25% of patients had narrowing of the esophagus (5). All of these patients had carcinoma of the lung. It is likely that more patients would show morphologic abnormality if survival were longer in the patients receiving radiotherapy in doses above 4500 rad.

Radiation-induced strictures always occur within the irradiated portions of the esophagus. The appearance is usually that of a benign stricture with smoothly tapered margins and minimal irregularity in the area of narrowing (Fig. 8-12). Angulation may occur at or near the stricture, suggesting fixation to adjacent mediastinal structures. Obstruction of the esophagus, of varying extent, may result from the strictures. Ulceration occurs occasionally in the irradiated esophagus. Such ulcers heal poorly and may portend development of an esophageal fistula.

Differential Diagnosis

When abnormal motility is the only finding there are no pathognomonic signs indicating that radiation is the cause of the swallowing disturbance. The history of recent irradiation is invaluable in evaluating the changes. Under the appropriate clinical circumstances, distinction from opportunistic infections of the esophagus, primarily candidiasis, can be quite difficult. Esophagoscopy may be necessary.

When stricture is seen following radiotherapy, radiation is the most likely cause. Occasionally persistent or recurrent tumor may cause stricture. The smooth appearance of the narrowed area is quite helpful in this circumstance, though esophagoscopy may at times be necessary to exclude tumor.

Clinical Correlation

Most patients receiving mediastinal irradiation develop some dysphagia or burning in the chest during treatment. The changes generally occur approximately three weeks into treatment (of approximately 3000 rad). In most patients these symptoms are relieved with conservative management and resolve.

Generally, only patients who complain of persistent symptoms are examined by barium swallow, and radiographic abnormalities are usually pres-

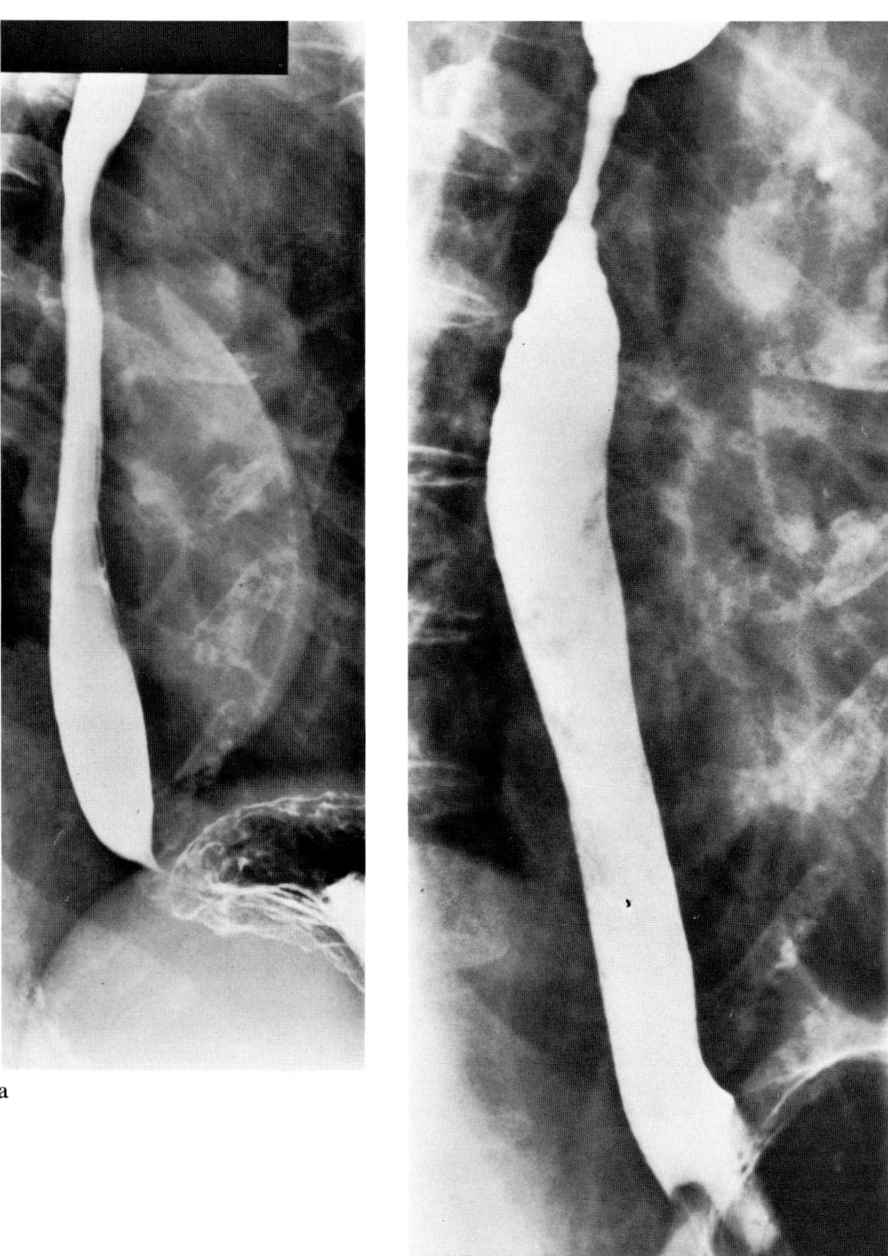

Fig. 8-12, a and b. **Esophageal stricture following radiotherapy and chemotherapy.** A 48-year-old female with immunoblastic sarcoma who had received multiple courses of combined chemotherapy including adriamycin prior to radiotherapy. She received 3000 rad to the mediastinum. **a** Normal esophagogram six months prior to radiotherapy. **b** Esophageal stricture is evident seven months following completion of radiotherapy.

ent. The frequency with which minimal radiographic changes will be found in patients with less pronounced symptoms is not known. It is likely that more morphologic abnormalities will be found using double-contrast techniques to examine the esophagus than are noted in single-contrast studies.

Bony Thorax

Radiation-induced changes in the bony thorax are most often seen in women who have received radiotherapy for breast cancer. This is a reflection of the number of women who have developed breast cancer, the frequency with which radiotherapy is included in their therapy, and the likelihood of the women surviving. Such changes were first described by Paul and Pohle (1) and Slaughter (2) in 1942. The bony changes to be described can be extrapolated to any radiation-induced bone injury.

Pathologic Changes

The exact nature of the pathologic changes in adult human bone is not completely understood. Most of the information concerning early radiation-induced bone injury has been derived from animal experimentation. While experience in humans generally is in keeping with animal experimentation, available human material generally reflects end-stage disease, obtained at resection of involved bones or at autopsy. The underlying changes are most likely related to osteocyte death, with or without partial recovery and later vascular damage (3). Damage to the vascular system is probably the major cause of radionecrosis of bone (4).

Factors Influencing the Radiographic Appearance

Volumes and Fields

Larger fields are more likely to include bony structures and their blood supply and in general are more likely to result in osseous damage. Knowledge of the portals used is of great value, as bony changes are confined to those bones included within them. This is frequently an extremely helpful differential diagnostic feature.

Dose

The energy absorption in bone of 250 kVp x-rays is approximately two times that of ^{60}Co photons (1.25 MeV). For this reason the frequency of radiation damage has markedly decreased with megavoltage irradiation. The threshold dose for osseous injury with megavoltage irradiation is thought to be approximately 4000 rad (5). A minimal safe dose has not been established. In evaluating radiation osteitis, dose information alone is not sufficient. The quality of the radiation and technique by which it was administered must also be known. Montague (6) has shown that higher doses per fraction may produce significant osseous changes that do not correlate with nominal standard-dose values.

Timing

While radiation changes have been observed as early as one year after completion of therapy, they are usually minimal at this time (7). Changes are not usually seen until two years after therapy has ended. Fractures are not usually seen until two to three years after therapy (8).

Radiographic Findings

The reported frequency of radiation changes in the bones of the thorax varies considerably (3,7,9–11). Following orthovoltage irradiation for cancer of the breast, the range reported has been from less than 1% (3) to over 20% (9). Our feeling is that the higher range approaches the true frequency. The rate of fractures following megavoltage irradiation has been lower. A 4% incidence of fractures following five-days-a-week therapy (6) and a 5% incidence of fractures (7) have been reported.

Howland et al. (7) have suggested that the term *postirradiation atrophy* be adopted rather than *radiation osteitis* or *radionecrosis* for the usual changes and that *osteitis* and *necrosis* be reserved for use only when either is indeed the case. They report identifying atrophy with varying amounts of demineralization in all patients three years after treatment with orthovoltage therapy. Langlands et al. (9) describe osteoporosis in 33.6% of irradiated patients and in 19.2% of control patients (women who had a radical mastectomy but no postoperative radiation). It is very likely that a high percentage of patients will show some demineralization in the irradiated fields if radiographs designed particularly for bony detail are obtained rather than trying to evaluate these changes on regular chest radiographs. In addition to demineralization, there may be coarsening of the trabecular pattern, small "cystic" areas, and thickening of the cortex. These changes may be the final appearance unless infection or fracture supervenes.

Fractures may develop in the ribs, clavicles, or humeri. The fractures are often spontaneous or follow minimal trauma (Figs. 8-13 and 8-14). Healing of fractures may be quite slow, and they occasionally remain ununited. Delayed fracture healing following irradiation has been demonstrated experimentally and is felt to be on a vascular basis (12). Significant bony resorption can also occur, with disappearance of bones, usually anterior ribs (Fig. 8-14).

Dystrophic calcifications may appear adjacent to the fractures and be emphasized by resorption of the involved bones. The absence of a soft component aids in distinguishing these areas of calcification from radiation-induced sarcomas.

Changes may progress about the shoulder joint with eventual flattening of the humeral head and concomitant changes in the glenoid fossa that resemble severe degenerative changes or even neuropathic disease with marked fragmentation (Fig. 8-14c and d).

Differential Diagnosis

The primary differential diagnostic consideration is to distinguish radiation osteitis from invasive or metastatic bone destruction. In radiation osteitis the bony changes are within the radiotherapy portals. Identifying changes only in those bones irradiated, such as the humerus, scapula, clavicle, and ribs, points strongly to a radiation cause. The fact that radiation change takes years rather than months after therapy to develop is also extremely helpful. Also helpful is the absence of symptoms or only minimal symptoms with radiation osteitis. Metastatic disease is more frequently symptomatic.

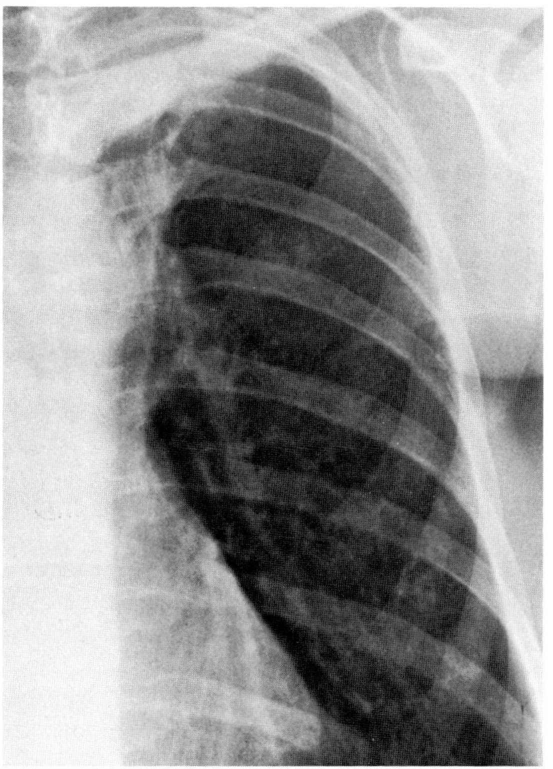

Fig. 8-13. Rib fractures following radiotherapy. A 50-year-old female treated six years previously with radiotherapy following radical mastectomy. She received 5000 rad to the chest wall, internal mammary nodes, supraclavicular area, and axilla (^{60}Co). Ununited fractures are present in the anterior second, third, fourth, fifth, and sixth ribs. On a radiograph a year prior, these fractures could be identified, and no obvious healing has occurred. Radiation fibrosis is seen in the left apex.

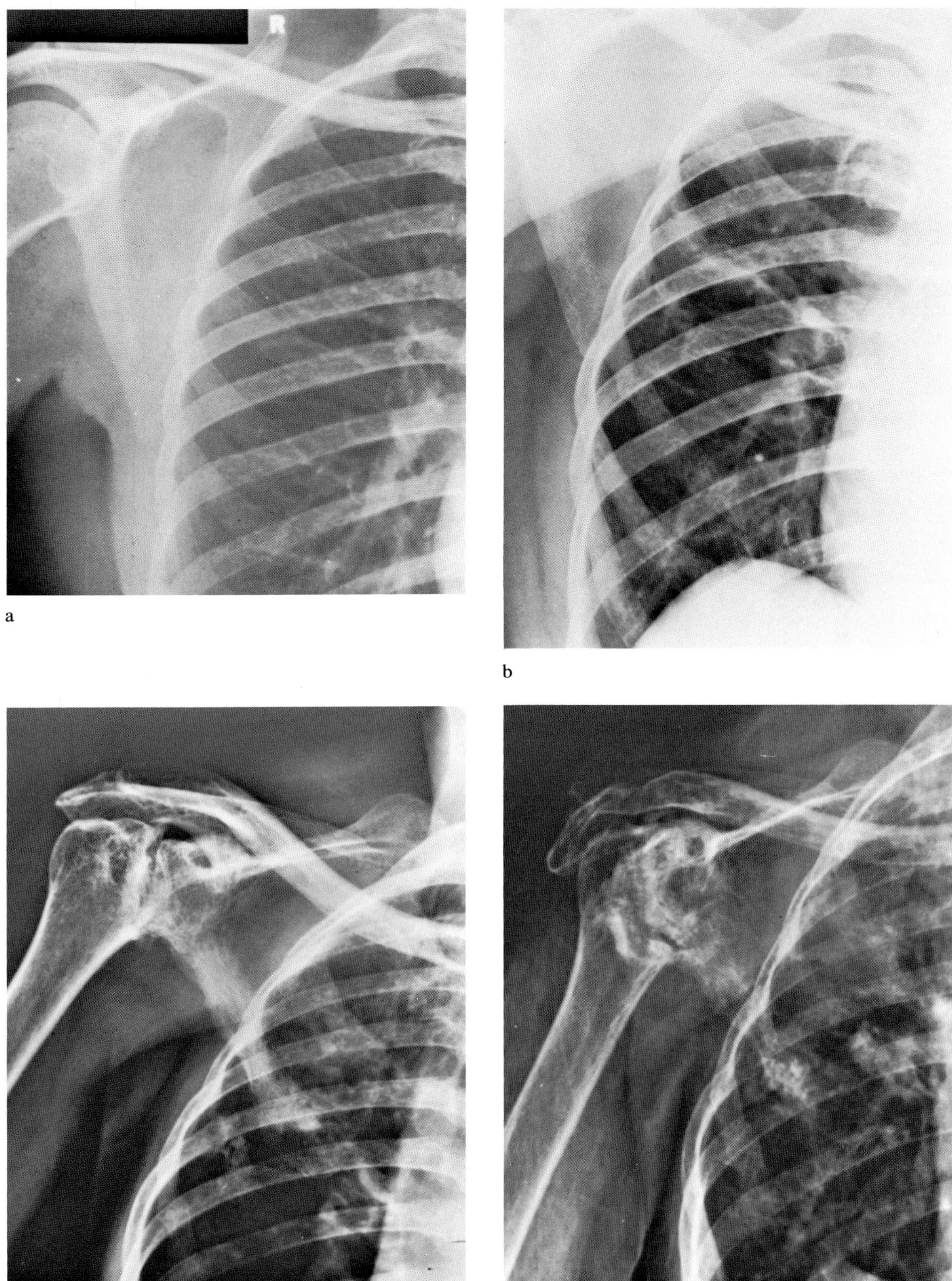

Fig. 8-14, a–d. Extensive bony changes following radiotherapy. At age 35, this female received preoperative radiotherapy for carcinoma of the breast. She received 4500 rad to the internal mammary nodes and 4000 rad to the axilla and supraclavicular area (250 kVp). **a** Pretreatment appearance of the right shoulder and upper rib area. **b** Four years following radiotherapy, ununited fractures of the right third, fourth, and fifth anterior ribs are present. **c** Seven years postradiotherapy, the fractures of the ribs have not healed. Flattening of the humeral head has occurred. Also seen is coarsening of the trabecular pattern in the distal clavicle and glenoid. **d** Twenty years after radiotherapy the shoulder joint is destroyed. The changes in the ribs have progressed markedly, with resorption of the anterior aspects of the third, fourth, and fifth ribs. Postradiotherapy changes are present in all the treated bones. Dystrophic calcifications are seen in the region of the fourth anterior rib. Five years after this study the patient was alive and well with slight progression of these bony changes.

Radiation-induced sarcomas occasionally occur. These are often associated with gross bony destruction, the presence of a soft-tissue mass, and somewhat less frequently tumor matrix production. Radiation-induced sarcomas develop on an average eight to ten years following radiotherapy, though occasionally they are found sooner and not infrequently much later (13). Rapid change in an area of radiation osteitis should make one suspicious of the development of a sarcoma (14). Prior radiographs are of great help. Radiation-induced sarcomas are frequently associated with the development of pain. When trauma or infection is superimposed on radiation osteitis, differentiation from sarcoma may prove quite difficult if not impossible.

References

Lung

1. Groover TA, Christie AC, Merritt EA: Observations on the use of the copper filter in the roentgen treatment of deep-seated malignancies. South Med J 15:440–444, 1922.
2. Hines LE: Fibrosis of the lung following roentgen-ray treatments for tumor. JAMA 79:720–722, 1922.
3. Tyler AF, Blackman JR: Effect of heavy radiation on pleurae and lungs. J Radiol 3:469–475, 1922.
4. Evans WA, Leucutia T: Intrathoracic changes induced by heavy radiation. AJR 13:203–220, 1925.
5. Desjardins AU: The reaction of the pleura and lungs to roentgen rays. AJR 16:444–453, 1926.
6. Bennett DE, Million RR, Ackerman LV: Bilateral radiation pneumonitis, a complication of radiotherapy of bronchogenic carcinoma (report and analysis of seven cases with autopsy). Cancer 23:1001–1018, 1969.
7. Warren S, Spencer J: Radiation reaction in the lung. AJR 43:682–701, 1940.
8. Jennings FL, Arden A: Development of radiation pneumonitis. Arch Pathol 74:351–360, 1962.
9. Jacobsen VC: The deleterious effects of deep roentgen irradiation on lung structure and function. AJR 44:235–249, 1940.
10. Jennings FL, Arden A: Development of experimental radiation pneumonitis. Arch Pathol 71:437–446, 1961.
11. Cohen Y, Gellei B, Robinson E: Bilateral radiation pneumonitis after unilateral lung and mediastinal irradiation. Radiol Clin (Basel) 43:465–471, 1974.
12. Ross WM: The radiotherapeutic and radiological aspects of fibrosis of the lungs. Thorax 11:241–248, 1956.
13. Rubin P, Casarett GW: Clinical Radiation Pathology. Philadelphia: WB Saunders Co, 1968.
14. Smith JC: Radiation pneumonitis. Case report of bilateral reaction after unilateral irradiation. Am Rev Respir Dis 89:264–269, 1964.
15. Gross NJ: Pulmonary effects of radiation therapy. Ann Intern Med 86:81–91, 1977.
16. Bate D, Guttman RJ: Changes in lung and pleura following two-million-volt therapy for carcinoma of the breast. Radiology 69:372–283, 1957.
17. Holt JA: The acute radiation pneumonitis syndrome. J Coll Radiol Aust 8:40–47, 1964.
18. Libshitz HI, Brosof AB, Southard ME: The radiographic appearance of the chest following extended field radiation therapy for Hodgkin's disease. Cancer 32:206–215, 1973.
19. Libshitz HI, Southard ME: Complications of radiation therapy: the thorax. Semin Roentgenol 9:41–49, 1974.
20. Libshitz HI, North LB: Lung. *In* Libshitz HI (ed): Diagnostic Roentgenology of Radiotherapy Change. Baltimore: Williams & Wilkins, 1979, Chap 3, pp 33–46.
21. Deeley TJ: The effects of radiation on the lungs in the treatment of carcinoma of the bronchus. Clin Radiol 11:33–39, 1960.
22. Kaplan HS, Stewart JR: Complications of intensive megavoltage radiotherapy for Hodgkin's disease. Natl Cancer Inst Monogr 36:439–444, 1973.
23. Littman P, Davis LW, Nash J, Tefft M, Borns P, Lepanto P: The hazard of acute radiation pneumonitis in children receiving mediastinal radiation. Cancer 33:1520–1525, 1974.
24. Cassaday JR, Richter MP, Piro AJ, Jaffe N: Radiation-adriamycin interactions; preliminary clinical observations. Cancer 36:946–949, 1975.
25. Donaldson SS, Glick JM, Wilbur JR: Adriamycin activating a recall phenomenon after radiation therapy. Ann Intern Med 81:407–408, 1974.
26. McInerney DP, Bullimore J: Reactivation of radiation pneumonitis by adriamycin. Br J Radiol 50:224–227, 1977.
27. Wara WM, Phillips TL, Margolis LW, Smith V: Radiation pneumonitis: a new approach to the determination of time-dose factors. Cancer 32:547–552, 1973.
28. Kaplan HS: Latent radiation injury of lungs or heart activated by steroid withdrawal. Ann Intern Med 80:593–599, 1974.
29. Parris TM, Knight JG, Hess CE, Constable WC: Severe radiation pneumonitis precipitated by withdrawal of corticosteroids: a diagnostic and therapeutic dilemma. AJR 132:284–286, 1979.
30. Braun SR, doPico GA, Olson CE, Caldwell W: Low-dose radiation pneumonitis. Cancer 35:1322–1324, 1975.
31. Lamoureux KB: Increased clinically symptomatic pulmonary radiation reactions with adjuvant chemotherapy. Cancer Chemother Rep, Part 1, 58:705–708, 1974.
32. Oppedal T, Kolbenstvedt A: Pulmonary contraction following ^{60}Co irradiation of mammary carcinoma. Acta Radiol (Ther) (Stockh) 15:329–336, 1976.
33. Lichtenstein H: X-ray diagnosis of radiation injuries of the lung. Dis Chest 38:294–297, 1960.
34. Berdon WE, Baker DH, Boyer J: Unusual benign and malignant sequelae to childhood radiation therapy. AJR 93:545–556, 1965.
35. Farmer W, Ravin C, Schachter EN: Hyperlucent

lung after radiation therapy. Am Rev Respir Dis 112:255–258, 1975.

36. Fleming JAC, Filbee JF, Wiernik G: Sequelae to radical irradiation in carcinoma of the breast. Br J Radiol 34:713–719, 1961.

37. Libshitz HI, Banner MP: Spontaneous pneumothorax as a complication of radiation therapy to the thorax. Radiology 112:199–201, 1974.

38. Twiford TW, Zornoza J, Libshitz HI: Recurrent spontaneous pneumothorax after radiation therapy to the thorax. Chest 73:387–388, 1978.

39. Bachman AL, Macken K: Pleural effusions following supervoltage radiation for breast carcinoma. Radiology 72:699–709, 1959.

40. Brereton HD, Johnson RE: Calcification in mediastinal lymph nodes after radiation therapy of Hodgkin's disease. Radiology 112:705–707, 1974.

41. Wyman SM, Weber AL: Calcifications in intrathoracic nodes in Hodgkin's disease in the chest. Radiology 93:1021–1024, 1969.

42. Evans RF, Sagerman RH, Ringrose TL, Auchincloss JH, Bowman J: Pulmonary function following mantle-field irradiation for Hodgkin's disease. Radiology 111:729–731, 1974.

43. Pagani JJ, Libshitz HI: CT manifestations of radiation change in the chest: preliminary observations. J Comput Assist Tomogr 6(2):243–248, 1982.

Heart

1. Blumenfield H, Thomas SF: Chronic massive pericardial effusion following roentgen therapy for carcinoma of the breast. Radiology 44:335–340, 1945.

2. Botti RE, Driscol TE, Pearson OH, Smith JC: Radiation myocardial fibrosis simulating constrictive pericarditis. Cancer 22:1254–1261, 1968.

3. Catterall M: The effect of radiation upon the heart. Br J Radiol 33:159–164, 1960.

4. Cohn KE, Stewart JR, Fajardo LF, Hancock EW: Heart disease following radiation. Medicine 46:281–298, 1967.

5. Connolly DC, Burchell HB: Pericarditis: a ten year survey. Am J Cardiol 7:7–13, 1961.

6. Vaeth JM, Feigenbaum LZ, Merrill MD: Effects of intensive irradiation on the human heart. Radiology 76:755–762, 1961.

7. Vinke B: The incidental effect on the heart of x-irradiation. Acta Med Scand 172:711–713, 1962.

8. Duane RJ, Rottino A: Constrictive pericarditis caused by Hodgkin's disease. NY State J Med 67:288–290, 1967.

9. Kagan AR, Morton DL, Hafermann MD, Johnson RE: Evaluation and management of radiation-induced pericardial effusion. Radiology 92:632–634, 1969.

10. Masland DS, Rotz CT, Harris JJ: Postradiation pericarditis with chronic pericardial effusion. Ann Intern Med 69:97–102, 1968.

11. McReynolds RA, Gold GL, Roberts WC: Coronary heart disease after mediastinal irradiation for Hodgkin's disease. Am J Med 60:39–45, 1976.

12. Morton DL, Kagan AR, Roberts WC, O'Brien KP, Holmes EC, Adkins PC: Pericardiectomy for radiation-induced pericarditis with effusion. Ann Thorac Surg 8:195–208, 1969.

13. Stewart JR, Cohn KE, Fajardo LF, Hancock EW, Kaplan HS: Radiation-induced heart disease. Radiology 89:302–310, 1967.

14. Westerhof PW, van der Putte SCJ: Radiation pericarditis and myocardial fibrosis. Eur J Cardiol 4:213–218, 1976.

15. Catterall M, Evans W: Myocardial injury from therapeutic irradiation. Br Heart J 22:168–174, 1960.

16. Gimlette TMD: Constrictive pericarditis. Br Heart J 21:9–16, 1959.

17. Macleod CA, Schwartz H, Linton DB: Constrictive pericarditis following irradiation therapy. JAMA 207:2281–2282, 1969.

18. Ali MK, Kahlil KG, Fuller LM, Leachman RD, Sullivan MP, Loh KK, Gamble JF, Shullenberger CC: Radiation related myocardial injury. Cancer 38:1941–1946, 1976.

19. Fajardo LF: Radiation-induced coronary artery disease. Chest 71:563–564, 1977.

20. Stewart JR, Fajardo LF: Radiation-induced heart disease. Front Radiation Ther Onc 6:274–288, 1972.

21. Stewart JR, Fajardo LF: Radiation-induced heart disease. Radiol Clin North Am 9:511–531, 1971.

22. Pierce RH, Hafermann MD, Kagan AR: Changes in the transverse cardiac diameter following mediastinal irradiation for Hodgkin's disease. Radiology 93:619–624, 1969.

23. Stewart JR, Fajardo LF: Dose response in human and experimental radiation-induced heart disease. Radiology 99:403–408, 1971.

24. Hill CA: Heart. In Libshitz HI (ed): Diagnostic Roentgenology of Radiotherapy Change. Baltimore: Williams & Wilkins, 1979, Chap 4, pp 47–54.

25. Fajardo LF, Eltringham JR, Stewart JR: Combined cardiotoxicity of adriamycin and X-radiation. Lab Invest 34:86–96, 1976.

26. Merrill J, Greco FA, Zimbler H, Brereton HD, Lamberg JD, Pomeroy TC: Adriamycin and radiation: Synergistic cardiotoxicity. Ann Intern Med 82:122–123, 1975.

27. Green B, Zornoza J, Ricks JP: Eccentric pericardial effusion after radiation therapy of left breast carcinoma. AJR 128:27–30, 1977.

28. Lawson RAM, Ross WM, Gold RG, Blesovsky A, Barnsley WC: Postradiation pericarditis. J Thorac Cardiovasc Surg 63:841–847, 1972.

29. Hurst DW: Radiation fibrosis of pericardium, with cardiac tamponade. Can Med Assoc J 81:377–380, 1959.

30. Iqbal SM, Hanson EL, Gensini GG: Bypass graft for coronary arterial stenosis following radiation therapy. Chest 71:664–666, 1977.

Esophagus

1. Northway MG, Libshitz HI, West JJ, Withers HR, Mukhopadhyay AK, Osborne BM, Szwarc IA, Dodd GD: The opossum as an animal model for studying radiation esophagitis. Radiology 131:731–735, 1979.

2. Phillips TL, Ross G: Time-dose relationships in the

mouse esophagus. Radiology 113:435–440, 1974.
3. Jennings FL, Arden A: Acute radiation effects in the esophagus. Arch Pathol Lab Med 69:407–412, 1960.
4. Goldstein HM, Rogers LF, Fletcher GH, Dodd GD: Radiological manifestations of radiation-induced injury to the normal upper gastrointestinal tract. Radiology 117:135–140, 1975.
5. Seaman WB, Ackerman LV: The effect of radiation on the esophagus: a clinical and histologic study of the effects produced by the betatron. Radiology 68:534–541, 1957.
6. Goldstein HM: Esophagus, stomach, and duodenum. *In* Libshitz HI (ed): Diagnostic Roentgenology of Radiotherapy Change. Baltimore: Williams & Wilkins, 1979, Chap 6, pp 69–83.
7. Horwich A, Lokich JJ, Bloomer WD: Doxorubicin, radiotherapy, and oesophageal stricture. Lancet 2:561–562, 1975.
8. Chabora BM, Hopfan S, Wittes R: Esophageal complications in the treatment of oat cell carcinoma with combined irradiation and chemotherapy. Radiology 123:185–187, 1977.
9. Greco FA, Brereton HD, Kent H, Zimbler H, Merrill J, Johnson RE: Adriamycin and enhanced reaction in normal esophagus and skin. Ann Intern Med 85:294–298, 1976.
10. Newburger PE, Cassady JR, Jaffe N: Esophagitis due to adriamycin and radiation therapy for childhood malignancy. Cancer 42:417–423, 1978.
11. Boal DKB, Newburger PE, Teele RL: Esophagitis induced by combined radiation and adriamycin. AJR 132:567–570, 1979.

Bony Thorax

1. Paul LW, Pohle EA: Radiation osteitis of the ribs. Radiology 38:543–549, 1942.
2. Slaughter DP: Radiation osteitis and fractures following irradiation: with report of five cases of fractured clavicle. AJR 43:877–895, 1942.
3. Parker RG: Tolerance of mature bone and cartilage in clinical radiation therapy. Front Radiation Ther Onc 6:312–331, 1972.
4. Kim JH, Chu FCH, Pope RA, Woodard HQ, Bragg DB, Shidnia H: Time dose factors in radiation induced osteitis. AJR 120:684–690, 1974.
5. Meyer JE: Thoracic effects of therapeutic irradiation for breast carcinoma. AJR 130:877–885, 1978.
6. Montague ED: Experience with altered fractionation in radiation therapy of breast cancer. Radiology 90:962–966, 1968.
7. Howland WJ, Loeffler RK, Starchman DE, Johnson RG: Postirradiation atrophic changes of bone and related complications. Radiology 117:677–685, 1975.
8. de Santos LA, Libshitz HI: Adult bone. *In* Libshitz HI (ed): Diagnostic Roentgenology of Radiotherapy Change. Baltimore: Williams & Wilkins, 1979, Chap 11, pp 137–150.
9. Langlands AO, Souter WA, Samuel E, Redpath AT: Radiation osteitis following irradiation for breast cancer. Clin Radiol 28:93–96, 1977.
10. Serna GM: Osteoradionecrosis. Mo Med 64:997–1000, 1967.
11. Ackerman LV: An evaluation of the treatment of cancer of the breast at the University of Edinburgh (Scotland), under the direction of Dr Robert McWhirter. Cancer 8:883–887, 1955.
12. Green N, French S, Rodriquez G, Hays M, Fingerhut A: Radiation-induced delayed union of fractures. Radiology 93:635–641, 1969.
13. de Santos LA, Libshitz HI: Growing bone and radiation-induced neoplasia. *In* Libshitz HI (ed): Diagnostic Roentgenology of Radiotherapy Change. Baltimore: Williams & Wilkins, 1979, Chap 12, pp 151–166.
14. Bragg DG, Shidnia H, Chu FCH, Higinbotham NL: The clinical and radiographic aspects of radiation osteitis. Radiology 97:103–111, 1970.

9 Iatrogenic Disorders of the Esophagus

John Braver

Iatrogenic complications have increased as a result of the more aggressive, modern therapeutic and diagnostic interventions. This is as true for the esophagus as it is for other organs; in fact, in some respects the esophagus is more vulnerable than many other organs, as we shall see shortly. It is difficult to quantitate these complications precisely, but some idea of the scope of the problem comes from studying endoscopic and surgical data: endoscopic perforations occur in less than 1% of cases (1,2); postsurgical complication rates of 20%, 30%, or even 40% are not uncommon (2,3). It is thus likely that most radiologists will encounter some iatrogenic complication related to the esophagus in their daily practice. We will consider the potential complications under the following categories: those related to (a) endoscopy/biopsy, (b) surgery, (c) dilatation, (d) indwelling tubes, (e) drugs, (f) miscellaneous. We will not consider the important subject of radiation-induced complications here; they have been fully dealt with elsewhere in this volume.

Before considering the various complications, a brief review of esophageal anatomy will help demonstrate why this is a vulnerable organ and how and why damage to the esophagus can be manifest elsewhere in the thorax.

Anatomy/Relationships

The esophagus is a muscular tube measuring some 20–25 cm in length. It is the narrowest portion of the gastrointestinal tract, and certain anatomic relationships further limit its distensibility. The esophagus proper begins in the neck at approximately the level of the sixth cervical vertebra; this portion is considered the cervical esophagus. The cervical esophagus is squeezed between the trachea anteriorly and the cervical spine posteriorly. The first potential area of narrowing occurs at the level of the upper esophageal sphincter—the cricopharyngeus muscle. This muscle normally functions sequentially during swallowing to prevent reflux back into the pharynx. It is part of the inferior constrictor muscle, the bulk of which lies superior to the cricopharyngeus. Not only is this portion of the esophagus relatively narrow, but there are areas of potential muscular weakness both superior and inferior to the cricopharyngeus where trauma is more likely to cause perforation (Fig. 9-1).

As the esophagus passes through the thorax, it remains between the trachea anteriorly and the spine posteriorly. The esophagus begins in the midline, swings to the left of the trachea in the neck, crosses to the right of the descending aorta below the level of the arch, and eventually winds up back on the left side by crossing anterior to the aorta just above the diaphragm. As the esophagus descends through the thorax it lies posterior, and closely adherent, to the left atrium. One anatomic point of importance is that the esophagus is in contact with pleura for a considerable distance on the right side. On the left side, the aorta is interposed between the esophagus and the pleura except for a short distance just above the diaphragm as the esophagus swings to the left of the aorta. Obviously a process involving the middle esophagus can more easily spread to involve the right pleural space and lung because the aorta

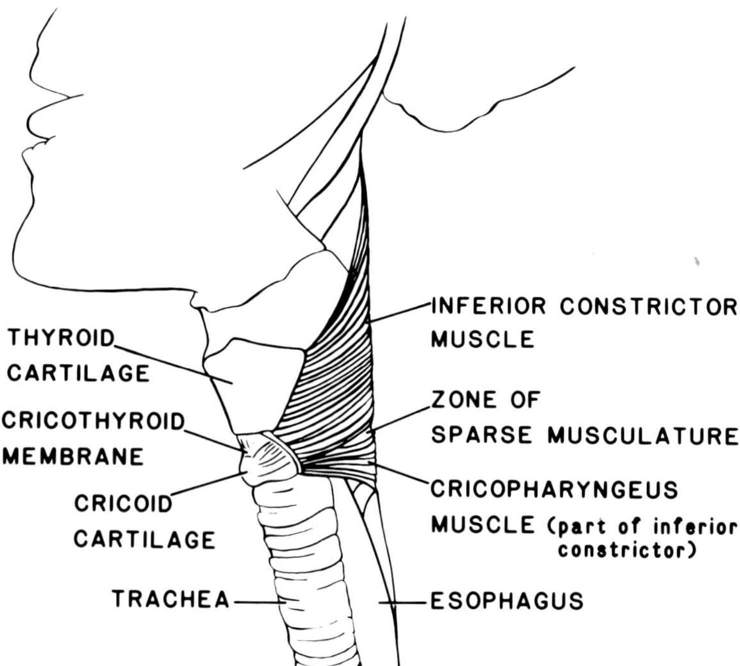

Fig. 9-1. Cricopharyngeal area of cervical esophagus. This is a potential weak spot where trauma can occur relatively easily.

forms a barrier to the pleura on the left. If a process occurs just above the diaphragm, however, it is more likely to manifest in the left hemithorax (Fig. 9-2). The clinical implications will become apparent shortly.

We have already discussed the relative area of narrowing and weakness in the proximal esophagus. Other areas of potential narrowing occur: at the level of the carina where the left mainstem bronchus crosses ventrally, and at the level of the

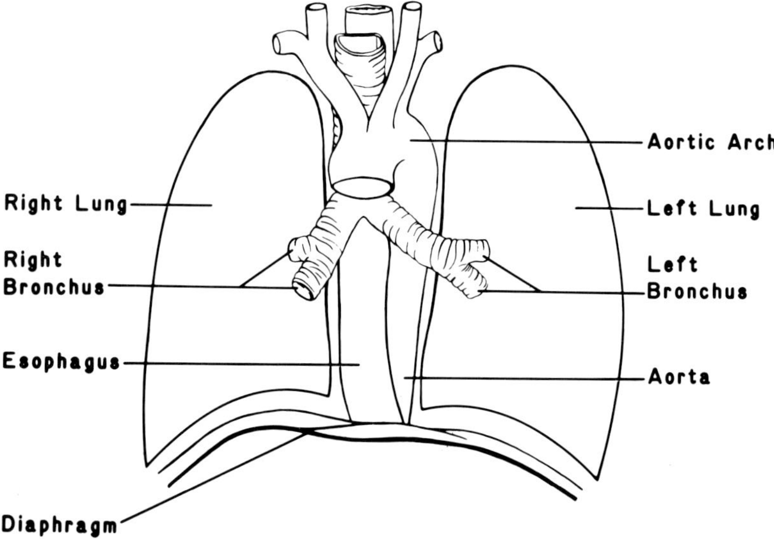

Fig. 9-2. Anatomic relationships of the thoracic esophagus. Note that the relationship of the esophagus to the pleura is different on the right and left sides. The aorta is an interposed barrier on the left side between the esophagus and the pleura.

hiatus. There is some controversy about whether large cardiac chambers can cause *symptomatic* esophageal narrowing, but no one can argue that the esophagus can be narrowed by a huge left atrium.

The intimate relationship of the vagus nerve trunks to the distal esophagus has particular relevance to surgery. The left and right vagus nerves run laterally along the esophagus until they encircle it at the level of the hiatus. Since they are so intimately related to the esophageal adventitia, the wall of the esophagus can be damaged when the nerves are dissected off the esophagus during vagotomy.

Clinical Approach

Trauma to the esophagus frequently is silent in the early stages. It doesn't remain that way for long, and by the time it becomes obvious, the patient is frequently moribund. The clinical and radiologic challenge is to diagnose injury early enough to institute corrective therapy. The key to doing this is to have *a high index of suspicion* for esophageal injury. As we shall see, certain patients are at high risk for iatrogenic esophageal injury, especially those who have undergone instrumentation of various types, who have had surgery, radiation, etc., and their films deserve extra-careful scrutiny. It has already been stressed that certain areas of the esophagus have more potential for being injured than others, and the radiologist should pay special attention to these vulnerable areas when evaluating films of high-risk patients.

Let's assume you want to evaluate a patient in a high-risk category for esophageal injury. How do you proceed most expeditiously? Something approaching 10% of patients will have a normal chest x-ray, but since the majority *will* demonstrate some abnormality, plain radiographs are a rational starting point. Although exact causation may still be obscure, plain films can frequently confirm, localize, and often lateralize an acute esophageal process, which can be extremely helpful in directing the contrast study that will follow.

Plain films of the soft tissues of the neck, PA and lateral chest, and erect chest/upright abdomen should be obtained as soon as a diagnosis is entertained. Most authors report positive findings in the great majority of cases (up to 90%). Plain films are useful to (a) confirm perforation, (b) localize and lateralize in many cases the site of perforation, and (c) document extension of the perforation and complications in periesophageal tissues. Whether or not plain-film findings are positive depends on location and extent of perforation and the time that has elapsed since injury. This last point is most important. If films are taken *immediately* following a perforation, no abnormality may be detected, resulting in a false-negative interpretation. Evidence of mediastinitis takes several hours to develop, and even subcutaneous emphysema may not be visible for at least an hour following injury (1).

Most reported series (1,2,4–7) agree that iatrogenic perforations (usually endoscopic) account for most esophageal perforations. These are most likely to occur in the normal esophagus in the cervical area and in the distal esophagus; in both regions there are areas of anatomic narrowing and weakness of the esophageal wall. The other area where the esophagus is narrowed, in the region of the left mainstem bronchus, is the third most common site of iatrogenic perforation. In the diseased esophagus, of course, perforation will frequently be at, or close to, the site of pathology (e.g., a tumor). Cervical perforations are likely to cause localized subcutaneous emphysema, which, if present, can be readily detected on soft-tissue films of the neck. It should be noted that dissection of air and even fluid into the mediastinum can occur with even these high perforations and should be searched for on chest films.

Perforations of the thoracic esophagus can present a number of radiologic findings in addition to cervical emphysema (which in this case is due to dissection of mediastinal air superiorly). Mediastinal emphysema is a dramatic finding but will not be present in all cases (1) (Fig. 9-3). Mediastinal widening and bowing forward of the trachea, due to both mediastinitis and accumulation of fluid, take several hours to develop. Perforation of the thoracic esophagus will be manifest in the chest cavity (as opposed to mediastinum) only when the mediastinal pleura has been violated. Since the thin mediastinal pleura ruptures in most cases, many plain films will ultimately show pneumothorax, pleural effusion, or hydropneumothorax (5).

Which side these changes occur on gives some clue as to the site of perforation. This becomes

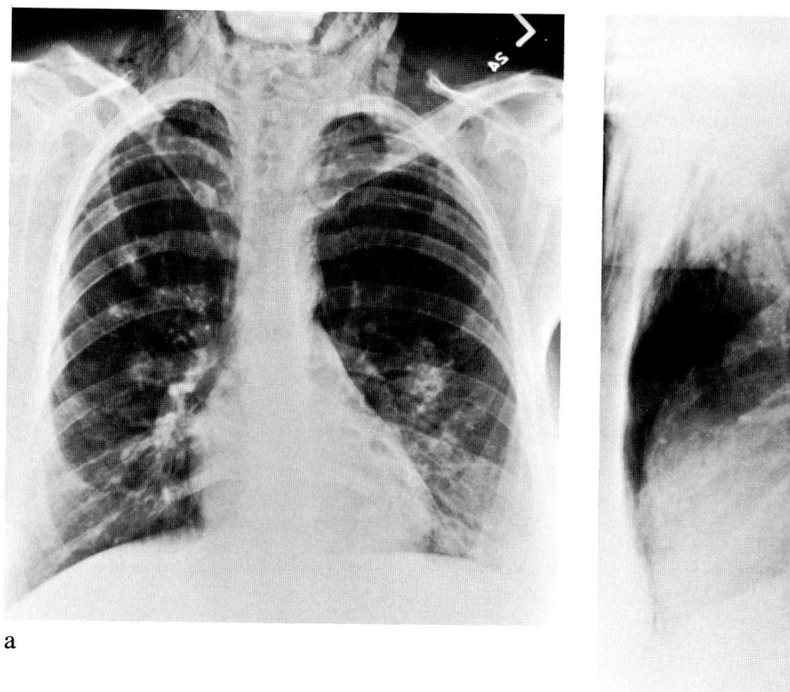
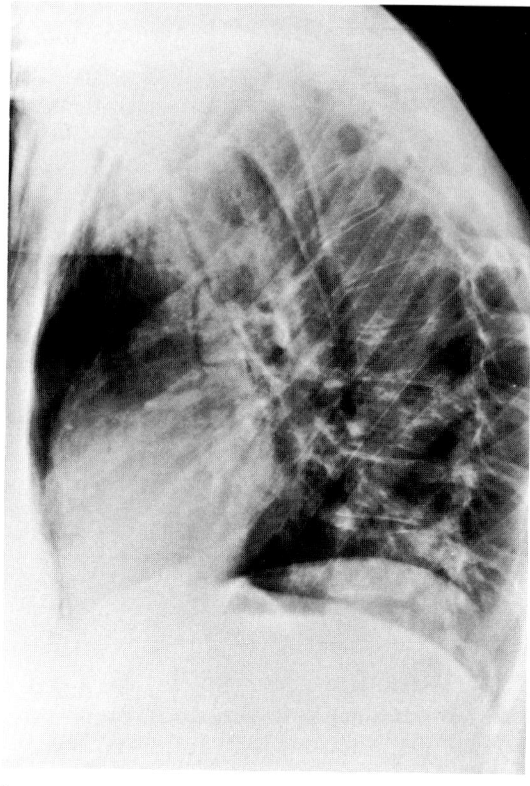

Fig. 9-3, a and b. **Excellent example of mediastinal and subcutaneous emphysema.** Unfortunately, not all cases of thoracic esophageal perforation will be this obvious. **a** Anteroposterior view. **b** Lateral view.

clear when we review the anatomy. Since the right pleura is in direct contact with most of the thoracic esophagus, perforation of the right lateral esophagus will manifest in the right chest. A very distal perforation will manifest in the left chest, because only at this level is the esophagus in contact with the *left* mediastinal pleura (Fig. 9-4). Perforations of the anterior or posterior wall of the esophagus, or on the left wall in the midesophagus where the pleura is protected by the interposed aorta, will be confined to the mediastinum. Pleural effusion without rupture (transudates) can eventually occur on either side secondary to mediastinal infection, but this occurs slowly and is a late sign.

After plain films have been obtained, it is necessary to perform a contrast study immediately, *whether or not* the plain films suggest perforation. There are several important reasons for this. First, even if the plain films are positive, it is helpful to confirm a leak and establish its exact site and extent so proper surgical therapy can be instituted promptly. The full extent of a perforation and subsequent dissection of air and fluid contents is often greater than initially realized. The contrast study must be performed *promptly*. Appleton et al. report several cases in which the leak had sealed by the time the study was performed and proper diagnosis was impeded (5). Most importantly, since some 10% or more of perforations will not be manifest on plain films, a contrast study is mandatory even with negative films because the consequences of untreated perforation are so catastrophic.

The ideal contrast agent should be well tolerated, easily administered, offer good definition of pathology, and induce no complications. Whether to use water-soluble contrast or dilute barium has engendered some debate. At first glance it would appear that water-soluble contrast agents are ideal. Unfortunately, few things in medicine are as simple as they first appear. Water-soluble agents are advocated because they are thought not to potentiate the inflammatory process caused by contents leaking from the esophagus, but there are several

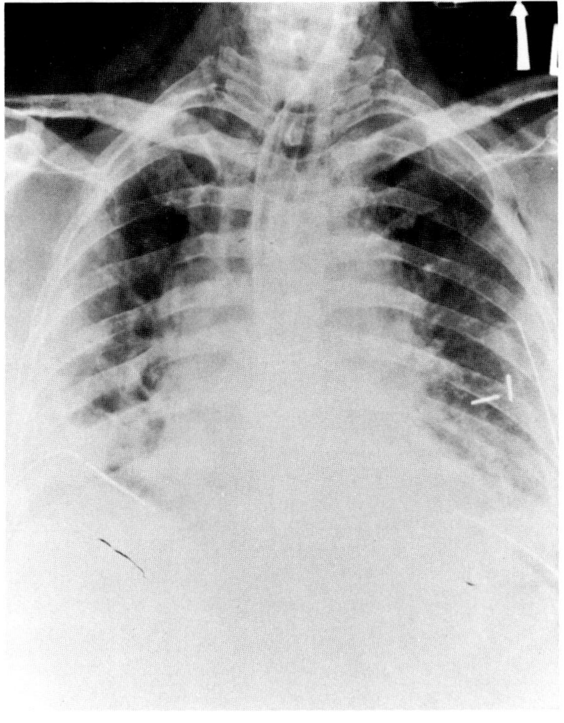
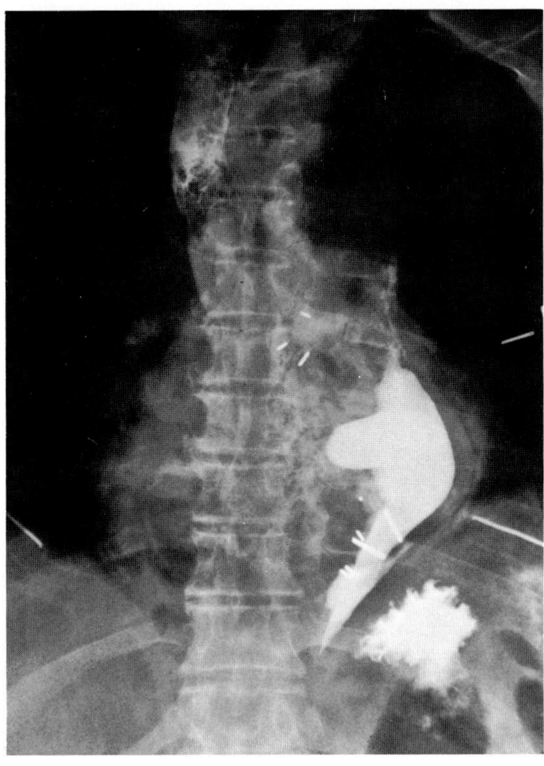

Fig. 9-4, a and b. Older male who developed vomiting following a meal. a Chest x-ray shows widened mediastinum and cervical subcutaneous emphysema. **b** Barium examination demonstrates distal perforation which is commonly into the left chest in Boerhaave's syndrome for the anatomic reasons described in the text.

potential drawbacks to these substances which may effect their diagnostic usefulness. They are not particularly palatable and frequently difficult for ill patients to swallow. This, coupled with the fact that they are potentially lethal if aspirated, makes extreme caution necessary in using them to study these gravely ill patients. One other drawback that should be noted is the frequent lack of definition when using these substances, which can hamper precise localization of the leak.

Barium preparations would seem to offer many advantages. Barium is relatively palatable, safe if aspirated, and unquestionably gives good radiographic definition. The controversy centers mainly around how safe barium is when it leaks out of the esophageal lumen. Those who believe it unsafe state that it potentiates mediastinal infection. They make this claim, however, largely by extrapolating from experience with barium-potentiated fecal peritonitis following colonic perforation. Vessal et al. (8) performed animal experiments and concluded that this extrapolation is not justified when applied to the mediastinum. In their experiments there was no increased lethality, when barium and flora were introduced into the mediastinum, over water-soluble contrast agent and flora. In fact, there was even some evidence that barium retarded the infectious process. One other argument advanced in favor of using barium is that a demonstrable leak (especially in the thoracic esophagus) is grounds for immediate surgical intervention, and barium can be removed at surgery. It would thus appear that dilute barium is safe to use and in fact has such an advantage in giving better definition that it is the superior agent.

Many radiologists would advocate a first swallow with water-soluble contrast followed by dilute barium if no obvious leak is demonstrated. If communication with the tracheobronchial tree is suspected, an oily contrast medium that is well tolerated by the respiratory tract, such as propyliodone (Dionosil), can be used safely.

Several authors have stressed proper technique in the radiography of perforations. A few films in the supine position following a swallow of contrast may not be adequate to exclude a perforation. Films should be exposed with the patient in different positions, e.g., lying on both sides and even prone in addition to the standard supine views. Parkin advocates horizontal beam radiography as an important adjunct (1).

Now let's look at specific causes of iatrogenic perforation.

Endoscopy

Endoscopy is a commonly performed procedure and is *the most common cause of iatrogenic perforation of the esophagus.* It was hoped that this complication would diminish with the introduction of flexible fiberoptic endoscopes, but this has not happened; the incidence of this complication continues to rise. Parkin (1) tabulated data from a number of series and showed that endoscopy accounted for over half the cases of iatrogenic perforation of the esophagus. Fortunately, the numbers of cases are small considering the total numbers of procedures performed—less than 1% in all series reported.

We have already explained where and why these perforations are likely to occur—in the cervical area, the distal esophagus near the hiatus, and the bronchial segment. If there is a pathologic process (tumor, stricture, hernia, or esophagitis), perforation in or near the lesion can occur regardless of where it is located. Biopsy combined with the endoscopy can increase the risk, particularly in the area of disease. It should be stressed that perforations can occur deceptively easily, and the endoscopist may not even be aware of the traumatic episode at the time that it occurs.

Not all endoscopic complications involve perforation. Impaction of the flexible endoscope is an example. The endoscope is advanced into the stomach, retroflexed, and if withdrawn in the flexed position can impact in the esophagus.

Surgery

Operations on or near the esophagus probably rank just after endoscopy as the most common cause of iatrogenic esophageal injury. Operations on the esophagus such as tumor resection or repair of hiatus hernia and operations near the esophagus such as vagotomy are examples of commonly performed procedures during which the esophagus can be unintentionally injured. Strictures and tumors, depending on size, location, and pathology, may be removed and the esophagus reanastomosed to itself or an interposition of bowel, usually colon but occasionally small intestine, performed. The interposed bowel can be placed in any of several locations, commonly retrosternally (Fig. 9-5). Complications following such reconstructive surgery occur either soon after surgery or at some time remote from surgery. Postsurgical breakdown of the anastomosis with resultant leak is an early and rather frequent complication. Calenoff and Norfray (3) indicate that this complication occurs in the cervical area in 40% of cases. These same authors report late strictures in the anastomotic region in one-third of cases. Distal esophageal anastomoses are additionally at risk for stricture formation because of alkaline reflux. Other operations, such as tracheoesophageal fistula repair in infants, can also be complicated by leaks at the anastomotic site early and strictures later in life (Fig. 9-6).

There are numerous operations for repair of hiatus hernia, and perforations soon after surgery are a known complication of these operations too. Stricture formation at this level may be due to operative technique when the hiatus is made too tight.

Even operations near the esophagus can cause esophageal complications. The intimate relationship of the vagus nerve trunks to the distal esophagus has already been discussed. One complication of vagotomy is perforation of the distal esophagus. Another type of complication associated with this procedure has been reported by Rogers (9). He describes the radiologic diagnosis of a transient phenomenon which he calls postvagotomy dysphagia. Within the first week or two following vagotomy, the patient experiences dysphagia following resumption of a solid diet. The disorder results from denervation of the lower esophageal segment and is manifested by a smooth, tapered, persistent narrowing of the distal few centimeters of esophagus. Normal proximal esophageal motility is preserved. This process is self-limited and removal of solid food and resumption of liquids for a couple of weeks is the only required therapy. He cautions that *persistent* dysphagia may indicate other, less common lesions—for example, fibrosis, esophagitis, or hematoma.

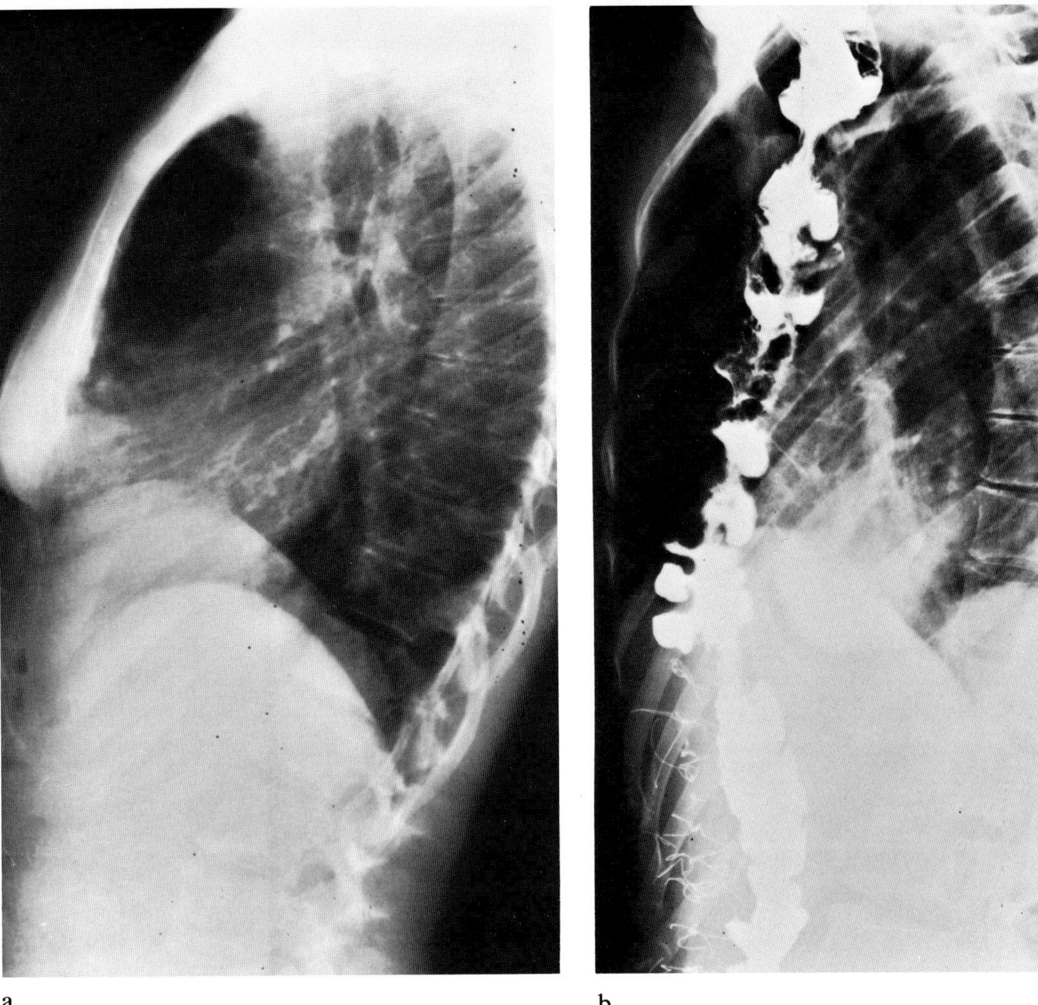

Fig. 9-5, a and **b. Colonic interposition.** This conduit lies in the usual retrosternal position. **a** Lateral chest x-ray demonstrates air-filled colon behind sternum. **b** Barium examination of same patient.

Surgery on adjacent organs can sometimes cause esophageal complications, and such have been reported following tracheostomy, especially when performed under emergency conditions.

following pneumatic dilatation. A somewhat ironic complication of *successful* dilatation is recurrent stricture caused by the induction of free gastro-esophageal reflux.

Dilatation

Dilatation of an esophageal stricture can be complicated by further damage to the esophagus. Perforation of the esophagus has occurred following both mechanical bouginage and pneumatic dilatation (Fig. 9-7), as well as following the Heller myotomy procedure. Submucosal hemorrhage causing esophageal obstruction can also occur

Tubes

The modern-day critically ill patient sprouts tubes from every orifice. The irony of many lifesaving therapeutic interventions is that they carry with them a not inconsiderable complication rate of their own.

A variety of tubes that traverse the esophagus, from small pediatric feeding tubes to large-bore

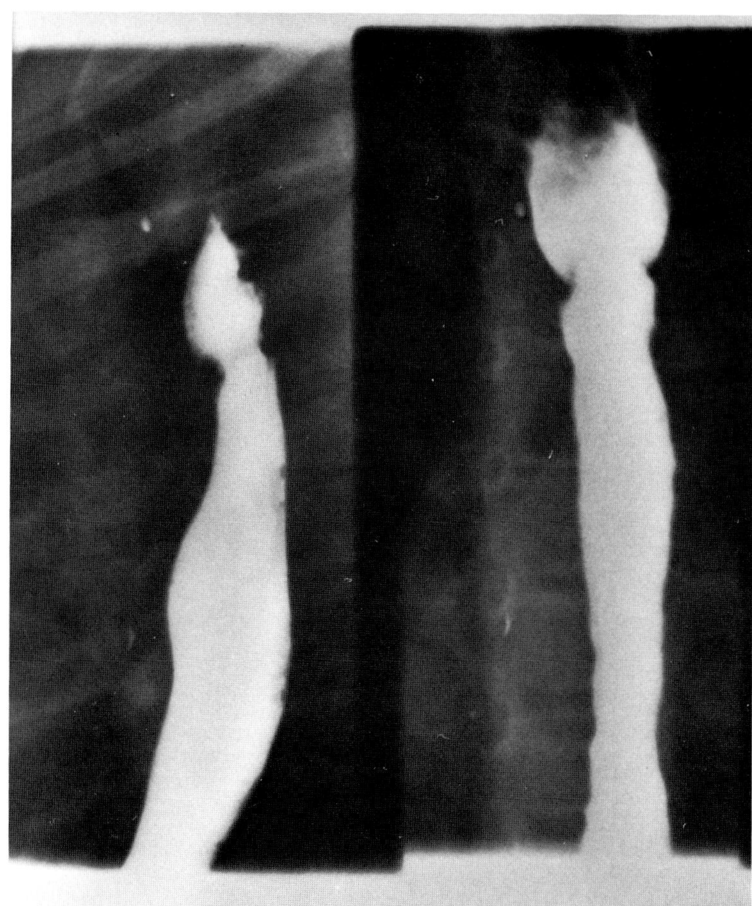

tubes such as the Sengstaken-Blakemore, can cause esophageal injury. Perforation of the hypopharynx or upper esophagus in the neonate with even thin, flexible tubes used for suction or for feeding can occur rather easily. Free perforation or false passage can occur (Fig. 9-8). In a recent review, Ghahremani et al. (10) remind us that the soft flexible nature of nasogastric tubes has engendered a certain amount of complacency regarding their use and inattention to possible complications. Although perforation of the adult esophagus by these flexible tubes is much less likely than in the neonate, it can happen, particularly in the pharyngeal and cervical regions.

Nonperforating complications are also seen. We have seen several hematomas of the esophagus caused by traumatic nasogastric intubation (Fig. 9-9). Strictures can occur following nasogastric intubation. These are thought to occur because the tube, which traverses the gastroesophageal junction, promotes reflux, which leads to stricture for-

mation. It is somewhat surprising to learn that stricture formation can be initiated after the tube has been in place for as few as five days (11). Mucosal erosions have also been described.

Other less common problems, such as knotting of tubes making removal difficult or impossible, have been reported. The larger tubes, such as the Sengstaken-Blakemore, have been known to cause esophageal laceration and rupture; this complication is frequently related to improper positioning and control of the balloon (Fig. 9-10). Ghahremani (10) also discusses complications related to placement of relatively large-caliber Celestin tubes for palliative treatment of nonresectable carcinomas.

As attempts at resuscitation of moribund patients become more vigorous, the rate of complications rises. A recent increase in esophageal injury following attempts at insertion of both endotracheal and esophageal airways, particularly when performed hastily under adverse field conditions, has been noted. Many of these complications occur

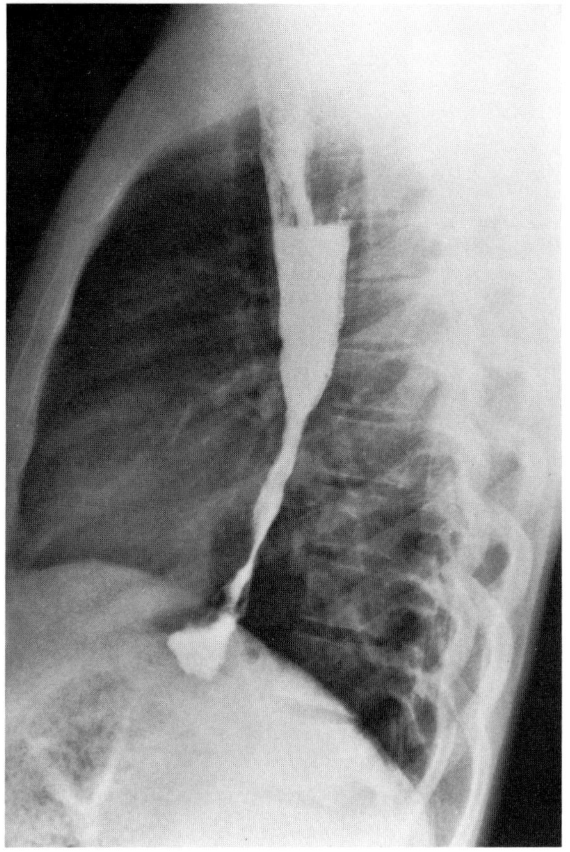

a

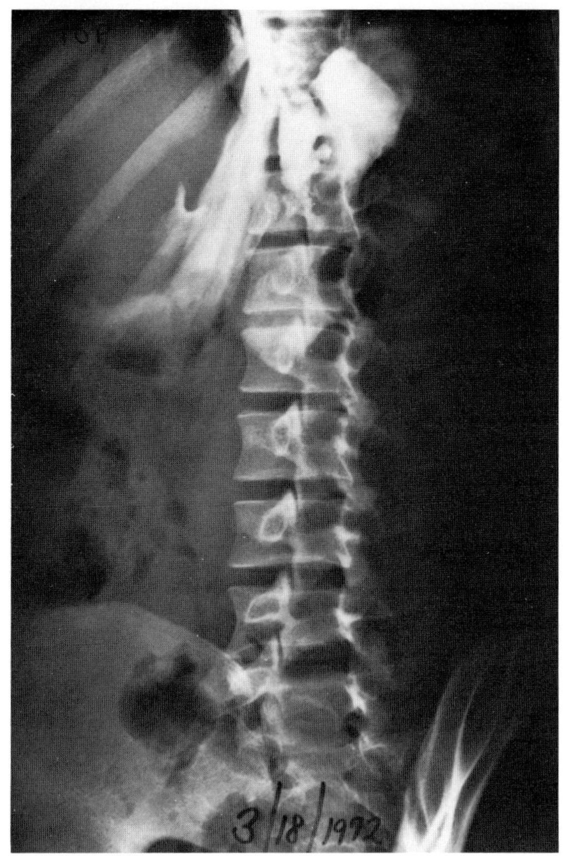

b

Fig. 9-7, a and b. Perforation following bouginage. a Predilatation. Note stricture in this 22-year-old male following repair of congenital esophageal atresia. **b** Water-soluble contrast examination postdilatation demonstrates contrast leaking from a posterior gastric perforation. (Courtesy of John Kirkpatrick, Children's Hospital Medical Center, Boston)

extrathoracically, particularly in the pharynx and cervical esophagus, but Pilcher (12) reports a case of a large rent in the thoracic esophagus caused by manipulation of an esophageal airway.

Drugs

No discussion of iatrogenic complications of any organ system would be complete without reference to drug-induced disease. The esophagus is not immune to modern pharmacologic intervention. Everyone is familiar with monilial esophagitis in immunosuppressed patients. It is important to stress that a normal esophagogram does not exclude the disease, especially early in its course. A number of roentgenographic findings, including spasm and linear ulcers, have been reported to be diagnostic (Fig. 9-11). The double-contrast technique utilizing high-density barium followed by water is an elegant way to diagnose subtle mucosal changes. Herpes esophagitis has also been reported in these iatrogenically compromised hosts. Steroids, long associated with gastric ulcer induction, can also cause esophageal ulcers (13). Potassium chloride preparations have been documented to cause gastrointestinal tract ulceration (and subsequent stricture formation), and the esophagus has not escaped this fate. Excessive anticoagulation is known to induce spontaneous gastrointestinal tract hemorrhage. This is most commonly seen in the small bowel, but Andress (14) reported a large esophageal submucosal hematoma in a woman on anticoagulant therapy (Fig. 9-12).

One final illustration should suffice to indicate the variety of drug-induced esophageal injuries.

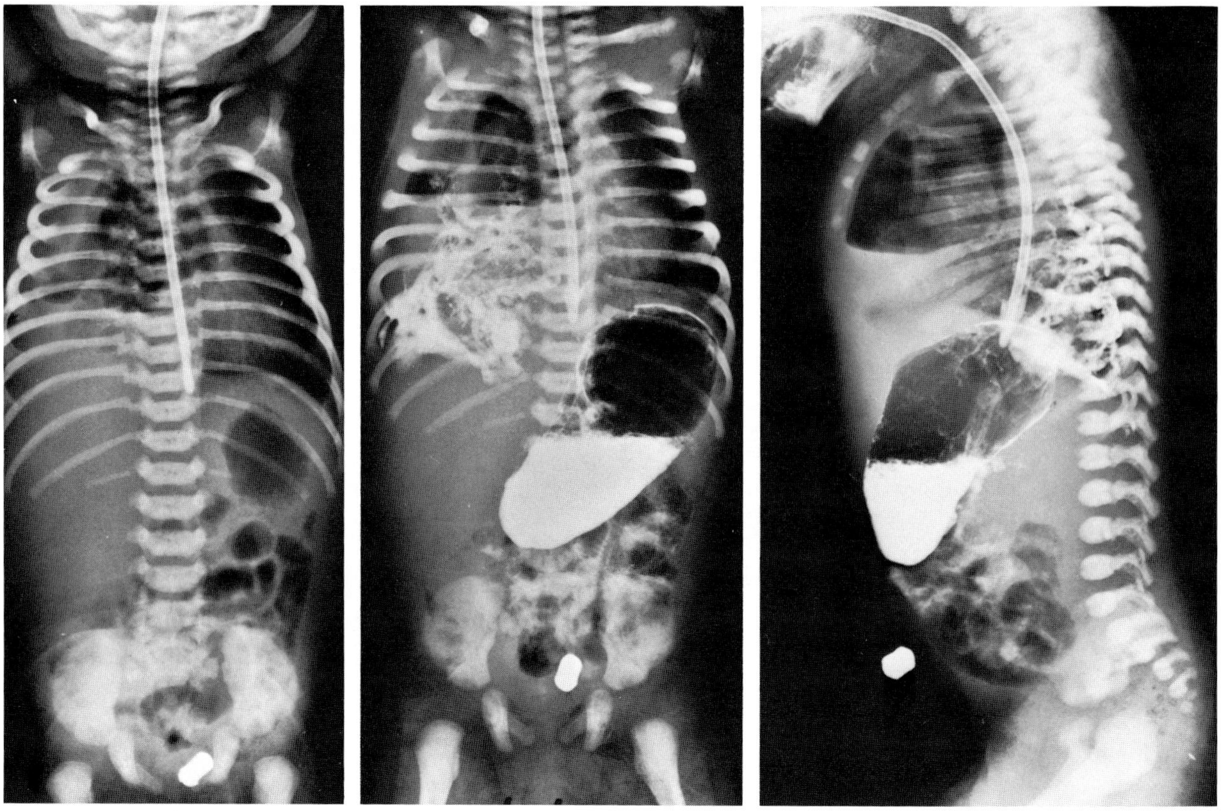

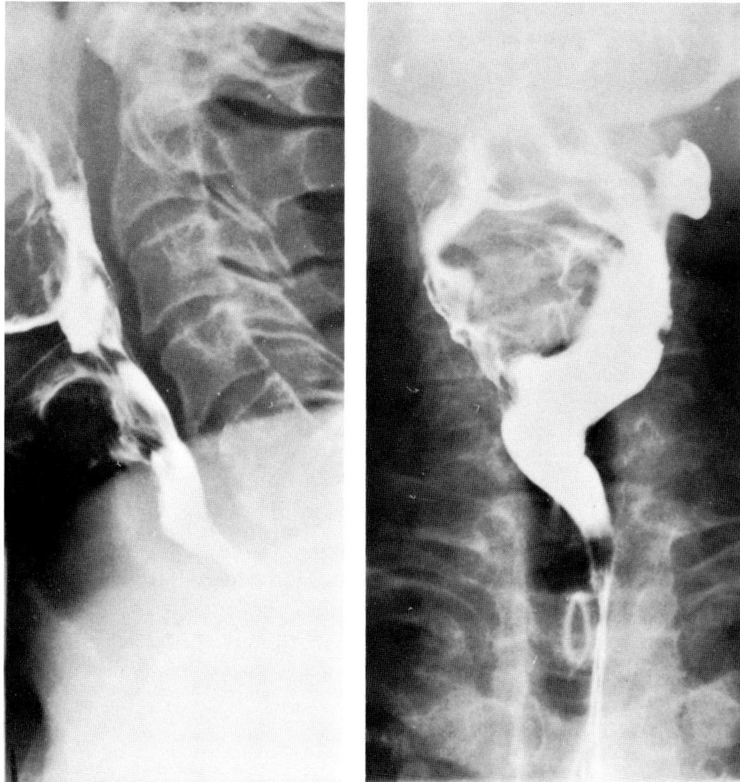

Fig. 9-8, a–c. Nasogastric tube passed in neonate to relieve abdominal distention. a Chest film a few days later shows opacification of the right lung base and air in the mediastinum. **b** PA film from esophagogram confirms rupture into the right pleural space. Even flexible tubes can cause perforation, especially in infants. (Courtesy of John Kirkpatrick, Children's Hospital Medical Center, Boston) **c** Lateral film from the same examination.

Fig. 9-9. Large pharyngeal hematoma following nasogastric intubation.

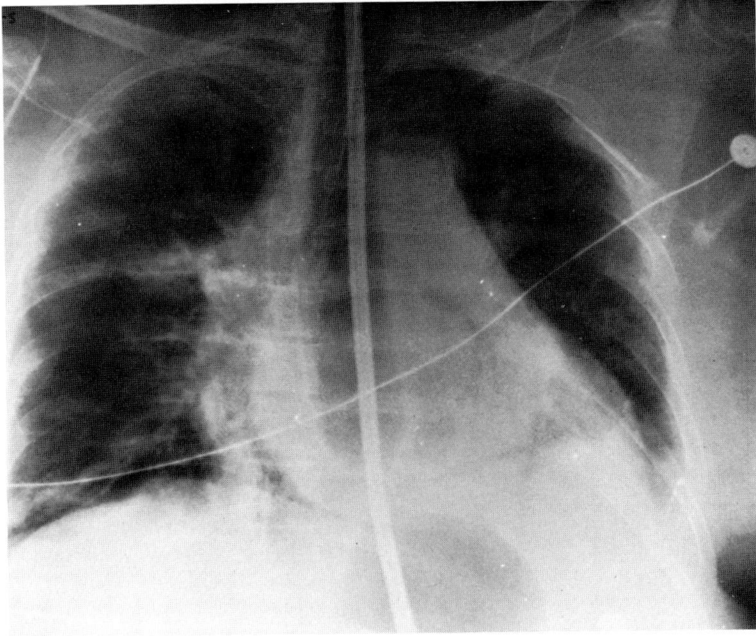

a

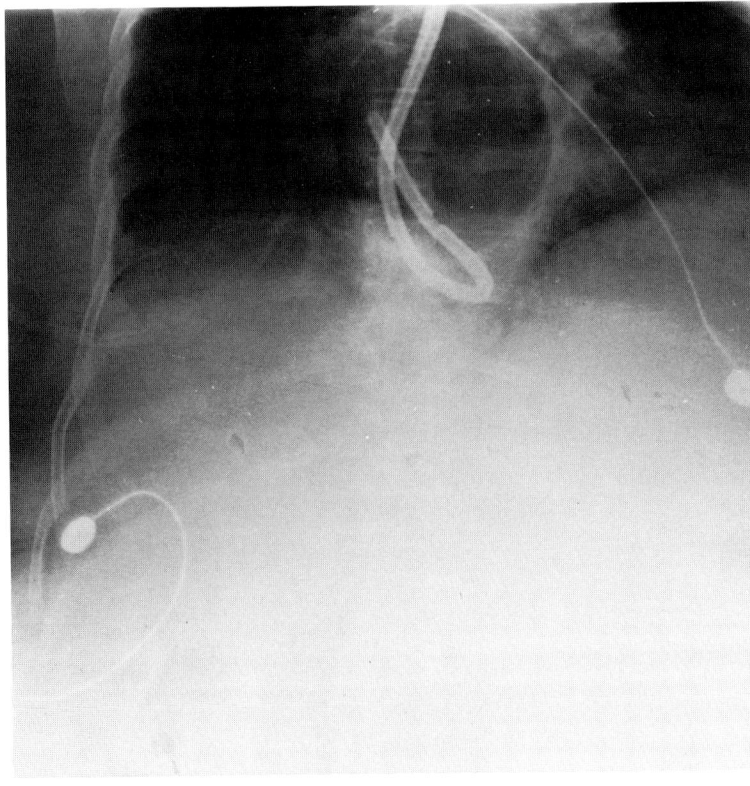

b

Fig. 9-10, a and b. **Malpositioned Sengstaken-Blakemore tube. a** Distal balloon of the Sengstaken-Blakemore tube properly positioned in the stomach. **b** The distal balloon has slipped superiorly and when inflated in the lower esophagus caused perforation.

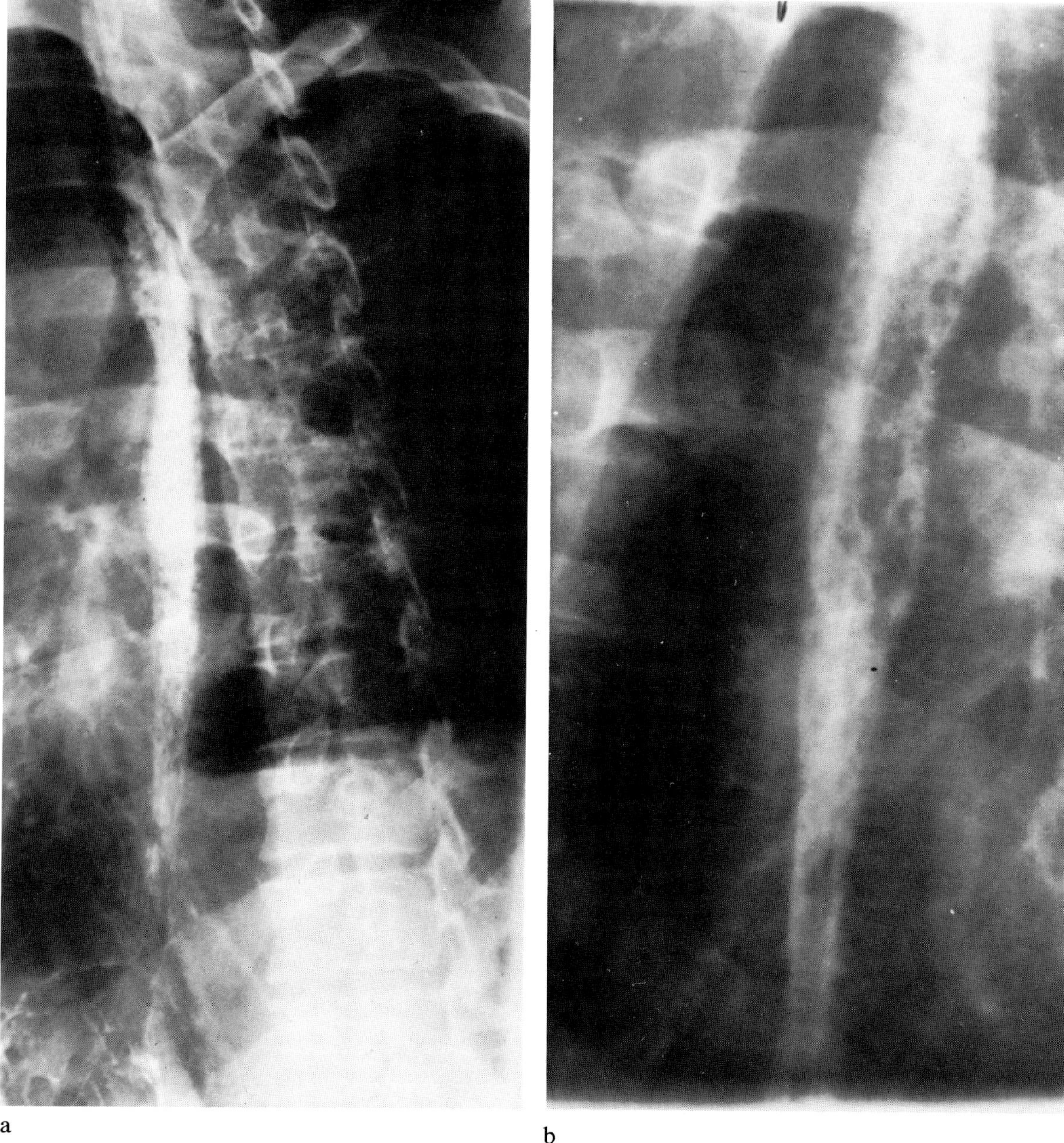

a

b

Fig. 9-11, a and b. Monilial esophagitis. a Note plaque formation and ulceration, described as characteristic. **b** Detailed view of **a.**

Impaction of a bolus of meat in the esophagus can cause complete esophageal obstruction. In an attempt to avoid endoscopic removal, pharmacotherapy with a proteolytic enzyme (papain, "meat tenderizer") has been successfully tried. Unfortunately the esophagus itself, as well as the meat, has occasionally been digested, with subsequent perforation.

Miscellaneous Complications

Other iatrogenic esophageal complications rarely occur. One of some interest, which may be underdiagnosed, is esophageal laceration secondary to the blunt trauma of cardiopulmonary resuscitation.

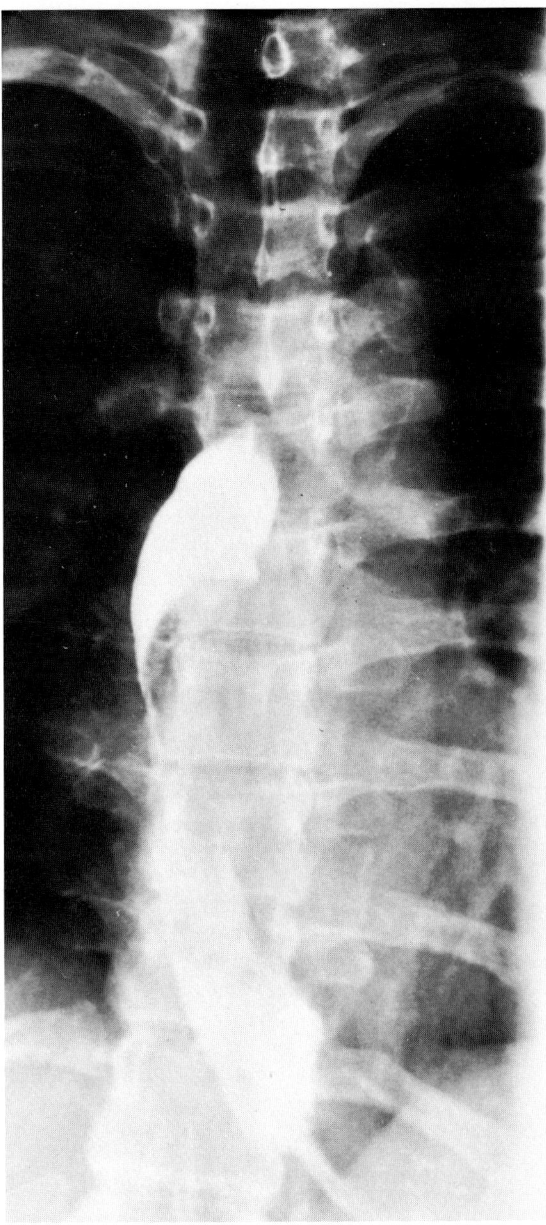

Fig. 9-12. Intramural hematoma of esophagus following anticoagulant therapy.

Summary

In this chapter we have shown how relatively vulnerable the esophagus is and how it can be involved in a wide variety of iatrogenic complications. Some complications are relatively benign; others, such as perforation, are highly lethal if not treated promptly and vigorously. Much of the trauma that has been described is symptomatically relatively silent early-on. As was pointed out, the person who directly or indirectly caused the trauma is frequently unaware that a potentially fatal complication has occurred. The radiologist may help save the patient by being the first to recognize the insult. To do this, the radiologist must be constantly alert to the possibility of esophageal injury, because, as we have shown, all findings short of actually demonstrating the perforation are relatively nonspecific. Diagnostic accuracy is increased when the radiologist diligently searches for potential complications in patients who are clearly at risk, e.g., those who have undergone endoscopy or surgery. A methodical search of plain films of the neck, chest, and abdomen, followed by a carefully performed contrast esophagogram will increase diagnostic accuracy and perhaps alleviate a potentially fatal outcome. It is a distressing fact, which all who care for patients must reckon with, that the incidence of iatrogenic complications involving the esophagus is not diminishing. We must make a greater effort to prevent those complications that can be prevented or to at least diagnose promptly those that cannot.

References

1. Parkin GJS: The radiology of perforated oesophagus. Clin Radiol 24:324–332, 1973.
2. Love L, Berkow AE: Trauma to the esophagus. Gastrointest Radiol 2:305–321, 1977.
3. Calenoff L, Norfray J: The reconstructed esophagus. AJR 125:864–876, 1975.
4. Berry BE, Ochsner JL: Perforation of the esophagus. J Thorac Cardiovasc Surg 65:1–7, 1973.
5. Appleton DS, Sandrasagra FA, Homer CDR: Perforated oesophagus: review of twenty-eight consecutive cases. Clin Radiol 30:493–497, 1979.
6. Meyers MA, Ghahremani GG: Complications of fiberoptic endoscopy. Radiology 115:293–300, 1975.
7. Calenoff L, Rogers LF: Radiologic manifestations of iatrogenic changes of the esophagus. Gastrointest Radiol 2:229–237, 1977.
8. Vessal K, Montali RJ, Larson SM, et al: Evaluation of barium and Gastrografin as contrast media for the diagnosis of esophageal ruptures or perforations. AJR 123:307–319, 1975.
9. Rogers LF: Transient post-vagotomy dysphagia: a distinct clinical and roentgenographic entity. AJR 125:956–960, 1975.
10. Ghahremani GG, Turner MA, Port RB: Iatrogenic intubation injuries of the upper gastrointestinal tract in adults. Gastrointest Radiol 5:1–10, 1980.
11. Banfield WJ, Hurwitz AL: Esophageal stricture as-

sociated with nasogastric intubation. Arch Intern Med 134:1083–1086, 1974.

12. Pilcher DB, DeMeules JE: Esophageal perforation following use of esophageal airway. Chest 69:377–380, 1976.

13. DeWitte C, Dory A, Sersté JP: Ulcere oesophagien iatrogene. J Belge Radiol 55:655–656, 1972.

14. Andress M: Submucosal haematoma of the oesophagus due to anticoagulant therapy. Acta Radiol 11:216–219, 1971.

10 Complications of Angiography in the Thorax

Michael A. Bettmann

Complications of angiography in the thoracic region are related to several different factors. A certain number of complications are inherent in the use of angiographic techniques, such as passage of guide wires through the right ventricle or injection of contrast media into coronary arteries. Other complications appear to be related to the skill and experience of the angiographer. Still others, such as acute congestive heart failure following pulmonary arteriography in patients with pulmonary hypertension, are essentially complications of the patient's disease process. This chapter will deal with the incidence of complications, the types of complications encountered, and the causes of various complications.

Incidence of Major Complications

Cardiac Angiography

The first major effort to examine complications of cardiac catheterization and coronary angiography was a cooperative study (1) in 1968; several other large, carefully performed studies have appeared subsequently (2–7). Both the techniques of angiography and the types of patients studied have changed with time, reflecting the evolution of therapy for heart disease. In the cooperative study, data were collected from 16 institutions over a two-year period. Of 12,367 studies, only 27% included coronary arteriograms and the bulk of these were performed at one institution; 41% of patients were studied for congenital heart disease

and 22.7% for rheumatic heart disease. Most subsequent large studies have concerned coronary angiography exclusive of other types of cardiac catheterization.

In the cooperative study (1), the overall mortality rate was 0.45% and the incidence of major complications was 3.6%. In examining separate age groups, the incidence of major complications was 15.4% in patients under 30 days of age, 6.6% between 1 and 12 months of age, and 3.0% in patients older than 1 year. In patients with no organic heart disease, the complication rate was 2.1%. Evaluated by procedure, the complication rate among patients undergoing right heart catheterization only, without angiography, was 1.9%; among those who had transseptal left heart catheterizations, 3.4%; and among those who had percutaneous left ventricular puncture, 3.1%. The mortality rate for coronary angiography was 0.9%. Clearly, those at highest risk were neonates, probably in large part because of the complex anomalies that led to the catheterization.

In a questionnaire survey in 1970–71 regarding complications of coronary angiography, Adams et al. (2) found an overall mortality rate of 0.45% and a complication rate of 4.1%, compared with rates of 0.9% and 1.9% in the collaborative study several years earlier. That is, although the overall complication rate was higher, the mortality rate had been cut in half. An interesting finding in Adams' study was the significant difference in both morbidity and mortality between the femoral and brachial approaches. Mortality was 0.13% in those studied via the brachial approach and 0.78% in those studied using the percutaneous femoral technique. Major complications such as myocardial infarction, arrhythmias, and hemorrhage were also more frequent when the femoral approach was used; arterial thrombosis was the only complication that occurred significantly more frequently in those studied via brachial artery cutdown (1.67% vs. 1.19%). In contrast, Judkins and Gander (4) reported an overall mortality rate of 0.4% using the percutaneous femoral approach exclusively.

In a subsequent survey, covering 89,079 coronary arteriograms performed during 1973–74, Adams and Abrams (6) found that the mortality rate had dropped to 0.14%, a statistically significant change. The reason for this change was the striking drop in mortality with the femoral approach, to the point that mortality from the two approaches was not significantly different (0.16% femoral vs. 0.12% brachial). Similarly, the overall incidence of severe complications had fallen from 4.1% to 3.1%. As will be dealt with in more detail subsequently, the overall complication rate, including death, was not altered by heparinization of patients during the procedure.

In a more recent cooperative study of patients undergoing coronary arteriography (7), the overall mortality rate among 7553 patients was 0.20%, slightly higher than in Adams' second study (6) but dramatically less than in earlier studies. All deaths occurred in patients with arteriographic findings of severe coronary artery disease. In contrast to earlier studies, the brachial approach increased the risk of death by a factor of 3.6 as compared with the femoral approach (0.50% incidence vs. 0.15%, p <0.05). The overall complication rate in this series had decreased to 1.08%, from 2%–4% in earlier studies. Again, heparinization did not appear to lessen the incidence of complications.

Cerebral Angiography

In contrast to the complication and mortality rates from coronary angiography and, earlier, cardiac catheterization in general, the complication rates of cerebral angiography have ranged up to 18–26% (8,9), particularly using direct carotid puncture rather than the percutaneous femoral approach. In a more recent study, however, in patients studied exclusively via the percutaneous femoral approach, no deaths were encountered in 5000 patients, and the incidence of major compli-

cations was 1.4% (10). A similar range in the complication rate of percutaneous subclavian venous line placement has been found; depending on technique and experience, the incidence has ranged from no complications (11) to 9.9% (12), but is usually in the range of 0.2%–1.2% (13,14). Extending from these data as well as from other surveys concerning cerebral angiography and coronary angiography, estimates can be made of the range of complications that might be expected. That is, using catheter technique and the percutaneous femoral approach, major complications of thoracic angiography would currently be expected to occur in 1%–2% of patients in most institutions. Death would be expected in less than 0.4% of cases. Factors that alter these expectations will be discussed subsequently.

Types of Complications and Predisposing Factors

Many of the complications encountered in cardiac and thoracic angiography are obvious, but others are noted only when carefully looked for. It must be emphasized that even occult complications may be important.

Mortality

The single most important complication is, obviously, death. In most series, death is classified as due to angiography if it occurs up to 24 hours following the procedure. Death does occur related to thoracic aortography but is very unusual. During coronary angiography, the risk of death is increased markedly by the presence of left main coronary artery disease. In one study (7), the relative risk of death was 6.3 times greater in patients with significant stenosis of the left main coronary artery than in those without it (0.76% vs. 0.12%). The same study indicated that left ventricular dysfunction increases the risk of death: those patients with an ejection fraction of 30%–50% had a mortality rate of 0.46%, and those with an ejection fraction greater than 50% had a mortality rate of 0.07%. The relative risk of death for patients with an ejection fraction under 30% as compared with normal was 9 times greater. Other factors that increased risk were the presence of systemic hypertension, congestive heart failure, and resting, frequent ventricular premature contractions. These factors increased the risk of death 4.2, 5.3, and 6.8 fold respectively.

Myocardial Infarction

Myocardial infarction is probably the next most significant complication, and has ranged in reported incidence from 0.09% (5) to 2.6% (15), with the most recent series reporting an incidence of about 0.2% (7,16). Predisposing factors for myocardial infarction are not clear, although arrhythmias and severe coronary artery disease are important. In patients studied within 30 days of an acute myocardial infarction, the incidence of a myocardial infarction during coronary angiography was about 1% (1 of 92 patients) (17), an incidence clearly higher than that in all patients undergoing coronary angiography. None of the patients with an uncomplicated postmyocardial infarction course, however, had significant angiographic complications.

Vascular Dissection or Perforation

Vascular perforations or major dissections occur with any catheter use. In the 1968 cooperative study (1), the incidence of perforation was 0.8%, probably far higher than is encountered currently. The largest number of these perforations occurred with attempts at transseptal left atrial puncture, as reflected in the fact that 33% of the (unintentional) perforations involved the right atrium; 21% were of the right ventricle. Currently, transseptal catheterizations are relatively rare, and when performed by investigators with experience, the incidence of complications is low—on the order of 1%, which is far lower than in the cooperative study. The bulk of perforations that occur now are probably of the right ventricle, usually in the outflow tract during attempted passage of a catheter into the pulmonary artery. Another relatively common cause of right ventricular perforation is attempted transvenous endomyocardial biopsy.

Coronary Artery

Major dissections or vessel occlusions occur most dramatically in the coronary arteries (18–21). In one study of coronary occlusion during coronary angiography (18), the overall incidence was 0.4%, approximately half due to dissection and half to embolization. Out of 7 dissections that occurred in 2981 patients, 4 occurred with Sones catheters and 3 with Judkins catheters. As will be discussed subsequently, 8 coronary occlusions in all occurred with the Judkins technique, all in the first 414 patients and none in the subsequent 490. Such dissections have been reported in thoracic vessels other than coronary arteries. A case of a dissection of the innominate artery has been reported (22), due to a guide wire used with a Sones catheter. The dissection led to a mediastinal hematoma and an arteriovenous fistula, which was repaired surgically. In another case, a false aneurysm of an anomalous right subclavian artery developed following a difficult right brachial artery catheterization, presumably due to a local vessel wall dissection (23).

Pseudoaneurysm Formation

Pseudoaneurysms and bleeding of major arteries secondary to dissection occur with some frequency. In one study (24) of retrograde brachial artery catheterization, there was a 0.01% incidence of bleeding leading to large hematoma formation. In a recent survey (25) of arterial complications, 27% of the deaths that occurred were due to aortic dissection or aneurysm rupture, although at least some of these patients had these processes prior to angiography. Local hemorrhage and pseudoaneurysm formation at the puncture site are relatively common but also relatively milder types of complications, and will be discussed subsequently.

Arrhythmias

Arrhythmias are another serious complication, essentially independent of catheter insertion site. They are encountered most frequently during right heart catheterization, due to the irritability of the right ventricle, and during coronary angiography, particularly in patients with severe coronary artery disease. Patients with left bundle-branch block are at particular risk during right heart catheterization, as right bundle-branch block is a fairly common occurrence during catheter passage to the pulmonary outflow tract (26–28), and thus complete heart block may ensue. In the Cooperative Study (1), the incidence of arrhythmias deemed serious was 1.2%. It must be kept in mind that most of these patients did not undergo coronary angiography. In studies of patients who had coronary arteriography, the incidence of major arrhythmias has ranged from 1.2% (2) to, more recently, 0.6% (7,16). Ventricular tachycardia occurred in 2% of patients (2 of 92) who underwent coronary arteriography within 30 days of an acute myocardial infarction. Both of these patients, however, had experienced ventricular irritability during convalescence. In 5000 cerebral angiograms, no serious arrhythmias were encountered (10). In assessing complications of all types of arteriograms (25), the reported incidence of arrhythmias was 0.06%.

Other Local Complications

Many additional complications are related, directly or indirectly, to the site of catheter insertion. The incidence of hemorrhage, pseudoaneurysm formation, local occlusion, and distal embolization depends, in part, on which vessel is punctured. The overall incidence of local hemorrhage or pseudoaneurysm is in the range of 0.16% or less (7,16). These two complications are rarely life-threatening, but are disquieting and often require surgical intervention. Hemorrhage is generally obvious on examination and is dealt with by local control and blood replacement. On occasion, when very large catheters have been used or multiple catheter exchanges have been performed, surgical exploration and closure are necessary for control. Pseudoaneurysm formation may be related to excessive catheter manipulation or large catheter size, but more importantly to inadequate or incorrect compression of the arterial puncture site. Pseudoaneurysms are not usually evident for days to weeks after a procedure. They most often present as a pulsatile mass in the groin, noted by either the patient or the physician. As the danger of rupture is great, rapid surgical repair is indicated.

Local occlusion of a punctured artery or embolization distal to the puncture site occurs in 0.72% (7) to 1.1% (6) of patients undergoing coronary angiography. Interestingly, the incidence of local occlusion or embolism among all angiographic procedures appears to be lower (about 0.2%) (25).

Cerebral embolism occurs in about 0.09% of coronary arteriograms (2,7), 0.23% of all angiograms performed from the femoral approach and 0.61% performed via the axillary approach, and, more directly, in 0.9% of catheter cerebral angiograms.

Renal Function Abnormalities

Renal function abnormalities occur following any procedure in which currently available radiopaque contrast agents are used. The incidence of detectable renal failure following renal angiography has been reported to be as high as 10%, although it is probably a good deal lower (29). Renal failure occurs almost invariably in patients with preexisting compromise of renal function, and less often in patients with marked congestive heart failure (29–31). Rare cases of transient renal failure have been seen following contrast administration in patients with normal renal function, generally unrelated to the amount of contrast used. In one study of renal biopsies of normal patients following contrast administration, osmotic nephrosis of the tubules was frequently seen (32). This finding, however, is relatively nonspecific and probably of little importance. Contrast studies are particularly fraught with danger in azotemic diabetics, as this group may be more prone to develop marked deterioration of renal function (30). In patients with underlying azotemia the severity of worsening of renal function appears to be related to the amount of contrast used, but renal function almost invariably returns to baseline levels (33).

Acute renal failure following the administration of contrast agents to patients with multiple myeloma has long been recognized. This complication, due to precipitation of Bence-Jones protein, is related to the hypertonicity and hyperviscosity of the currently available contrast media. If the patient is well-hydrated and the amount of contrast agent is limited, this complication can be largely eliminated.

Allergy-like Reactions

Allergy-like reactions to contrast agents occur more than twice as often following intravenous as following intraarterial administration (5.6% vs. 2.3%) (34). The mildest of these reactions, urticaria, is by far the most common. Other types of reactions, such as laryngeal edema, respiratory collapse, and anaphylaxis, are very rare, although clearly disquieting. In one large series of patients undergoing urography, the overall incidence of acute allergic-like reactions was 1.72%, including a 0.12% incidence of cardiovascular or respiratory reactions (35).

Causes of Complications

The major causes of complications are underlying disease, age, lack of experience, puncture site, prolonged examination time, thrombosis, and technical factors associated with catheters, guide wires, and contrast agents.

Underlying Disease

As several studies have shown, the incidence of complications varies with the patient group. The incidence of complications among patients undergoing coronary angiography is much higher if the patients are studied within one month of a myocardial infarction (3% vs. 1%) (7,17).

Similarly, the presence of unstable angina at the time of coronary angiography increases the risk of a nonfatal myocardial infarction 3.4 times (7). Patients with left main coronary artery stenosis also seem, in most studies, to be at particular risk of severe complications. In the CASS study (7), the relative risk of death was 6.3 times as great in the presence of significant left main coronary disease as in the general population. Other studies have also demonstrated that a higher percentage of complications occurs in this group of patients (5,6), with a mortality rate as high as 10%–15% (36–38). The CASS study also indicated that the most significant single risk factor predisposing to death associated with coronary angiography was the presence of three-vessel disease. This conferred a relative risk 15.6 times that of the general population.

In patients undergoing cerebral angiography, the incidence of complications in patients with cerebrovascular disease was two to three times that in patients with tumors, headaches, or seizures (39). Earlier studies (40,41) gave similar results, although in those studies the relationship of com-

plications to underlying vascular disease was even more striking, probably because of technical and experiential factors. In the early Cooperative Study (1), the incidence of major complications in all patients was 3.6%, but this fell to 2.1% in patients without organic heart disease. It appears, therefore, that one major cause or predisposition to significant complications is underlying atherosclerotic disease. As indicated by the cooperative study and implied by other studies (7,17,25), the incidence of complications also increases as the general health of the patient deteriorates.

Age

Age is similarly an important factor. Patients at each end of the age spectrum have a higher rate of complications for the same procedure. Again, from the Cooperative Study, the incidence of major complications was 15.4% in patients under 30 days old, 6.6% between 30 days and 1 year, and 3% in all other patients. These rates are higher than currently encountered, but the trend remains unchanged. In patients undergoing catheter cerebral angiography, the incidence of complications was greater for patients over 40, and appeared to increase further with advancing age (42). Above 60 years of age, the incidence of complications was clearly greater than in younger patients, regardless of underlying disease. In the CASS study (7), the average age of patients who died following coronary angiography was 10 years greater than the mean patient age, and the age of patients who suffered postprocedure myocardial infarctions was 5 years greater.

Physician Experience and Training

The experience of the physician performing the procedure is an important consideration in complications, even though the significance of this factor is not entirely clear. Comparing complications from one group or hospital to another is difficult, as sensitivity to the occurrence of complications, technique of angiography, as well as the experience of the physicians all vary widely. These factors, and others, play a role in explaining the wide range of reported incidences of complications for the same procedure (43,44). The total number of procedures performed may not in itself play a central role in reducing complications: the CASS study of 7553 coronary arteriograms (7) showed a difference in complication rate between hospitals, but no relationship between the number of cases per year and the complication rate. Other, earlier studies of coronary angiography demonstrated that there *was* an inverse correlation between number of cases performed and the incidence of complications (2,6,45), although there was also a clear difference among certain hospitals handling approximately the same number of cases. In a study of complications of percutaneous placement of a subclavian venous line, it was found that operators who had performed fewer than 50 such procedures had a complication rate of 8.1%. Those who had performed 50 or more, however, had no complications (11). Thus operator intelligence, attitude, skill and training may be more important than actual cumulative number of cases performed. A study of complications of catheter cerebral arteriography helps to clarify the role of training: the overall complication rate was 4.5 times as high in training as in nontraining institutions (10). Further, the incidence of complications in nontraining hospitals was more than twice as great when the studies were done by nonneuroradiologists as when neuroradiologists performed the studies. This is a strong argument for the role of training, possibly as distinct from total experience.

A retrospective survey of complications of all types of angiography (25) disclosed what on the surface are conflicting results but probably are consistent. The incidence of complications was lower in teaching than in nonteaching institutions, and in nonteaching institutions the percentage of complications decreased as the number of cases increased. The relative rate among angiographers vs. nonangiographers was not assessed. The higher incidence of complications in nonteaching institutions may reflect the common practice of general radiologists, or even nonradiologists, performing angiographic procedures. This practice is more common with general angiography than with neuroradiology. Thus both of these studies (10,25) probably indicate that the incidence of complications is inversely correlated with the degree of training. Further, as the incidence of complications in both types of hospitals decreased with increasing number of cases, it appears likely that experience per se was operative. This does not appear to be true with neuroradiologists, as their training is generally adequate in a training institution. The same probably holds for coronary angiographers.

In both studies, the overall incidence of major as distinct from minor complications—major permanent complications in Mani et al. (10) and death in Hessel et al. (25)—was essentially the same regardless of type of hospital or number of cases. While minor complications, then, can be reduced by training and, to a lesser extent, by experience, these studies do not indicate whether major complications are at an irreducible minimum due to underlying disease or whether other, alterable factors are still important.

A further interesting study which helps to explain this point as well as the role of experience concerns the initial use of the percutaneous femoral technique for coronary arteriography at a large teaching hospital (18). Coronary artery occlusion occurred in 8 patients out of the first 414, in the first three and a half years the technique was used. In the subsequent 490 patients studied with this technique, over the ensuing 18 months, no coronary occlusions were encountered. Although systemic heparinization was used in the second period and not in the first, it is likely that experience, in the form of improved catheter technique, was the major reason for the decrease in complications. As will be discussed subsequently, heparin appears to play a role in decreasing local complications but probably does not influence the incidence of major ones.

Thus, as with other causes, it is impossible to entirely divorce one reason for complications from others. Experience may in fact not be as important a factor as training: increased patient load does not invariably lead to decreased complications, unless the number of procedures or the level of training is quite low.

Duration of Procedure

Length of procedure is another causal factor concerning which there are conflicting thoughts, but results of most studies are fairly conclusive. Many studies do not address the causal role of length of procedure, probably as it is frequently a somewhat imprecise measurement. Early studies of coronary angiography showed a clear relationship between increased duration of the procedure and increased complication rate (1,38). In a more recent study of complications of catheter cerebral angiography (42), there was a clearly higher incidence of complications when the duration of a procedure was greater than 80 minutes. This finding is less clear, however, when broken down: procedures tended to be longer in teaching hospitals, in which the overall complication rate was higher than in nonteaching institutions, but there was no clear relationship between duration and complication rate. In the nonteaching institutions, which had lower complication rates and generally shorter procedures, the complication rate increased when the duration was greater than 90 minutes. Again, the relationship between duration of procedure and complications may actually reflect the level of training of the angiographer, as well as underlying disease which led to a lengthier procedure (46). The effect of training is probably more significant than the length of the angiographic study.

Thrombus Formation and Embolism

Thrombosis as a cause of complications is another important consideration, one that is perhaps more easily evaluated due to the widespread use of heparin during coronary angiography beginning in about 1973. The incidence of thrombosis at the arterial puncture or cutdown site or on the catheter or guide wire varies over a wide range, from 0.2% (47) to 13% (48), and thrombus on the catheter following removal has been reported in over 50% of studies (45). It would seem logical that, since thrombi occurring on catheters and guide wires have been documented by many different methods (49–52), and since many patients undergoing angiography have friable, atherosclerotic vessels, careful systemic heparinization would be of value. It has been used essentially since the beginning for the brachial approach to cardiac catheterization, although initially it was not reported (53). The reason was, apparently, that 5000 units of heparin were administered intraarterially distal to the catheter, and it was felt that only local anticoagulation occurred. In fact, systemic heparinization was rapidly accomplished.

Approach

The early studies showed a marked increase in incidence of major complications using the percutaneous femoral technique for coronary angiography (Judkins approach) compared with the brachial artery cutdown technique (Sones method); the increased incidence generally was related to myocardial infarction, usually due to thrombosis, embolism, or dissection. Several studies, including that mentioned previously (18) and another sequential study (54), showed an initial high incidence of thrombotic complications with the Judkins technique, and then a marked reduction which seemed to coincide with the institution of routine systemic heparinization. This seemed good evidence that anticoagulation played an important role in coronary arteriography. As with other causes of complications, however, the conclusions become muddied by other results. The more recent studies of coronary angiography also show a decreased incidence of complications related to the percutaneous femoral (Judkins) approach (6,7), but this decrease in complications is clearly not related solely to the use of anticoagulation: the same degree of reduction was observed in laboratories that used heparin as in those that did not, and the incidence of both death and myocardial infarction was almost identical in the two settings. The incidence of local thrombosis, however, did decrease with heparinization.

In angiography of vessels other than the coronaries, there is good evidence that systemic heparinization decreases symptomatic arterial occlusion, nonocclusive thrombi, and fibrin coating of the catheter (55). Among factors other than systemic heparinization which may play a role in decreasing thrombosis are shorter duration of use of thrombogenic guide wires and catheters, frequent catheter flushing with heparinized saline, alterations in catheter manufacture, and general improvement in catheter technique.

Thrombus formation, then, is an important factor in causing complications, although its relationship per se to the major complications, specifically death and myocardial infarction, is still not clear. Systemic heparinization is generally indicated in coronary angiography because heparin does clearly lower complications at the catheter site, and complications of heparin use during procedures are very unusual. Frequent catheter flushes with heparinized saline is possibly as useful and is sufficient in general angiography. The usual dose is 3000–7000 units for systemic heparinization and 2000–4000 units per liter of saline for all flushing solutions.

Guide Wires and Catheters

Thrombus Formation and Embolism

As regards thrombogenicity of different guide wires and catheters, experimental evidence does not provide clear results. Benzalkonium-heparin coating of guide wires, in a dog model, appeared to increase the time between wire insertion and thrombus formation, and Teflon-coated wires developed thrombi more rapidly than did uncoated steel wires (50). However, it was found that levels of fibrinopeptide A, a cleavage product of the conversion of fibrinogen to fibrin, were higher with benzalkonium-heparin-coated Teflon wires than with either stainless steel or just Teflon-coated wires in the critical first four minutes following wire insertion (52). This study also used a canine model.

The clinical implications of these studies are not clear. Teflon coating of guide wires is often used to facilitate passage through catheters. Heparin coating of wires is probably of minor importance, at least in comparison to technique: it is far more important to limit the time a wire guide is in the vascular tree than it is to use heparin coating.

Catheter materials also differ in thrombogenicity. One study found that following coronary angiography, both polyethylene and polyurethane catheters had external surface irregularities by electron microscopy, and both had a high incidence of thrombus on the external surface (51). Polyurethane catheters, however, had more thrombus internally than did polyethylene, consistent with the increased incidence of irregularities of the inner surface. It was theorized, from this study, that external thrombi are probably related to complications at or distal to the puncture site, whereas internal irregulatities may lead to complications such as cerebral embolization or myocardial infarction. As the thrombosis on the catheter surface is probably related to general biocompatibility and specifically to surface irregularities, improved catheter manufacture, rather than change in material or systemic heparinization, may help decrease the incidence of complications. Heparin coating of catheters has been suggested, but a study of benzalkonium-heparin-coated catheters indwelling in the axillary artery for chemotherapy infusion showed a high incidence of partial or complete thrombotic occlusion (56). The incidence was no lower than with standard catheters (57).

In practical terms, then, the important factors in preventing thrombotic-embolic complications are very careful attention to technique: short-duration usage of guide wires, frequent catheter flushes with heparinized saline, and the use of catheters of as high quality as is available.

Site of Arterial Puncture

Percutaneous Approaches

A significant cause of complications is the arterial entry itself, particularly in patients with extensive vascular disease. In reviewing all types of angiography, the incidence of complications was found to be higher using the percutaneous axillary approach than the percutaneous femoral (25). The incidence of complications using the translumbar approach was intermediate. Whether these differences reflect the inherent complications of the technique, the underlying disease, or the experience of the angiographer is unclear. The high number of femoral punctures with the low incidence of complications suggests that experience plays a role. It might be speculated that the slightly lower incidence of complications using the translumbar compared with the axillary approach (2.89% vs. 3.29%), despite roughly the same number of procedures, may relate to both shorter procedure time and less catheter manipulation. It is interesting to note that the incidence of complications at the arterial entry site is lower for general than for coronary angiography (6,7,25). This difference also may reflect patient health, duration of procedure, or operator experience.

Percutaneous vs. Cutdown Approach

As regards the brachial cutdown (Sones) vs. the percutaneous femoral (Judkins) approach to coronary arteriography, the results of studies are striking. Early studies clearly indicated that the Sones approach had a lower complication rate (1,2). More recent studies, however, indicate that the Judkins method is safer, under most circumstances (6,7). Specifically, the incidence of complications using the brachial approach dropped slightly from an already low level between Adams et al. studies of 1971 (2) and 1974 (6). The complication rate from femoral studies, however, dropped markedly and became less than from the brachial approach. This drop was not related to case volume alone, as low-volume institutions using the femoral approach had a lower complication rate than high-volume institutions using the brachial technique. In the CASS study (7) of 1979, there was a higher mortality rate with the brachial than with the femoral approach. The rate equalized in comparing centers using only the brachial approach. However, if both techniques were used, mortality with the femoral technique remained low while that from the brachial technique was high. These differences were not related to underlying risk factors, to volume of procedures in the institution, or to heparinization. Heparinization, as in the Adams et al. study (6) of 1974, was shown to have no protective effect.

Contrast Material

Contrast agents themselves are a cause of complications. In the vast majority of cases, these complications are minor and of no significance. As noted previously, the incidence of major complications from intravenous contrast use is 0.12%, and the incidence is somewhat lower with arterial use (34,35). Most of these reactions are readily reversible and have no long-term sequelae. Many angiographers use, as a pretreatment, steroids and diphenhydramine (benadryl) in patients who have a history of a reaction to intravascular contrast injection (58). However, reactions have been encountered (59) despite this pretreatment. Further, Lalli has provided a compelling argument for the role of psychogenic factors and also for careful reassurance of the patient, no pretreatment, and readiness to treat any reaction (59–61). This appears to be a more rational and functional approach.

Cardiac complications related to contrast agents are in essence ubiquitous with intracoronary or ventricular injection: minor electrocardiographic and pressure alterations always occur with the currently used hypertonic, hyperviscous contrast agents (62). These complications, however, are rarely more than transient. They are important to keep in mind, particularly in patients with severely compromised myocardial function or potentially severe compromise. This latter group includes patients with tight left main coronary artery stenosis and those with tight aortic stenosis. It is likely that the newer contrast agents such as metrizamide, hexabrix or iohexol, which are far less hypertonic than current ones, will cause fewer of these cardiac effects (63–65).

Percutaneous Transluminal Angioplasty

A final important cause of complications is the use of percutaneous transluminal angioplasty. In the thorax, the major role of this exciting procedure has been and probably will remain treatment of proximal, discrete coronary artery stenoses. As occurred with coronary arteriography (2,6,7), and probably with any new, major procedure, there is a "learning curve." That is, the initial complication rate generally decreases with time. Currently, although the success rate in coronary artery dilatation is 63%, the incidence of major complications is slightly greater than 10% (66). Considering the availability of coronary artery bypass surgery as a backup and the incidence of complications and morbidity of this operation, the complication rate of angioplasty is not unacceptably high. It can be anticipated, however, that the incidence will decrease with improved technique and increased experience.

Is There an Irreducible Number of Complications?

The question must be raised as to whether there is an irreducible minimum number of complications which will occur during angiography in the thorax. Two early studies explored the rate of complications of "nonangiography" (67,68), that is, complications that occurred in patients who were scheduled for angiography but then had the procedure canceled. In both studies, the incidence of serious complications (death and myocardial infarction) was essentially the same in the angiography and nonangiography groups. This suggested that, due to underlying disease, a certain number of complications must be expected as naturally occurring events which coincidentally occur during or immediately following angiography. It is important, however, to realize that there has been a clear decrease in the incidence of complications comparing earlier (1–4) with more recent studies (6,7,10).

Conclusions

The final judgment on the complications of angiography of the thorax must take into account many factors and many, often conflicting studies. The major variables that currently affect the complication rate, and are probably of equal importance, are age and health of the patient, experience, skill and judgment of the angiographer, and catheter insertion site. Under the category of skill, experience, and judgment of the angiographer fall the proper choice and use of guide wires, catheters, and type of examination. Of lesser importance, but still relevant, is duration of the procedure and type of contrast agent. Anticoagulation is also in this category, although it probably is not important to distinguish between systemic heparinization and frequent flushing with heparinized saline. It is clearly important to be aware of the types of complications that occur and to be ready to treat them when they begin. The type of institution is probably of importance only insofar as the institution has proper equipment to perform the procedure and handle complications (such as embolization, arrhythmias, or acute myocardial infarction) and an angiographer of sufficient skill, judgment, and experience to plan, perform, and interpret the procedures.

References

1. Braunwald E, Gorlin K, McIntosh, HI et al: Summary, cooperative study on cardiac catheterization. Circulation 37 (Suppl 111):93–101, 1968.
2. Adams DF, Fraser DB, Abrams HL: The complications of coronary arteriography. Circulation 48:609–618, 1973.
3. Chahine RA, Herman MV, Gorlin R: Complications of coronary arteriography: comparison of the brachial to the femoral approach. Ann Intern Med 76:882, 1972.
4. Judkins MP, Gander MP: Prevention of complications of coronary arteriography. Circulation 45:599, 1974.
5. Bourassa MG, Noble J: Complication rate of coronary arteriography. A review of 5250 cases studied by percutaneous femoral technique. Circulation 53:106, 1976.
6. Adams DF, Abrams HL: Complications of coronary arteriography: a follow-up report. Cardiovasc Radiol 2:89–96, 1979.
7. Davis K, Kennedy JW, Kemp HG Jr, et al: Complications of coronary arteriography from the collaborative study of coronary artery surgery (CASS). Circulation 59:1105–1112, 1979.
8. Coddon DR, Krieger HP: Circumstances surrounding complications of cerebral angiograms. Am J Med 25:580–589, 1958.
9. Olivecrona H: Complications of cerebral angiography. Neuroradiology 14:175–181, 1977.
10. Mani RL, Eisenberg RL, McDonald EJ Jr, Pollock JA, Mani JR: Complications of catheter cerebral arteriography: analysis of 5000 procedures. I. Criteria and Incidence. AJR 131:861–865, 1978.
11. Bernard RW, Stahl WM: Subclavian vein catheterization: a prospective study. I. Non-infectious complications. Ann Surg 173:184–190, 1971.
12. Borja AR: Current status of infraclavicular subclavian vein catheterization. Ann Thorac Surg 13:615–624, 1972.
13. Brinkman AJ, Costley DO: Internal jugular venipuncture. JAMA 223:182–183, 1973.
14. Mitchell SA, Clark RA: Complications of central venous catheterization. AJR 133:467–476, 1979.
15. Watson WJ, Lee GB, Amplatz K: Biplane selective coronary arteriography via percutaneous transfemoral approach. AJR 100:332, 1967.
16. Grossman W: Complications of cardiac catheterization: incidence, causes and prevention in cardiac catheterization and angiography. In Grossman W (ed): Cardiac Catherization. Philadelphia: Lea & Feibiger, 1980, pp 25–35.
17. Turner JD, Rogers WJ, Mantle JA, Rackley CE, Russell RO Jr: Coronary angiography soon after myocardial infarction. Chest 77:58–64, 1980.
18. Guss SB, Zir LM, Garrison HB, Dagett WM, Block PC, Dinsmore RE: Coronary occlusion during arteriography. Circulation 52:1063–1068, 1975.
19. Meller J, Friedman S, Dack S, Herman MV: Coronary artery dissection—a complication of cardiac catheterization without sequelae: case report and review of the literature. Cathet Cardiovasc Diagn 2:301, 1976.
20. Silverman JF, Guekow W, Pfeifer JF: Iatrogenic dissection of the coronary arteries: a complication of selective coronary arteriography and the transfemoral percutaneous approach. Circulation 38:678, 1968.
21. Hass JM, Peterson CR, Jones RC: Subintimal dissection of the coronary arteries: a complication of selective coronary arteriography and the transfemoral percutaneous approach. Circulation 38:678, 1968.
22. van Heeckeren DW, Botti RE, Cohen AM: Innominate arterial arteriovenous fistula complicating retrograde brachial arterial catheterization. Am J Cardiol 44:566–568, 1979.
23. Chiavacci WE, Bucciarelli RL, Victorica BE: Aneurysm of the subclavian artery: complication of retrograde brachial catheterization. Cathet Cardiovasc Diagn 2:93–96, 1976.
24. Campion BC, Frye RL, Pluth JR, Fairbairn JF, Davis GD: Arterial complication of retrograde brachial arterial catheterization. Mayo Clin Proc 46:586–592, 1971.
25. Hessel SJ, Adams DF, Abrams HL: Complications of angiography. Radiology 138:273–281, 1981.
26. Stein PD, Mathur VS, Herman MV, Levine HD: Complete heart block during cardiac catheterization of patients with pre-existent bundle branch block. Circulation 34:783, 1966.
27. Guptu PK, Haft JI: Complete heart block compli-

cating cardiac catheterization. Chest 61:185, 1972.

28. Wennerold A, Christianson I, Lindeneg O: Complications in 4413 catheterizations of the right side of the heart. Am Heart J 69:173, 1965.

29. Older RA, Miller JP, Jackson DC, Johnsrude IS, Thompson WM: Angiographically induced renal failure and its radiographic detection. AJR 126:1039–1045, 1976.

30. Weinrauch LA, Healy RW, Leland DS Jr, Holdstein HH, Kassissieh SD, Libertino JA, Tallacs FJ, D'Elia JA: Coronary angiography and acute renal failure in diabetic azotemic nephropathy. Ann Intern Med 86:56–59, 1977.

31. Port FK, Wagoner RD, Fulton RE: Acute renal failure after angiography. AJR 121:544–550, 1974.

32. Moreau J-F, Droz D, Sabto J, Jungers P, Kleinknecht D, Hinglais N, Michel J-R: Osmotic nephrosis induced by water-soluble triiodinated contrast media in man. Radiology 115:329–336, 1975.

33. Milman N, Stage P: High-dose urography in advanced renal failure. Acta Radiol Scand 15:104–112, 1974.

34. Shehadi WH: Adverse reactions to intravascularly administered contrast media. A comprehensive study based on a prospective survey. AJR 124:145–152, 1975.

35. Witten DM, Hirsch FD, Hartman GW: Acute reactions to urographic contrast medium. Incidence, clinical characteristics and relationship to history of hypersensitivity states. AJR 119:832–840, 1973.

36. Cohen MV, Cohn PF, Herman MV, Gorlin R: Diagnosis and prognosis of main left coronary artery obstruction. Circulation 45 (Suppl I):1–57, 1972.

37. Lavine P, Kimbiris D, Segal BL, Linhart JW: Left main coronary artery disease: clinical, arteriographic and hemodynamic appraisal. Am J Cardiol 30:791, 1972.

38. Wolfson S, Grant D, Ross AM, Cohen LS: Risk of death related to coronary arteriography: role of left coronary arterial lesions. Am J Cardiol 37:210, 1976.

39. Mani RL, Eisenberg RL: Complications of catheter cerebral arteriography: analysis of 5,000 procedures. II. Relation of complication rates to clinical and arteriographic diagnoses. AJR 131:867–869, 1978.

40. Feild JR, Lee L, McBurney RF: Complications of 1,000 brachial arteriograms. J Neurosurg 36:324–332, 1972.

41. Pribram HFW: Complications of angiography in cerebrovascular disease. Radiology 85:33–37, 1965.

42. Mani RL, Eisenberg RL: Complications of catheter cerebral arteriography: analysis of 5,000 procedures. III. Assessment of arteries injected, contrast medium used, duration of procedure, and age of patient. AJR 131:871–874, 1978.

43. Bettmann MA, Salzman EW, Rosenthal D, Clagett P, Davies G, Nebesar R, Rabinov K, Ploetz J, Skillman J: Reduction of venous thrombosis complicating phlebography. AJR 134:1169–1172, 1980.

44. Albrechtsson U, Olsson CG: Thrombotic side effects of lower limb phlebography. Lancet I:723–724, 1976.

45. Formanek G, Frech RS, Amplatz K: Arterial thrombus formation during clinical percutaneous catheterization. Circulation 41:833–839, 1970.

46. Selzer A, Anderson WL, March HW: Indications for coronary arteriography. Risks vs. Benefits. Calif Med 115:1, 1971.

47. Saur H: Ein Überblick über die Komplikationen bei der indirekten (perkutunen katheter) Methode der Aortographie. A Kreislauffortschr 53:314, 1964.

48. Brenner J, Couch NP: Peripheral arterial complications of left heart catheterization and their management. Am J Surg 125:521–526, 1973.

49. Nachnani GH, Lessin LS, Motomiya T, Jensen WN: Scanning electron microscopy of thrombogenesis on vascular catheter surfaces. N Engl J Med 286:139–140, 1972.

50. McCarty RJ, Glasser SP: Thrombogenicity of guide wires. Am J Cardiol 32:943–946, 1973.

51. Bourassa MG, Cantin M, Sandborn EB, Pederson E: Scanning electron microscopy of surface irregularities and thrombogenesis of polyurethane and polyethylene coronary catheters. Circulation 53:992–997, 1976.

52. Casarella WJ, Wilner GD: Guide wire thrombogenicity measured by fibrinopeptide A radioimmunoassay. AJR 128:363–366, 1977.

53. Sones FM Jr, Shirey EK: Cine coronary arteriography. Mod Concepts Cardiovasc Dis 31:735–738, 1962.

54. Walker WJ, Mundall SL, Broderick HG, Prasad B, Kim J, Ravi JM: Systemic heparinization for femoral percutaneous coronary arteriography. N Engl J Med 288:826–828, 1973.

55. Antonovic R, Roesch J, Dotter CT: The value of systemic arterial heparinization in transfemoral angiography: a prospective study. AJR 127:223–225, 1976.

56. Tyler U, Forsberg L, Owman T: Heparinized catheters for long-term intra-arterial infusion of 5-fluorouracil in liver metastases. Cardiovasc Intervent Radiol 2:111–114, 1979.

57. Forsberg L, Hofstrom LO, Lunderquist A, Sundquist K: Arterial changes during treatment with intrahepatic arterial infusion of 5-fluorouracil. Radiology 126:49–52, 1978.

58. Zweiman B, Mishkin MM, Hildreth EA: An approach to the performance of contrast studies in contrast material-reactive persons. Ann Intern Med 83:159–162, 1975.

59. Lalli AF: Contrast media reactions: data analysis and hypothesis. Radiology 134:1–12, 1980.

60. Lalli AF: Urography, shock reaction and repeated urography. AJR 125:264–268, 1975.

61. Lalli AF: Urographic contrast media reactions and anxiety. Radiology 112:267–271, 1974.

62. Fischer HW, Thomson KR: Contrast media in coronary arteriography: a review. Invest Radiol 13:450–459, 1978.

63. Morris TW, Francis M, Fischer HW: A comparison of the cardiovascular responses to carotid injections of ionic and nonionic contrast media. Invest Radiol 14:217–223, 1979.

64. Higgins CB, Sovak M, Schmidt WS, Kelley MJ, Newell JD: Direct myocardial effects of intracoronary administration of new contrast materials with low osmolality. Invest Radiol 15:39–46, 1980.
65. Tragardh B: Coronary angiography with Iohexol and other contrast media in the dog. I. Electrocardiographic alterations. Acta Radiol Scand (Suppl) 362:14–24, 1980.
66. Levy RI, Mock MB, Willman VL, Passamani ER, Frommer PR: Percutaneous transluminal coronary angioplasty—a status report. N Engl J Med 305:399–400, 1981.
67. Baum S, Stein GN, Kuroda KK: Complications of "No Arteriography." Radiology 86:835–838, 1966.
68. Hildner FJ, Javier RP, Ramaswamy K, Samet P: Pseudo complications of cardiac catheterization. Chest 63:15–17, 1973.

11 The Radiologic Manifestations of the Complications of Cardiac Pacing

C. J. Tegtmeyer

Surgical implantation of a cardiac pacemaker to stimulate the heart is a well-established procedure of great benefit. Pacemakers now provide a better life for 1 in every 5000 persons in the United States and Canada. A malfunctioning pacemaker, however, is a hazard to well-being and to life. Once a pacemaker has been installed, the physician's attention is directed not only to the patient's illness but also to the unique complications of cardiac pacing. Careful radiologic studies are extremely helpful in the proper evaluation and care of patients with cardiac pacemakers (1–9). It is important that physicians thoroughly understand the extent to which radiologic studies can depict the functioning of and complications associated with pacemakers.

Normal Roentgenographic Findings

As in all of radiography, it is necessary to have a thorough understanding of what is normal in order to recognize the abnormal. It is also necessary to obtain properly exposed radiographs, using short exposure times to prevent blurring of the intracardiac portion of the electrode. The electrodes of an implanted pacemaker should be visible on chest films throughout their course. If the generator is implanted in the abdomen, an abdominal film is also necessary for a complete evaluation of the pacemaker. An overexposed film is needed to visualize the electrode and generator well.

The tip of the transvenous electrode should be somewhat to the left of the midline in the posteroanterior view (Fig. 11-1a). On the lateral film, the catheter tip is seen anteriorly behind the ster-

num (Fig. 1b). The electrode should follow a gently curved course through the vena cava, with a slight outward curve in the right atrial region. This provides enough catheter length to maintain slight pressure against the endocardium at the right ventricular apex and avoids displacement by patient movement. If the curve is too great, excessive pressure may result, and the electrode tip may perforate the myocardium or be ejected from the ventricle. If the lead is too short, with the electrode describing a nearly straight line, patient movement may cause displacement of the tip, and intermittent pacing or complete loss of capture may result. Sharp bends in the leads are undesirable because they cause excessive motion, resulting in metal fatigue and electrode fracture.

The terminals of epicardial electrodes are readily visualized on the chest film. The lead may be sutured to the myocardium or "screwed in" to the myocardium. A new "screw-in" lead is also available for transvenous insertion. The epicardial leads are usually brought down into the abdominal wall, and an overexposed abdominal film is necessary to fully evaluate the pacemaker.

Pacemaker complicatoins may be classified into two major categories: those related to improper function of the pacemaker, and those arising from the body's reaction to the implanted foreign material.

Pacemaker Complications Related to Pacemaker Malfunction

Failure of the pacemaker to elicit a ventricular response may result from

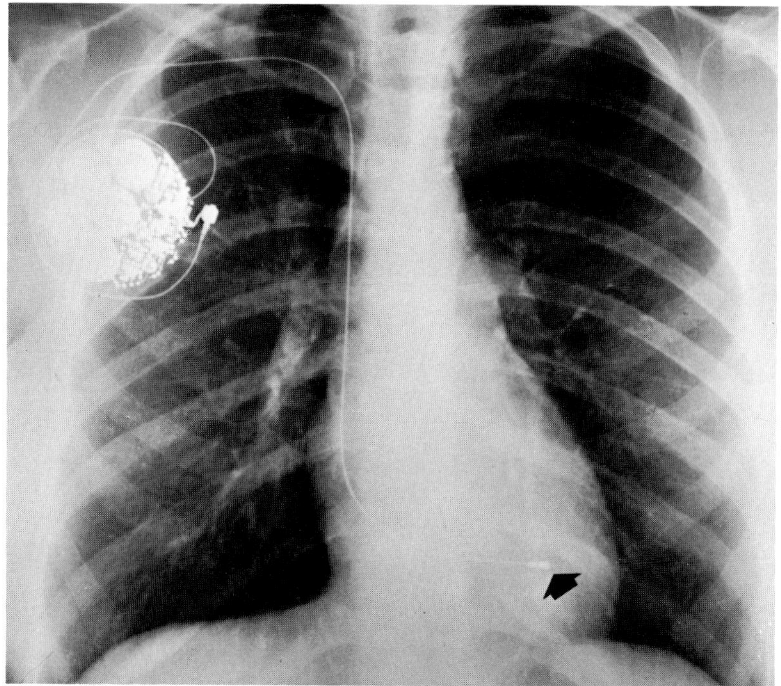

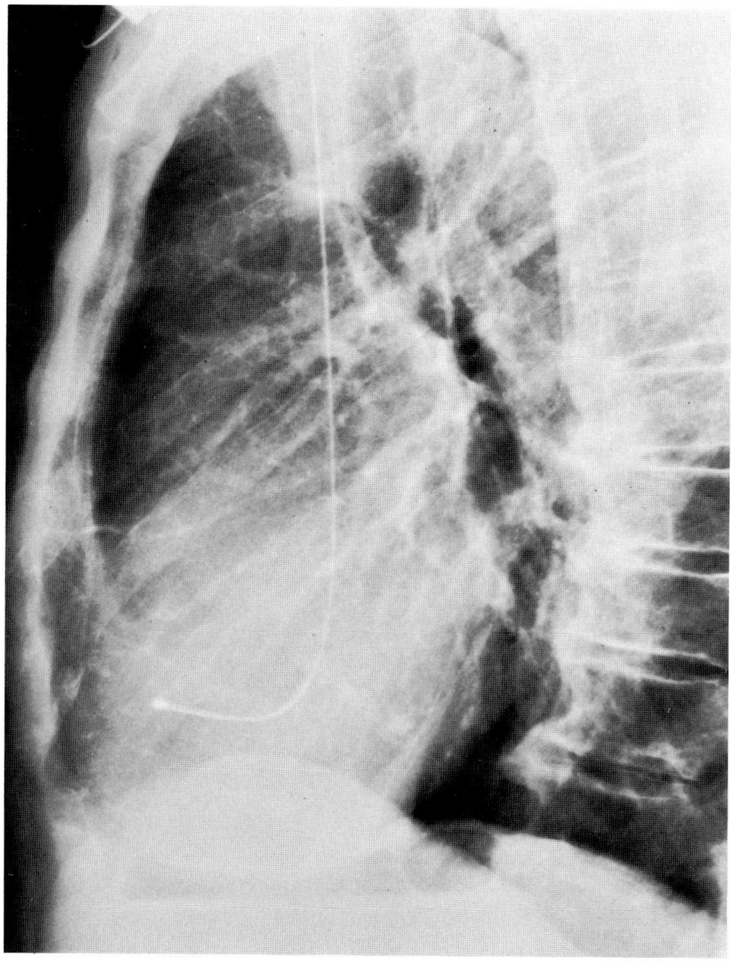

Fig. 11-1, a and **b. Normal transvenous lead. a** Posteroanterior radiograph demonstrates a normal transvenous lead traversing a smooth course through the right atrium to the apex of the right ventricle (*arrow*). (Tegtmeyer CJ: Am Fam Physician 14:66–75, 1976, with permission) **b** The tip lies anterior, behind the sternum, in the lateral view. (Tegtmeyer CJ: Am Fam Physician 14:66–75, 1976, with permission)

1. Exit block
2. Lead fracture
3. Electrode malposition and dislodgement
4. Electrode malposition (coronary sinus)
5. Electrode dislodgement by the pulse generator
6. Trauma
7. Myocardial perforation
8. Pulse generator or battery failure

Exit Block

A change in threshold amperage required to elicit a contraction accounts for some pacing failures when pacing systems are intact. This common cause of pacemaker failure is referred to as exit block. In this situation, the role of the roentgenogram is to confirm that the leads are intact and in their original position.

Lead Fracture

In the past, lead fracture was a major consideration, but electrodes constructed of metal alloys greatly reduced the incidence of lead fracture. Because reliable five- to ten-year batteries are now available, lead fracture has again become a problem. The diagnosis of fractured electrodes is best established by roentgen examination (10). High-density overpenetrated films are usually necessary to establish the diagnosis, and spot films may be very helpful. The usual sites of fracture are near the pulse generator, at sharp bends in the wire, or at the point where the leads are inserted into the epicardium (Fig. 11-2). A fractured electrode may cause only sporadic malfunction, because the fractured ends may have intermittent contact depending on the patient's position. Failure to demonstrate a complete break in the electrode does not completely exclude its presence, as the insulating sheath may hold the ends in close proximity, precluding detection on plain films. If the fracture site is not revealed on the chest films, fluoroscopy or cineroentgenography with the patient in various positions may be necessary to demonstrate the fracture (11).

A new problem has arisen with the development of bipolar polyurethane coaxial leads.* These leads

*Medtronic Inc., 3055 Old Highway Eight, Minneapolis, Minnesota 55440

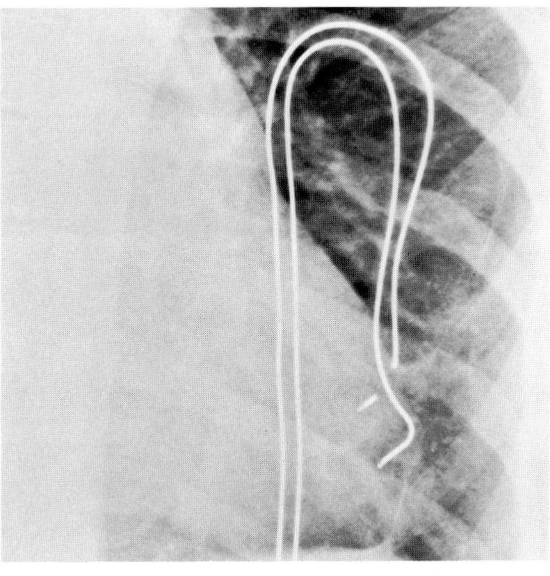

Fig. 11-2. Fractured epicardial lead. Posterolateral chest roentgenogram showing an epicardial lead with a fracture at its insertion into the epicardium.

are designed to reduce the diameter of the electrode. The design, however, requires separating the inner and outer coils for connection to the lead terminal pins. As a result, the radiographic picture of these leads is different (12) and may be misinterpreted as a fracture (Fig. 11-3a,b).

Electrode Malposition and Dislodgement

Electrode dislodgement is a common complication of transvenous cardiac pacing, occurring in 3% to 14% of patients. The tip of the lead may be inadvertently malpositioned at the time of insertion, or it may become dislodged later with subsequent failure to pace. Often, displacement can be anticipated when the electrode wire exhibits too little length (Fig. 11-4) or is markedly redundant, with a loop in its course. When chest roentgenograms on pacemaker patients are read, the position of the lead should always be reported. Occasionally, the malpositioned lead will capture, but at a higher threshold, resulting in premature battery failure.

Electrode dislodgement usually occurs in the early days or weeks after insertion. Displacement can often be corrected by repositioning the electrode under local anesthesia. Late displacement is uncommon because of the development of a fi-

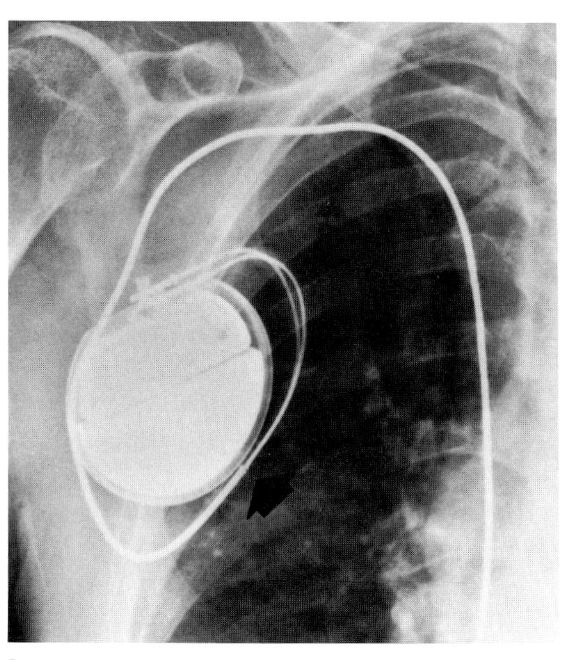

a

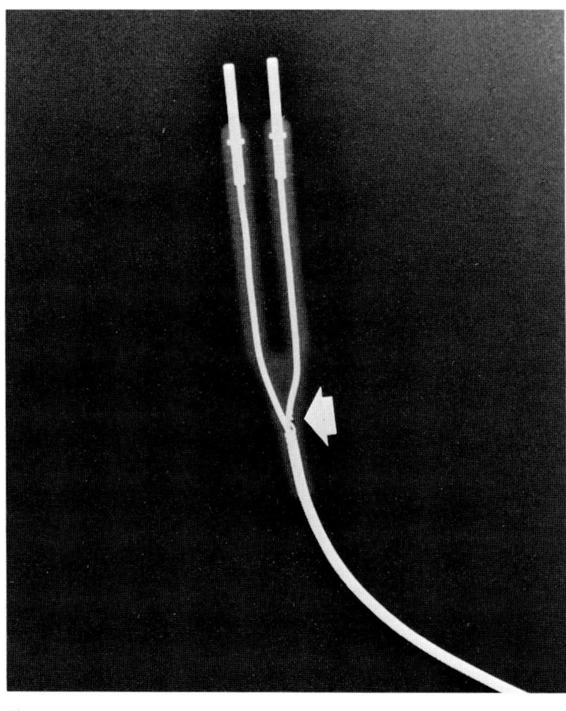

b

Fig. 11-3, a and **b. New coaxial lead simulating a fracture. a** The new bipolar polyurethane coaxial lead may simulate a fracture at the point where the inner and outer cores are separated (*arrow*). **b** Radiograph of coaxial lead demonstrating separation of inner and outer coils of lead. The straightened portion of the outer coil simulates a fracture (*arrow*).

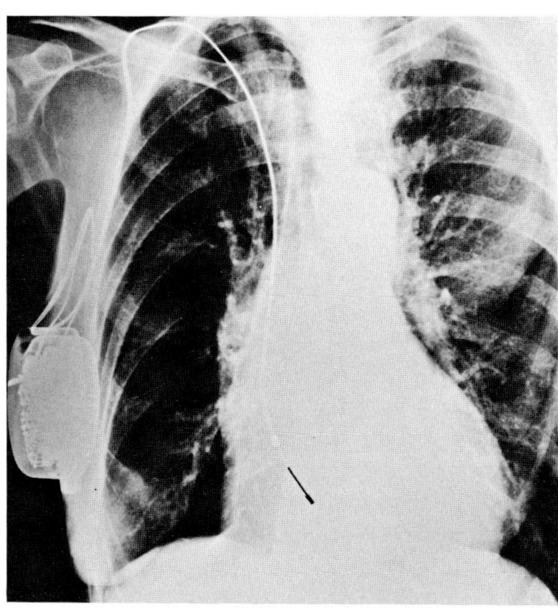

Fig. 11-4. Electrode malposition, lead too short. The posteroanterior radiograph reveals that this lead is too short. Ten days after this film was taken, the lead became dislodged and failed to pace. (Tegtmeyer CJ: Contemp Surg 1:79–88, 1972, with permission)

brous sheath, which forms a firm attachment between the electrode and the endocardium.

Dislocated intravenous electrodes have been reported in the right ventricular outflow tract or within the pulmonary artery. In other instances, the electrode tip may recoil into the right atrium or may loop within the body of the right ventricle. The displaced lead may stimulate the phrenic nerve, causing contractions of the diaphragm if it becomes dislodged into the superior vena cava (Fig. 11-5). Leads have also been seen in the inferior vena cava. The lead may inadvertently be placed in the left ventricle through the arterial system (Fig. 11-6).

The incidence of electrode dislocation is decreased with the increasing proficiency of the surgeon; i.e., proper positioning of the electrode at insertion decreases the frequency of this problem. Also, improved electrode tips, such as the "tined" lead and the new transvenous "screw-in" lead, hold the promise of further reducing the incidence of this problem.

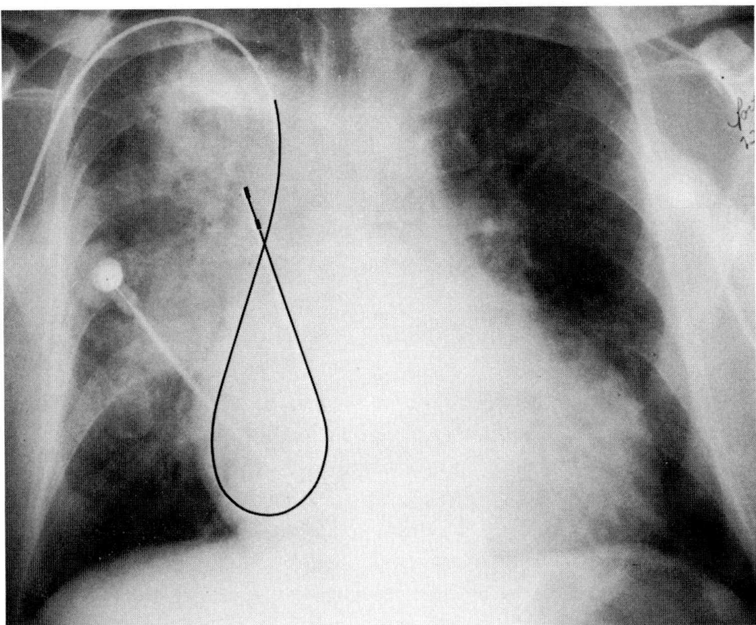

Fig. 11-5. Lead dislodgement. Anteroposterior roentgenogram of a patient in congestive failure. The pacemaker electrode has become dislodged. The lead has looped within the right atrium, and the tip is in the superior vena cava. (Tegtmeyer CJ: CRC Crit Rev Diagn Imaging 9:1–50, 1977, with permission)

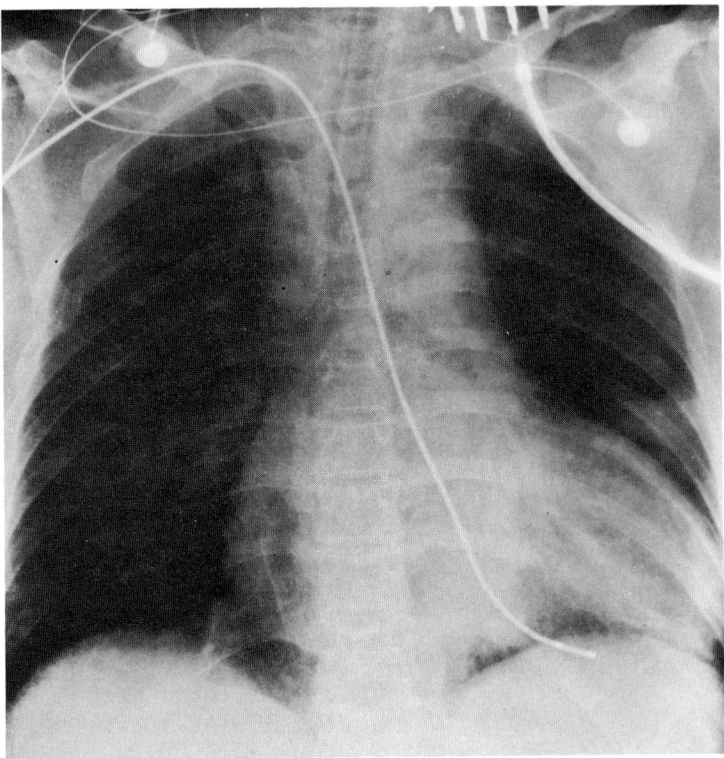

Fig. 11-6. Electrode malposition. The patient was in shock when this electrode was inserted. The electrode tip appears to be in the right ventricle. However, note the position of the electrode in the mediastinum. The lead has been inadvertently placed in the brachial artery and threaded into the left ventricle. (Tegtmeyer CJ: Clin Trends Cardiol 5:1, 3, 1975, with permission)

Electrode Malposition (Coronary Sinus)

The electrode may inadvertently be placed in the coronary sinus or one of its branches by the operator at the time of insertion (1,13,14). The diagnosis may be missed because of reliance on fluoroscopy and radiographs performed in the frontal plane only. Coronary sinus placement is suggested in the anteroposterior view if the tip of the electrode inclines upward and toward the left shoulder. This is not always the case, however. The lateral view is the best indicator of the true position of the lead. A lead that has been properly placed in the right ventricle runs anteriorly toward the sternum, whereas an electrode inserted in the coronary sinus system lies along the posterior border of the heart (Fig. 11-7a,b). A lead in the coronary sinus can point toward the sternum when advanced far enough (15). In this case, however, the posterior segment of the lead will be closer to the spine than normal. Failure to pace because of a higher threshold and shortened battery life are the complications of coronary sinus pacing.

A transvenous lead may be placed in the coronary sinus intentionally when atrial pacing is planned. The lead is usually inserted through the left cephalic vein, because of the gentle curve of the lead from this approach. This provides a clue that the electrode may have been intentionally implanted in the coronary sinus.

Electrode Dislodgement by the Pulse Generator

A change in position of the generator may cause traction on the lead and ultimately displace the electrode. The weight of a heavy pacemaker may cause it to migrate downward in a large pocket and result in retraction of the endocardial leads. Displacement of the transvenous leads may also result from traction on the lead produced by rotation of the pulse generator within an enlarged pocket (Fig. 11-8). Rotation can occur spontaneously; however, rotation is usually caused by the patient unconsciously twisting the generator within a capacious pocket. This phenomenon was first described by Bayliss (16) as the "pacemaker twiddler's syndrome." The electrode is wound on the pulse generator, as though a reel, retracting the tip of the lead out of the ventricle. If the pulse generator is rotated on its axis, the patient may twist the electrode into loops and retract it from the ventricle. Twisting the electrode imposes addi-

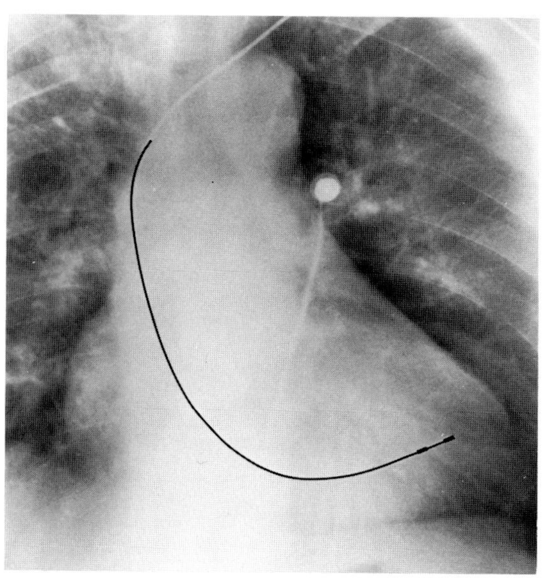

a

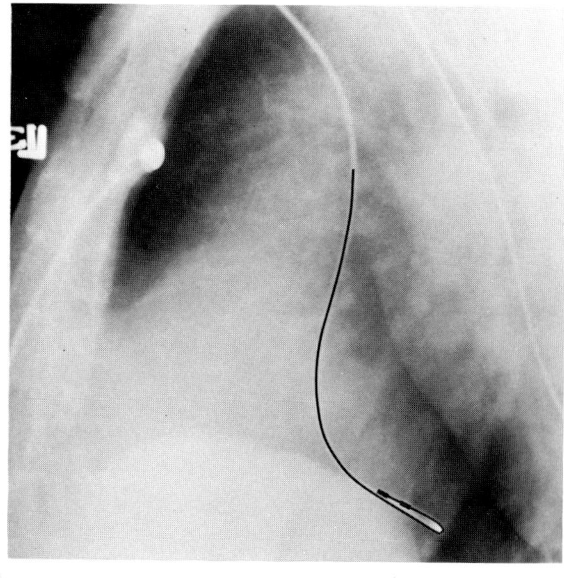

b

Fig. 11-7, a and b. Electrode malposition, coronary sinus. a This pacemaker electrode has been inadvertently inserted into the coronary sinus. The diagnosis is suggested in the anteroposterior view because the electrode tip inclines upward. **b** The lateral view confirms the diagnosis. The electrode lies along the posterior border of the heart. (Tegtmeyer CJ: CRC Crit Rev Diagn Imaging 9:1–50, 1977, with permission)

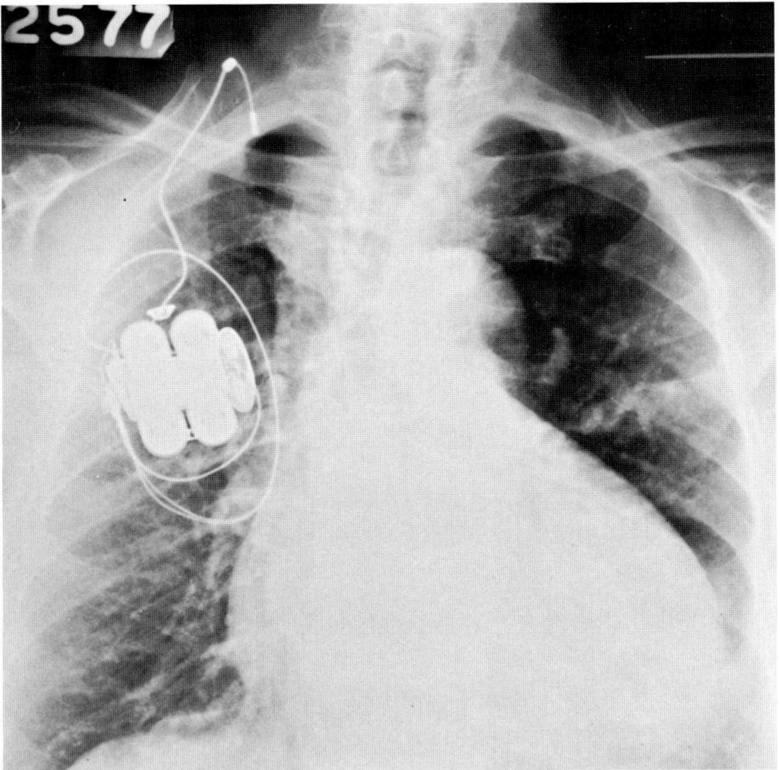

Fig. 11-8. Pacemaker twiddler's syndrome. The patient complained of twitching of her shoulder muscle. She had unknowingly twisted the generator on its axis. Note the lead coiled in the generator pocket.

tional strain, and it may fracture (17,18) (Fig. 11-9a–c).

Changes in generator position on serial films or the appearance of twists in the lead indicates that the generator pocket is too large. This eventually results in failure to pace because of electrode dislodgement or lead fracture. It is important to recognize that these changes are abnormal even if the tip of the electrode is still in the right ventricular apex.

Trauma

Patients with permanent pacemakers who sustain trauma present unusual clinical problems. Damage to the pacemaker system may be as critical as injury to the vital organs. Abrupt cessation of pacing may produce asystole, syncope, and even sudden death. Many patients, however, exhibit cerebral symptoms that may simulate cerebral trauma.

If the pacemaker is damaged following trauma, the damage usually takes one of two forms: lead fracture (19–21) (Fig. 11-10) or electrode dislodgement (20,22). Examination of the pacemaker should not be overlooked in patients involved in accidents. If the accident victim with an implanted pacemaker exhibits changes in mental status, irregularities or changes in pulse rate, overpenetrated posteroanterior and lateral chest films should be obtained to evaluate the pacemaker system. The potentially lethal complication of damage to the cardiac pacing system in trauma victims can be corrected if detected.

Myocardial Perforation

Bernstein et al. (23) reported a 7.1% incidence of myocardial perforation by transvenous electrodes. The true incidence may be higher, however, because many patients are clinically asymptomatic and pacing continues uneventfully, although at a higher threshold. This complication usually occurs at the time of insertion or during the first few days thereafter.

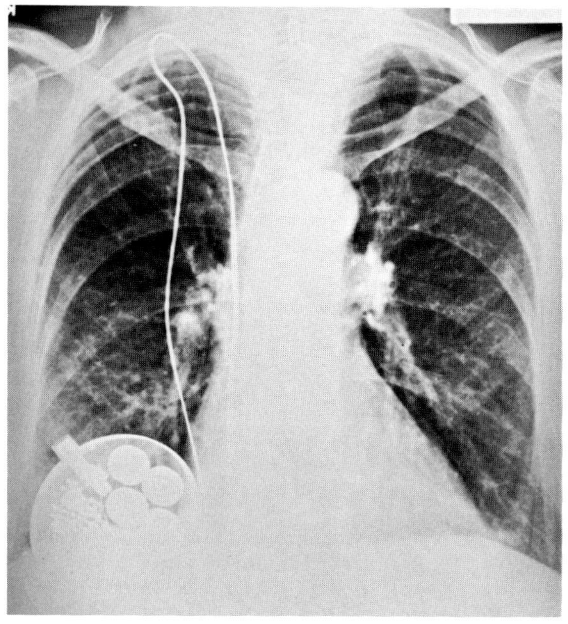

a

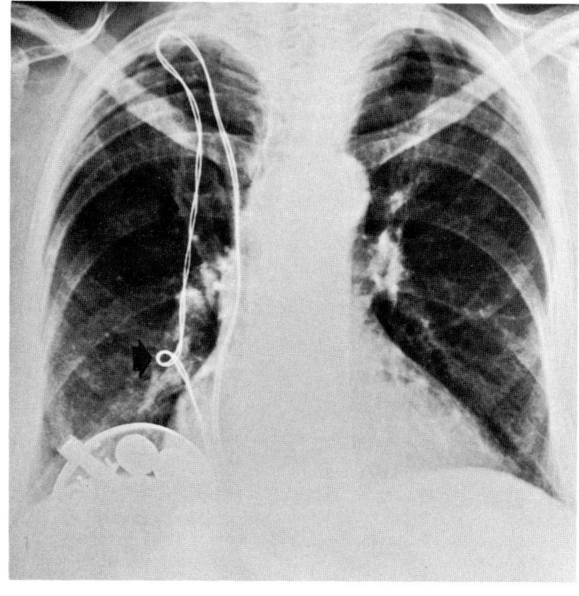

b

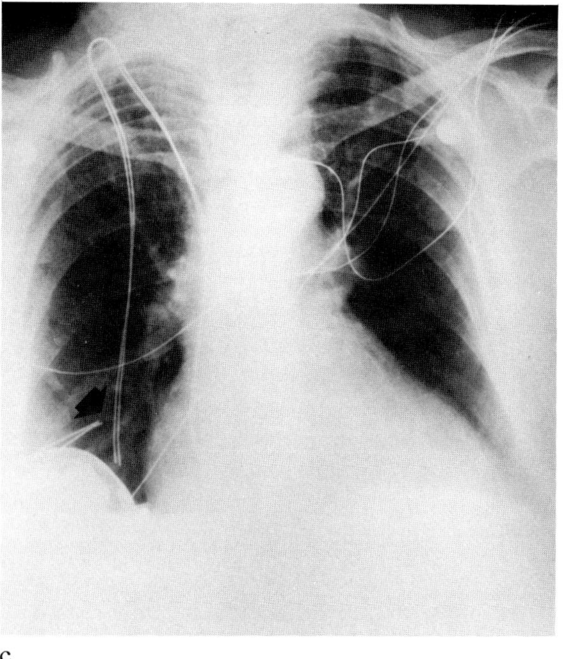

c

Fig. 11-9, a–c. Pacemaker twiddler's syndrome resulting in fractured lead. a Normal appearance of lead. The postimplantation frontal chest film demonstrates a normal transvenous lead in good position. (Tegtmeyer CJ, Deignan JM: AJR 126:1017–1018, 1976, with permission)

b Abnormal twisted lead. A follow-up radiograph obtained 13 days afer implantation shows the twisted endocardial leads (*arrows*). The electrode tip remains in good position, with normal pacing. The significance of the twisted leads was missed at this time. It indicates that the generator is rotating in a capacious pocket. (Tegtmeyer CJ, Deignan JM: AJR 126:1017–1018, 1976, with permission)

c Radiograph demonstrating fractured leads. A posteroanterior radiograph taken six months later reveals fractured transvenous leads (*arrow*). The patient stated that she had occasionally felt the pacemaker turn over in the pouch when she rolled over in bed. This caused increased tension on the leads and ultimately resulted in their fracture. (Tegtmeyer CJ, Deignan JM: AJR 126:1017–1018, 1976, with permission)

Perforation should be suspected when the pacemaker fails to sense or elicit a ventricular response. This failure may be continuous or intermittent, about half the patients with perforation however will continue to pace satisfactorily. An occasional patient will experience twitching of the diaphragmatic, intercostal, or abdominal muscles and, occasionally, pain or singultus. The ECG may show a change from the left bundle-branch block pattern of right ventricular pacing to a right bundle-branch block pattern due to stimulation of the left ventricle.

Roentgenograms may be diagnostic. There is usually no difficulty in identifying myocardial per-

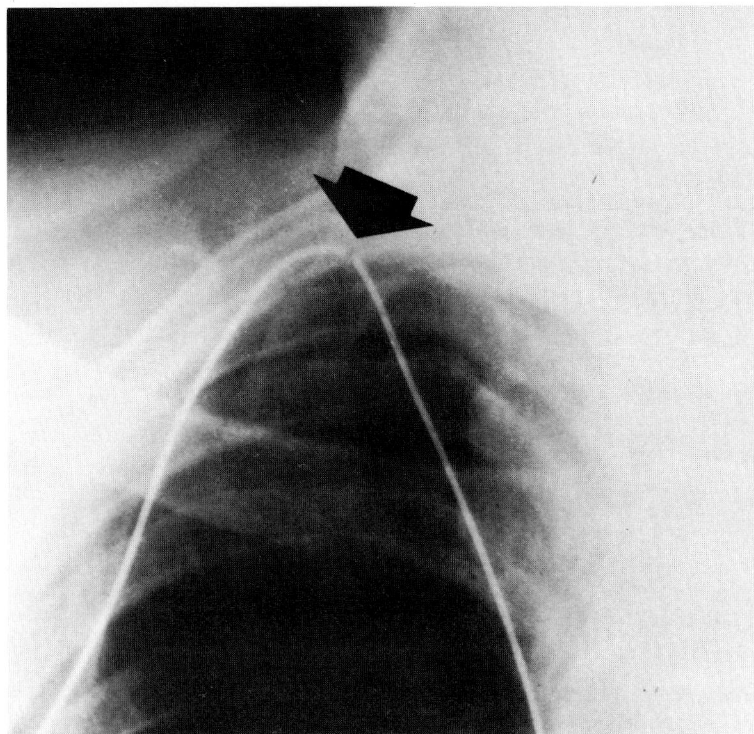

Fig. 11-10. Fractured transvenous lead due to trauma. The posteroanterior chest radiograph reveals a fractured transvenous lead (*arrow*). Two days prior to this film, the patient sustained an electric shock while trying to plug in her sewing machine. This event resulted in a sudden forced abduction and hyperextension of the right shoulder and upper extremity. Following this she complained of being tired and feeling weak and dizzy. Her pulse was found to be 32 per minute. (Tegtmeyer CJ, Bezirdjian DR, Irani FA, Landis JD: South Med J 74:378–379, 1981, with permission)

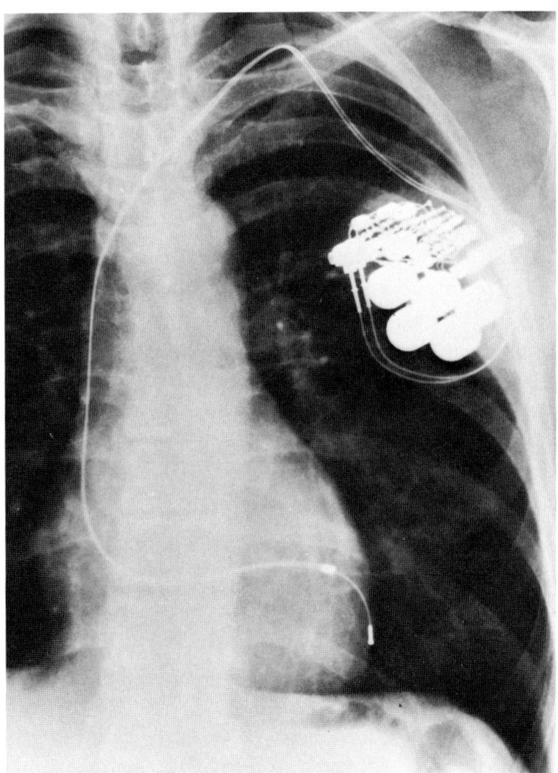

Fig. 11-11. Perforation of the myocardium by transvenous lead. Perforation of the myocardium by the electrode is evident on the posteroanterior film. Shortly after insertion this pacemaker failed to pace. The pacemaker subsequently recaptured the heart; however, the electrocardiogram changed to a right bundle-branch block pattern. (Tegtmeyer CJ: Am Fam Physician 14:66–75, 1976, with permission)

foration, since either the posteroanterior or lateral film will show the catheter tip lying outside the right ventricular cavity (Fig. 11-11). The right ventricular myocardium is only 4–5 mm thick, however, and the changes in the position of the electrode may be subtle. Lateral migration of the lead, noted when serial films are compared, is also a sign of perforation. In most cases, the electrode can be withdrawn under fluoroscopic control with little difficulty. Cardiac tamponade from pericardial bleeding has been reported, but it is uncommon.

Pulse Generator or Battery Failure

If the power source is separated from the generator, generator failure may occur, but it is relatively infrequent. Failure of the generator components is usually due to failure of a transistor, or connecting bridge or to a leak in the generator case. The radiograph is of little value in detecting component failure because the changes are usually too subtle to be recorded on the roentgenogram.

The majority of pulse generator failures, however, result from the depletion of the power supply. In the past, roentgenograms were employed to assess mercury batteries. The radiograph can detect a poor battery; however, electronic analysis is necessary to predict battery life. Since the middle of the 1970s, lithium power supplies have been implanted with increasing frequency because of their longer battery life. Today, roentgenographic evaluation of the power supply is of little value, because radiographic changes cannot be detected in the lithium batteries.

Complications Related to Pacemaker Insertion or Presence Within the Body

The complications associated with transvenous electrodes are related to inserting a foreign body into the heart and vascular system. Epicardial pacing may also be complicated by the body's reaction to the leads. The leads, however, are not situated within the vascular tree. Therefore, thrombosis and embolism are not hazards as in transvenous insertion. The major complications of epicardial pacing are those of thoracotomy and general anesthesia. The introduction of the sutureless, "screw-in" electrodes has reduced the incidence of these problems.

Air Embolus

Accidental venous air embolism can result from the fluctuation in intrathoracic pressures during respiration. Air embolism has been reported following the insertion of transvenous pacemaker leads in the neck. However, operators are aware of the problem, and care is taken to avoid this complication.

Venous Thrombosis

The complication of large-vein thrombosis and, in particular, subclavian-axillary thrombosis has occurred with varying frequency following permanent insertion of foreign bodies into the great veins. Autopsy studies showed that four to five days after implantation of pacemakers, there was marked thrombosis developing at the site of electrode implantation and along the leads. Seven months after implantation, thrombi were completely endothelialized, forming a sheath around the wire. By 26 months, thrombotic material had been resolved, and the electrodes were surrounded by a fibrous sheath (24).

Balau et al. (25) performed venograms in 49 patients following pacemaker implantation through the cephalic vein and found radiographic evidence of thrombi in 14. Despite this, clinically evident thrombosis remains uncommon following the insertion of transvenous cardiac pacemakers (26,27).

Superior vena cava obstruction may also result from the insertion of transvenous pacemaker electrodes (28,29), and transvenous cardiac pacing should be considered in the differential diagnosis of superior vena cava syndrome. The patients usually improve following treatment with anticoagulants without removing the leads.

Venography is a valuable study in patients with transvenous pacemakers who present with swelling of an arm or with superior vena cava syndrome. The axillary and subclavian veins are easily demonstrated by injecting contrast material through a 19-gauge scalp vein needle inserted into a vein on the medial aspect of the antecubital fossa (Fig. 11-12). Visualization of the superior vena cava is enhanced by simultaneously injecting contrast material into each arm.

Pulmonary Embolism

Pulmonary embolism is a rare complication of transvenous pacing. However, pulmonary emboli originating on transvenous electrodes have been implicated in the deaths of at least six patients (8). Although rare, pulmonary embolism should be considered in any patient with an implanted transvenous pacemaker who develops episodic dyspnea, tachypnea, and cyanosis.

Infection

The insertion of a foreign material inside the body carries with it a certain risk of infection. When the infection is localized, it presents as pain over the generator site. If the infection is not controlled, the generator may be extruded. Roentgen findings in such cases are similar to those that have been observed in other localized infections. The infection may travel along the lead to the myocardium, resulting in an increase in stimulation threshold and exit block. Septicemia, septic pulmonary emboli, and endocarditis have also been reported as

complications of cardiac pacing. Death may result from these complications.

Two cases of bronchocutaneous fistula resulting from infected pacemaker electrodes have been reported (30,31). In both cases, the infection traveled along retained epicardial leads after the infected pulse generator had been removed. A sinogram, obtained by injecting radiopaque contrast material into the cutaneous fistula, will delineate the extent of the fistula (Fig. 11-13a–c).

Extreme caution should be used when treating infected pacemakers. The infected pacemaker is not an ordinary wound infection because the pacing wires lead inward to the heart.

Summary

Electronic control of the heart has proven effective for patients with conductive defects, and it is estimated that more than 150,000 pacemakers have been implanted since the first self-contained unit was implanted in 1960. The introduction of this therapeutic modality, however, provides a new source of complications. After a pacemaker has been installed, the physician's attention must be directed not only to the patient's illness but also to the frailties of the pacemaker. The roentgenogram is a valuable resource in the management of patients with cardiac pacemakers.

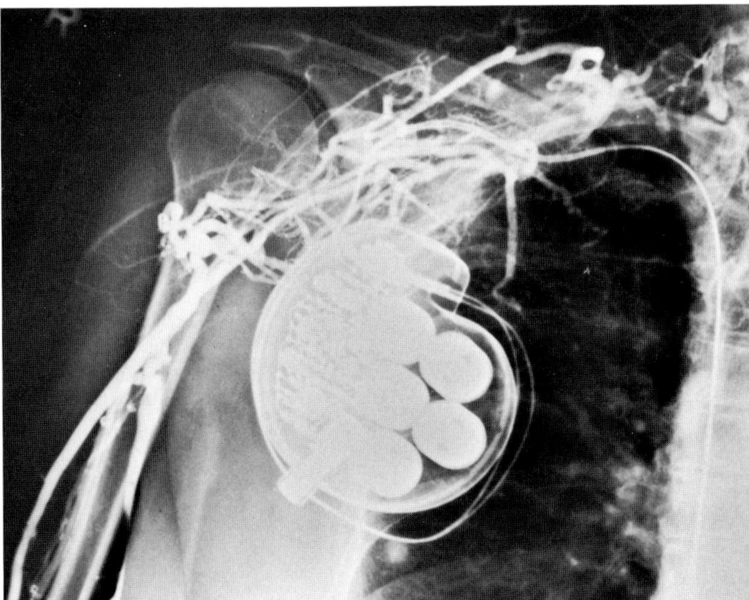

Fig. 11-12. **Venous thrombosis resulting from transvenous leads.** The patient developed a swollen painful arm three days after insertion of her pacemaker. The phlebogram demonstrates complete obstruction of the subclavian vein. Collaterals carry the contrast material around the obstruction. (Tegtmeyer CJ: Am Fam Physician 14:66–75, 1976, with permission)

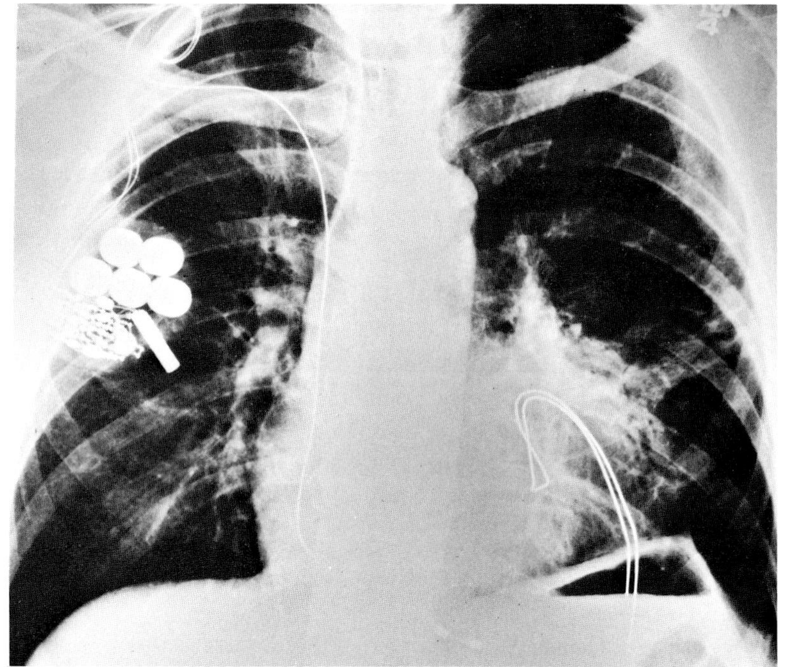

a

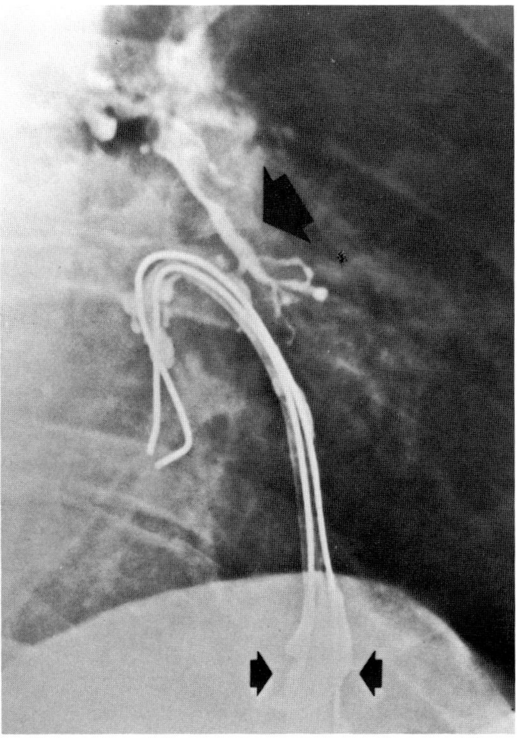

b

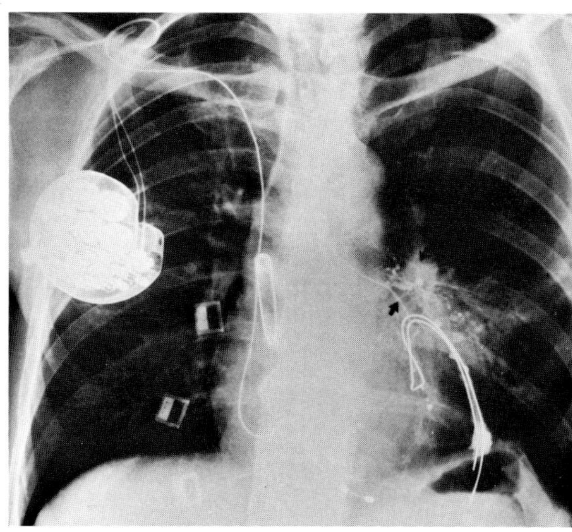

c

Fig. 11-13, a–c. Bronchocutaneous fistula, a complication of epicardial pacing. a Posteroanterior chest roentgenogram reveals an infiltrate in the lingula of a patient with a chronic productive cough. The proximal portion of the epicardial electrodes had been previously removed because of a persistent infection in the generator pocket. The functioning transvenous pacemaker is seen in good position. (Tegtmeyer CJ, Hunter JG Jr, Keats TE: AJR 121:614–616, 1974, with permission)

b A sinogram obtained by injecting contrast material into a persistently draining cutaneous fistula (*arrows*). The connection between the fistulous tract, which extends along the epicardial leads to the pericardium, and the lingular bronchus is demonstrated. (Tegtmeyer CJ, Hunter JG Jr, Keats TE: AJR 121:614–616, 1974, with permission)

c A follow-up chest film demonstrates the bronchocutaneous fistula and the lingular infiltrate (*arrows*). (Tegtmeyer CJ, Hunter JG Jr, Keats TE: AJR 121:614–616, 1974, with permission)

References

1. McHenry MM, Grayson CE: Roentgenographic diagnosis of pacemaker failure. AJR 109:94–100, 1970.
2. Rembert FM, Cooley RN: Implantable cardiac pacemakers: radiologic appearance. Tex Med 63:72–78, 1967.
3. Sorkin RP, Schuurmann BJ, Simon AB: Radiographic aspects of permanent cardiac pacemakers. Radiology 119:281–286, 1976.
4. Standen JR: The radiologist and the cardiac pacemaker. J Can Assoc Radiol 22:203–213, 1970.
5. Steiner RM, Morse D: The radiology of cardiac pacemakers. JAMA 240:2574–2576, 1978.
6. Tegtmeyer CJ: The roentgenology of cardiac pacemakers. Contemp Surg 1:79–88, 1972.
7. Tegtmeyer CJ: The complications and causes of cardiac pacemaker failure, a roentgen evaluation. Am Fam Physician 14:66–75, 1976.
8. Tegtmeyer CJ: Roentgenographic assessment of causes of cardiac pacemaker failure and complications. CRC Crit Rev Diagn Imaging 9:1–50, 1977.
9. Tegtmeyer CJ: The roentgenographic diagnosis of pacemaker failure and complications. *In* Morse D, Steiner RM: The Pacemaker and Valve Identification Guide. Garden City, New York: Medical Examination Inc, 1978.
10. Rosenbaum HD: Roentgen demonstration of broken cardiac pacemaker wires. Radiology 84:933–936, 1965.
11. Furman S, Escher DJW, Schwedel JW, Solomon N, Rubinstein B: Motion factors producing breaks in implanted cardiac leads. Surg Forum 15:248–249, 1964.
12. Medtronic, Inc. X-ray appearance of Medtronic models 6972 and 6990 U leads. Medtronic News 10:14–15, 1980.
13. Meyer JA, Millar K: Malplacement of pacemaker catheters in the coronary sinus. J Thorac Cardiovasc Surg 57:511–518, 1969.
14. Ragaza EP, Shapiro R: Radiologic recognition of unusual sites of a transvenous catheter pacemaker. J Can Assoc Radiol 21:214–216, 1970.
15. Kaul TK, Bain WH: Radiographic appearances of implanted transvenous endocardial pacing electrodes. Chest 72:323–326, 1977.
16. Bayliss CE, Beanlands DS, Baird RJ: The pacemaker twiddler's syndrome: a new complication of the implantable transvenous pacemaker. Can Med Assoc J 99:371–373, 1968.
17. Rodan BA, Lowe JE, Chen JTT: Abdominal twiddler's syndrome. AJR 131:1084–1085, 1978.
18. Tegtmeyer CJ, Deignan JM: The cardiac pacemaker: a different twist. AJR 126:1017–1018, 1976.
19. Kronzon I, Mehta SS: Broken pacemaker wire in multiple trauma: a case report. J Trauma 14:82–84, 1974.
20. Ohm O-J: Displacement and fracture of pacemaker electrode during physical exertion. Acta Med Scand 192:33–35, 1972.
21. Tegtmeyer CJ, Bezirdjian DR, Irani FA, Landis JD: Cardiac pacemaker failure: a complication of trauma. South Med J 74:378–379, 1981.
22. Lasky II: Pacemaker failure from automobile accident. Letter to the Editor. JAMA 211:1700, 1970.
23. Bernstein V, Rotem CE, Peretz DI: Permanent pacemakers: 8-year follow-up study. Ann Intern Med 74:361–369, 1971.
24. Huang TY, Baba N: Cardiac pathology of transvenous pacemaker. Am Heart J 83:469–474, 1972.
25. Balau J, Buysch KH, Marx E, Seling A, Knieriem H-J: Thrombose der Vena subclavia nach transvenoser Schrittmacher Implantation. Radiologe 11:50–57, 1971.
26. Rubio PA, Coan JD, Farrell EM, Berkman NL: Subclavian thrombosis secondary to transvenous pacing wire. South Med J 73:1547, 1980.
27. Williams EH, Tyers GFO, Shaffer CW: Symptomatic deep venous thrombosis of the arm associated with permanent transvenous pacing electrodes. Chest 73:613–615, 1978.
28. Branson JA: Radiology of cardiac pacemakers and their complications with three cases of superior vena caval obstruction. Aust Radiol 22.125–131, 1978.
29. Chamorro H, Rao G, Wholey MH: Superior vena cava syndrome: a complication of transvenous pacemaker implantation. Radiology 126:377–378, 1978.
30. Chua FS, Leininger BJ, Hamouda FA, PiFarre RF: Bronchopleura cutaneous fistula from infected pacemaker electrodes. Chest 63:284–286, 1973.
31. Tegtmeyer CJ, Hunter JG Jr, Keats TE: Bronchocutaneous fistula as a late complication of permanent epicardial pacing. AJR 121:614–616, 1974.

12 The Radiology of Prosthetic Cardiac Valves

Robert M. Steiner and Gary S. Mintz

Since Harken et al. in 1959 and Starr and Edwards in 1960 successfully implanted the first caged-ball valve prostheses in the aortic valve, continuous and dramatic improvement in operative mortality, the quality of the prosthetic devices, and the rate of postoperative complications has been achieved. At the present time, late deaths related to prosthetic valve implantation occur in approximately 10% of patients. Death is due in large part to intrinsic cardiac problems, such as myocardial infarction and arrhythmias, and also to complications directly related to the prosthesis itself. Life-threatening complications associated with cardiac valve implantation include thromboembolism, hemolysis, paravalvular or valvular insufficiency, infection, and those of anticoagulation (1).

The radiologist has a particularly important role in identifying the nature of the complications of prosthetic valve implantation using the tools of fluoroscopy, echocardiography, plain-film radiology, and angiography.

In this chapter an approach to the diagnosis of complications associated with prosthetic valve implantation will be offered together with comments on the evaluation of the patient with cardiac disease prior to surgery.

Selection of the Patient for Cardiac Valve Replacement

When cardiac valve disease is suspected clinically, a plain film of the chest will often yield important confirmatory information. A four-view cardiac series consisting of films in the erect posterior-anterior, lateral, and both right and left 45° oblique positions will outline the cardiac borders to best advantage. Thick barium sulfate is administered before each exposure to outline the esophagus, providing additional visualization of the cardiac borders. Barium is omitted in the left anterior oblique view so as not to obscure the area of the ductus arteriosus and the aorticopulmonary window. Fluoroscopy, preferably with videotape recording, supplements the four-view heart study. The presence or absence of annular or valve calcification and coronary artery calcification may be appreciated best by means of fluoroscopy, should calcification be present, additional studies, such as coronary arteriography, left ventricular angiography, and echocardiography may be needed. Calcification, especially of the mitral valve and annulus, will influence the type of surgery performed. Extensive calcification of the mitral valve leaflets or chordae will preclude mitral commissurotomy, which otherwise may be the procedure of choice. Successful mitral commissurotomy depends on the presence of a flexible, competent, noncalcified valve and is the preferable procedure for many surgeons because of the lower operative risk compared with valve replacement (1). Postoperative complications are reduced and chronic anticoagulation is avoided when commissurotomy is performed rather than mechanical valve replacement. It also appears that commissurotomy may delay valvular scarring and calcification and thus delay valve replacement. If a stenotic mitral valve is calcified, valve replacement is the procedure of choice in patients with New York Heart Association Functional Class III or greater (2,3).

The presence or absence of valve calcification is less important in a patient with severe aortic stenosis, since replacement will be recommended in all patients with significant aortic outflow tract obstruction, as determined by the patient's symptoms, echocardiography, and angiocardiography. Aortic valve commissurotomy is reserved for those patients with congenital aortic stenosis (2,3).

Patients with aortic insufficiency have a slower, more predictable rate of deterioration than those with aortic stenosis. Patients with aortic regurgitation who develop clinical signs of congestive failure have significant irreversible myocardial damage. Valve replacement is recommended when the patient is disabled with angina but before congestive failure ensues.

The sudden onset of severe aortic insufficiency may be related to aortic dissection or endocarditis. Such patients will require immediate replacement.

In mitral insufficiency, as in aortic insufficiency, the course of disease is prolonged and the patients may show increased heart size with few symptoms. Frequent chest films to monitor development of rapid cardiac enlargement, vascular redistribution, and other signs of left ventricular failure are helpful in determining when valve replacement must supersede medical treatment (3).

Radiologic Examination Following Valve Implantation

Once the native valve is replaced, the radiologist must be concerned with changes due to the many complications of prosthetic valves, including paravalvular insufficiency; structural changes of the base ring, struts, or occluder; evidence of obstruction due to tissue encroachment or thrombus formation; thromboembolic disease; infective endocarditis; and the effects of the use of chronic anticoagulants, including pulmonary and gastrointestinal hemorrhage.

Radiographic follow-up should include postsurgical videotape recording of prosthetic valve motion to act as a baseline study, as 10%–15% of patients develop alterations of function due to prosthetic failure within two years (2–9). Echocardiography is performed at the same time. The relative value of echocardiography and fluoroscopy in evaluation of prosthetic valve malfunction de-

pends on the type of valve implanted and its complications.

Evaluation of the chest when the patient has undergone cardiac valve replacement should include identification of the valve implanted, the number of valves implanted, and the position of the valves inserted, together with changes in the cardiac and mediastinal contour, in the search for complications or coexistent disease. Valve replacement is almost always performed through a median sternotomy. The presence of sutures or rib fractures suggesting right or left thoracotomy is usually related to other surgical procedures. For example, separation or fracture of the left posterior fifth and sixth ribs may be related to a previous mitral commissurotomy. A left thoracotomy in a patient with a prosthetic aortic valve may suggest that coarctation of the aorta was also present, and the mediastinotomy was done to replace an associated stenotic bicuspid valve (10). A right thoracotomy may be due to lung surgery, or mitral or tricuspid plication.

Radiographic Identification of Prosthetic Valves

There are over 40 cardiac prostheses distributed in the United States, with widely differing modes of action and complication rates. They are designed for the aortic, mitral, and tricuspid valves and also for use in intravascular conduits. Since operative notes may not be readily available, and since patients may not know the type of valve implanted, it is useful to be familiar with the distinguishing radiographic characteristics of each valve. The choice may be narrowed for the more common valves by using one of the published articles or guidebooks on prosthetic valve identification (1,3,11–13) (Fig. 12-1).

The major types of mechanical prostheses include the caged-ball valve, the low-profile caged-disc valve, the hinged-leaflet valve, and the cageless monocuspid tilting valve and tissue valves (Fig. 12-2).

Caged-Ball Valves

The caged-ball valves consist of an occluder of spherical shape and a base ring placed in the plane

RADIOLOGIC IDENTIFICATION OF COMMON CARDIAC PROSTHETIC VALVES AND THEIR ASSOCIATED COMPLICATIONS

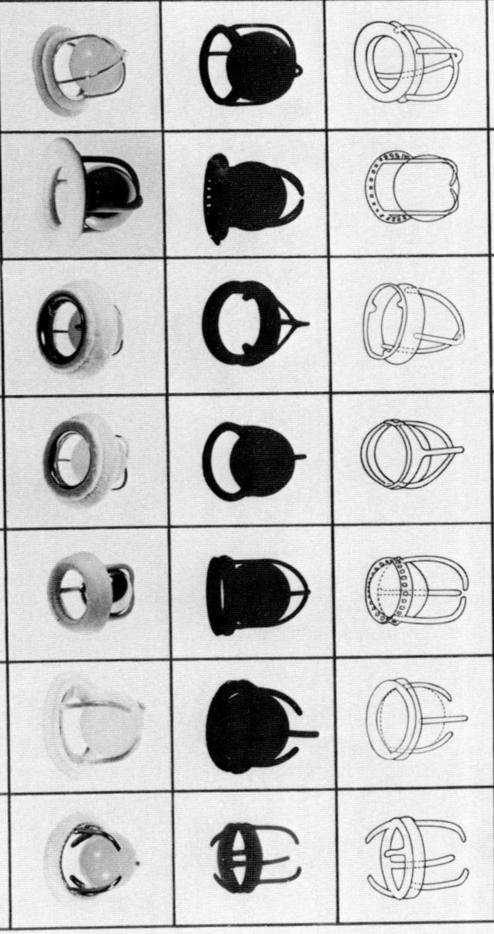

VALVE	SHAPE	X-RAY	X-RAY OUTLINE	MITRAL/ TRICUSPID	AORTIC	IDENTIFYING FEATURES	COMPLICATIONS
			BALL VALVES				
Starr-Edwards 6000				•		1. double donut 2. 4 thick struts joined at apex 3. radiolucent poppet (some with barium)	1. thromboemboli 2. ball variance 3. left ventricular incorporation of cage
6300				•		1. concave perforations 2. 4 thin struts not joined at apex 3. radiopaque poppet (in systole sits far from equator)	1. thromboemboli 2. bacterial endocarditis
1000					•	1. conical valve with 3 feet in orifice 2. 3 thin struts joined at apex 3. radiolucent poppet	1. thromboemboli 2. ball variance
1200					•	1. tapered support at each strut junction 2. 3 thin struts fused at apex 3. some barium poppets	1. thromboemboli 2. ball variance
2310					•	1. perforated concave valve base 2. 3 thin struts joined at apex after 12/69 3. radiopaque poppet (diastole sits close to equator)	1. close clearance model with poppet impacted in open position*
Braunwald-Cutter				•	•	1. open-ended cage 2. radiolucent poppet	1. thromboemboli 2. ball variance 3. hemolysis 4. cloth wear at apex 5. peri-valvular leaks
Smeloff-Cutter				•	•	1. open-ended cage 2. 3 struts 3. full-flow orifice ball valve 4. radiolucent poppet	1. thromboemboli 2. hemolysis 3. ball variance 4. open top buried in ventricular septum*

* characteristic for valve

Fig. 12-1. Prosthetic valve guide. The valves are identified by photographic and radiologic appearance. Asterisk indicates complications characteristic of valve. (Reprinted from Chun P, Nelson W: JAMA 237:401–403, 1977, with permission)

BALL VALVES continued							
VALVE	SHAPE	X-RAY	X-RAY OUTLINE	MITRAL/ TRICUSPID	AORTIC	IDENTIFYING FEATURES	COMPLICATIONS
MaGovern-Cromie				●	●	1. sutureless mechanical fixation prosthesis 2. open-ended cage 3. 3 struts 4. vertical fixation pins 5. radiopaque poppet	1. thromboemboli 2. hemolysis 3. ball variance
Debakey-Surgitool					●	1. closed-ended cage 2. 3 struts 3. serrated ring 4. radiolucent poppet	
LOW PROFILE VALVES A. DISC VALVES							
Starr-Edwards 6500				●		1. low profile cage 2. cross struts 3. radiopaque poppet 4. concave perforations	1. thromboemboli 2. cocking of disc
6520				●		1. low profile cage 2. cross struts 3. radiolucent poppet with radiopaque ring in poppet	
Kay-Shiley						1. single or double muscle guard 2. 2 parallel struts 3. radiolucent poppet	1. thromboemboli 2. sudden, unexpected, unexplained death 3. grooving and disc wear 4. restenosis with ingrowth` 5. perivalvular leaks 6. disc cocking, variance
Kay-Suzuki				●	●	1. close-ended cage 2. 4 struts 3. 4 short open base struts 4. double ring valve base 5. radiolucent poppet	1. thromboemboli 2. disc variance
Cross-Jones				●		1. open-ended cage 2. radiolucent poppet with radiopaque ring in poppet	1. thromboemboli 2. cocking of disc 3. disc variance

` characteristic for valve

DISC VALVES continued

VALVE	SHAPE	X-RAY	X-RAY OUTLINE	MITRAL/ TRICUSPID	AORTIC	IDENTIFYING FEATURES	COMPLICATIONS
Beall	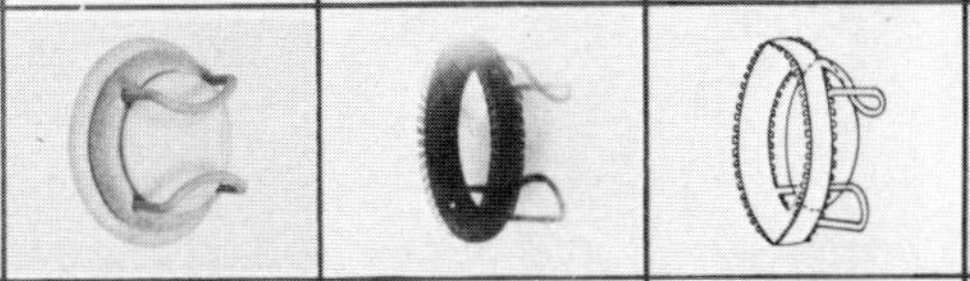			●		1. 2 parallel indented struts 2. radiopaque poppet	1. obstruction of prosthesis orifice by thrombus 2. cocking of disc 3. hemolysis 4. disc variance 5. gallstones*
Harken	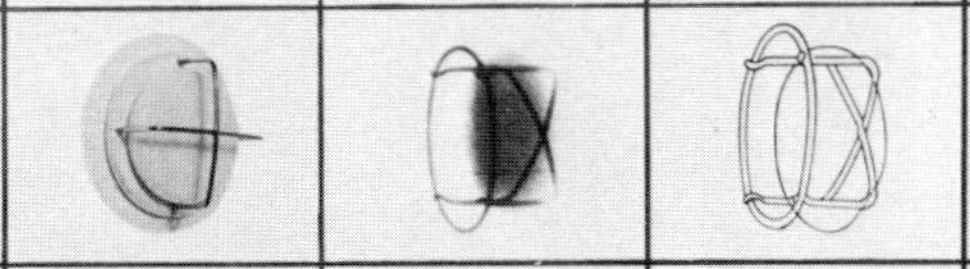				●	1. thin cross struts 2. radiopaque poppet	1. thromboemboli 2. disc variance
Cooley-Bloodwell-Cutter	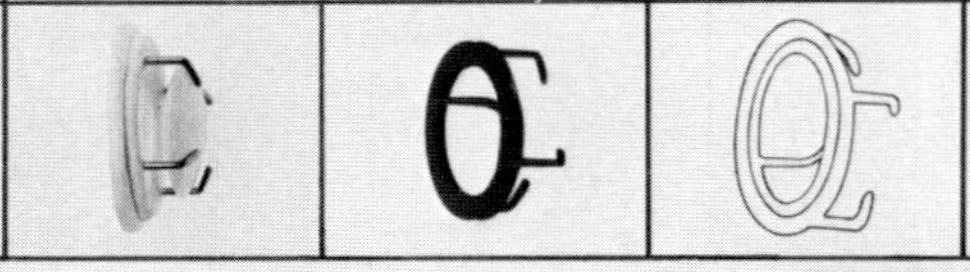			●		1. discoid valve 2. open-ended cage 3. 4 struts 4. radiolucent poppet	1. thromboemboli 2. prosthetic leaks 3. thrombotic valve occlusion
LOW PROFILE VALVES B. HINGED-LEAFLET VALVE							
Gott-Daggett	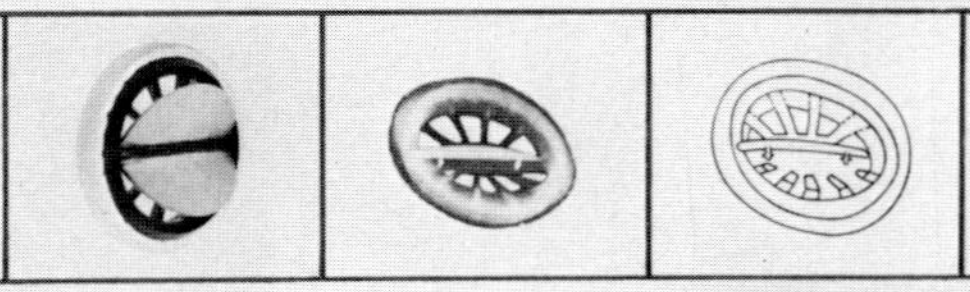				●	1. central cross strut 2. multiple projecting prongs from ring 3. radiolucent leaflets	1. thromboemboli 2. hemolysis 3. gallstones*
LOW PROFILE VALVES C. CENTRAL FLOW ECCENTRIC MONOCUSP VALVES							
Lillehei-Kaster	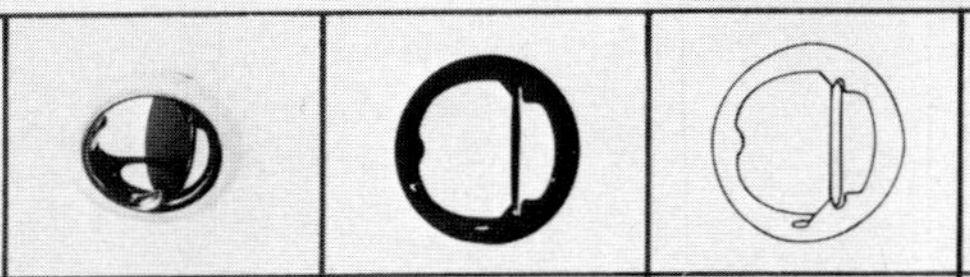			●		1. 2 teardrop-shaped pivots 2. 2 lateral disc guide-shields 3. radiolucent poppet	1. thromboemboli
Wada-Cutter	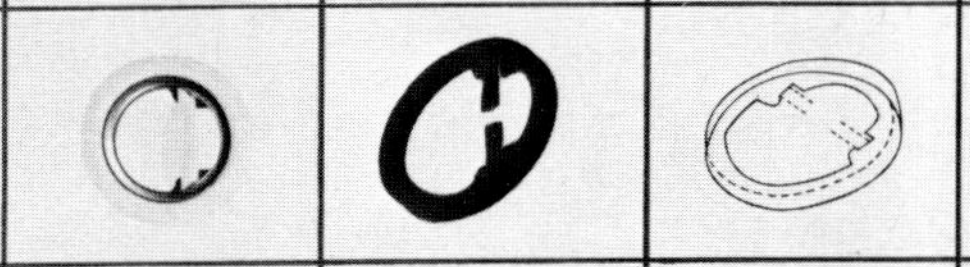			●	●	1. base ring with 2 notches 2. disc with 2 notches 3. radiolucent poppet	1. early disc wear 2. total valve thrombosis 3. thromboemboli 4. peri-basilar leaks with significant regurgitation
Bjork-Shiley	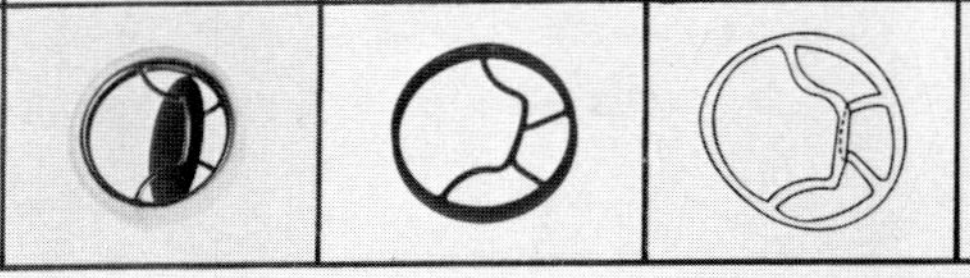			●	●	1. 2 eccentrically located support struts 2. radiolucent poppet	1. thromboemboli

*characteristic for valve

Fig. 12-1 (cont.)

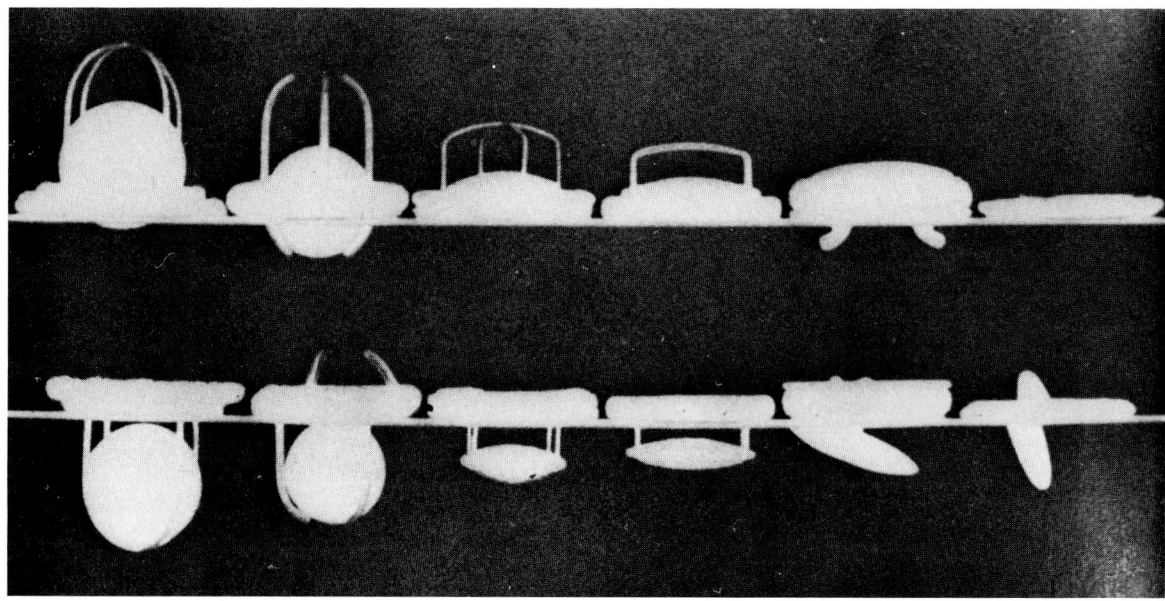

Fig. 12-2. Radiographs of the more common mechanical prosthetic valves. The upper row shows the valves in the closed position; the lower row shows the valves in the open position. From left to right are the caged-ball central occluding prosthesis with closed cage, caged-ball central occluding prosthesis with open cage, central occluding open-cage disc prosthesis, closed-disc prosthesis with flat cage, hinged-disc prosthesis, tilting-leaflet prosthesis.

of the valve annulus. The cage limits excursion of the occluder. The cage is composed of struts which join at the base ring. The valve may be open or closed at the apex of the cage (11) (Figs. 12-3, 12-4). The Starr-Edwards ball occluders were made of Silastic impregnated with barium to provide radiopacity (until 1974) and are now made of hollowed-out polished titanium metal to eliminate ball variance (14). The metal components are

covered with Teflon cloth to encourage development of a neointima (1,15). The early caged-ball prosthetic heart valves are the only completely silent mechanical prostheses, but the bulky high-profile design intrudes on a small left ventricle or small aortic root, occupying so much space that the flow rate may be compromised (1).

The more recent Starr-Edwards cloth-covered models have a lower thromboembolic rate, which

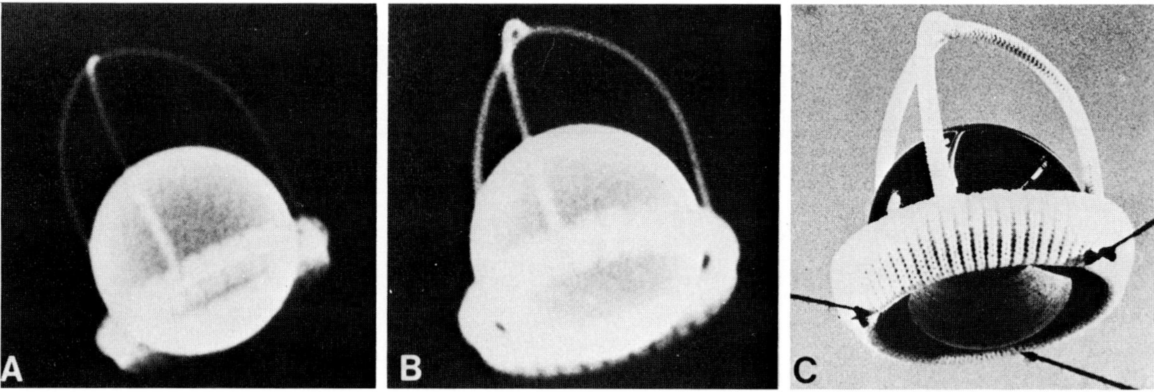

Fig. 12-3, a–c. Caged-ball prosthesis: Harken ball prosthesis in the aortic position. A in vitro AP radiograph; **B** in vitro lateral radiograph; **C** photograph in the lateral position. (Reprinted from Mehlman DJ, Resnekov L: Circulation 57:613–623, 1978, with permission)

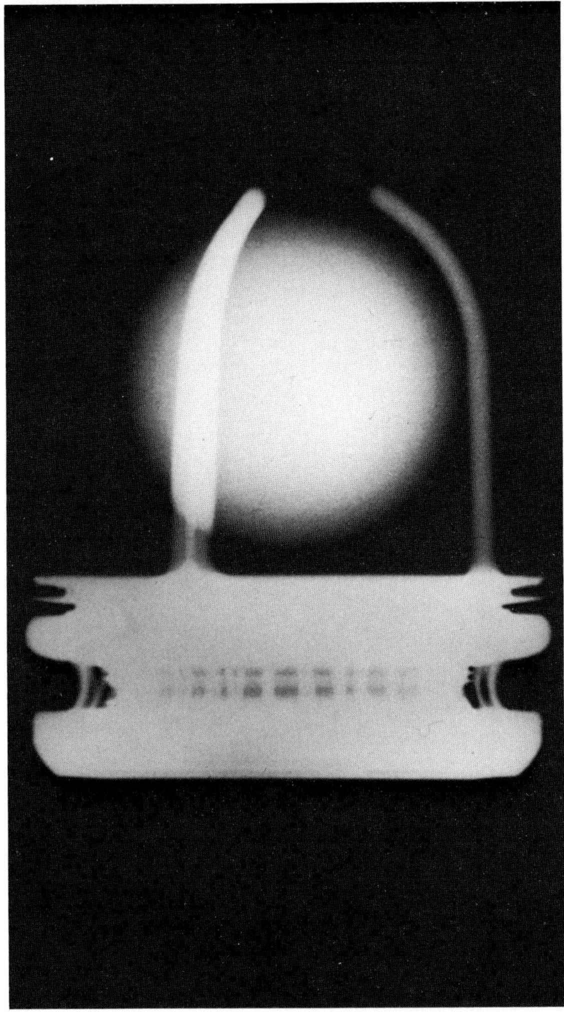

Fig. 12-4. Caged-ball prosthesis: Magovern-Cromie aortic valve. Numerous hooks emerge from the base ring. Three struts form an open-ended cage.

averages 3% per patient year at the mitral level and 1.5%–2% per patient year at the aortic level, in spite of chronic anticoagulation therapy.

The cloth-covered prostheses have a rougher surface, and as a result hemolysis is increased compared with valves with smooth exposed metal parts (1). The Starr-Edwards, the Braunwald-Cutter, the Harken, the Smeloff-Cutter, and the DeBakey-Surgitool valves are examples of the caged-ball type.

Caged-Disc Prosthesis

The lower-profile caged-disc prostheses include the Cooley-Cutter, Kay-Suzuki, Cross-Jones, Harken, Kay-Shiley, Beall, and Starr-Edwards 6500 models. The low-profile configuration has the advantage of reduced intrusion into a small outflow tract or chamber, but disc cocking and wear and a high incidence of thrombogenicity have been disadvantages with some of these models (Fig. 12-5).

Hinged-Disc Valves

In common use today is the hinged-disc valve, of which the Bjork-Shiley valve is the most commonly implanted. Other hinged-disc valves include the Hall-Kaster, Lillehei-Kaster, and Wada-Cutter (3,11,16) (Fig. 12-6).

The Bjork-Shiley concave-convex disc has a flat profile, so that when it is in the closed position it is within the framework of the sewing ring (Fig. 12-7). This is especially helpful in the patient with

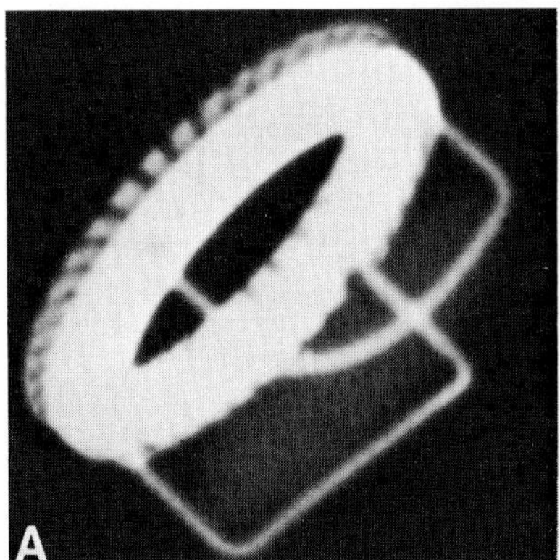
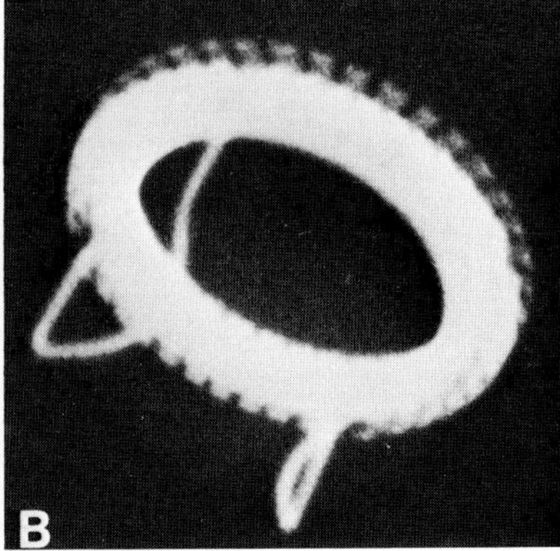
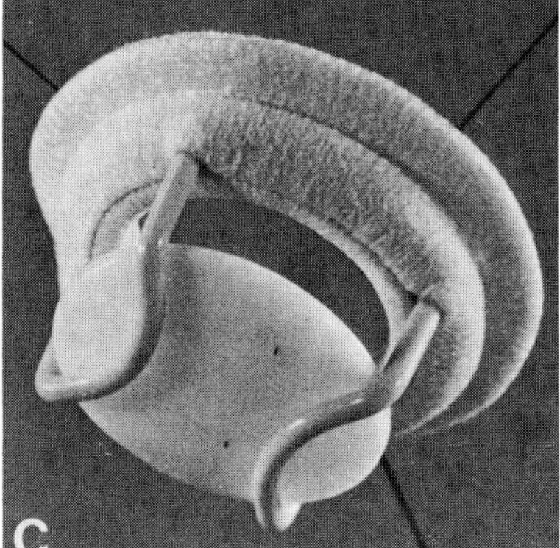

Fig. 12-5, a–c. Caged-disc prosthesis: Beall Model 103 in the mitral position. A AP radiograph; **B** left lateral radiograph; **C** photograph—note the serrated edges of the base ring and the radiolucent disc, which help to identify this model. (Reprinted from Mehlman DJ, Resnekov L: Circulation 57:613–623, 1978, with permission)

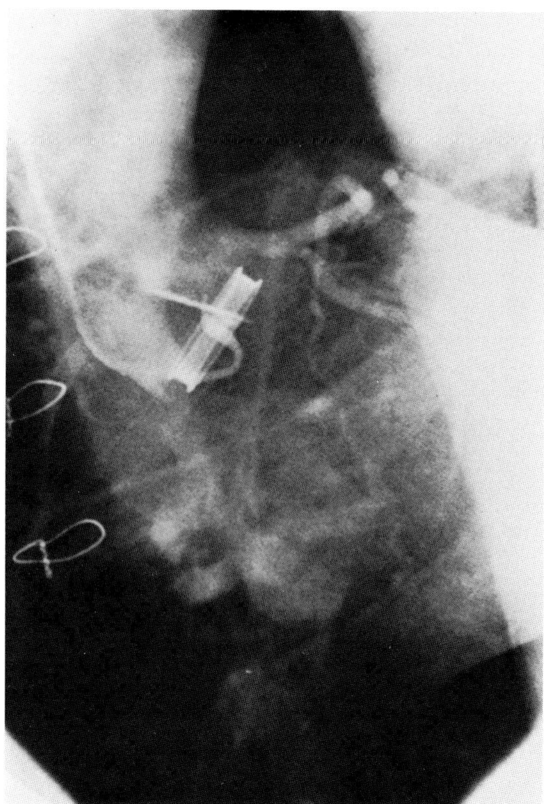

Fig. 12-6. Tilting-disc prosthesis: Hall-Kaster aortic prosthesis. The patient is undergoing aortography in the left anterior oblique position. No valvular insufficiency is noted.

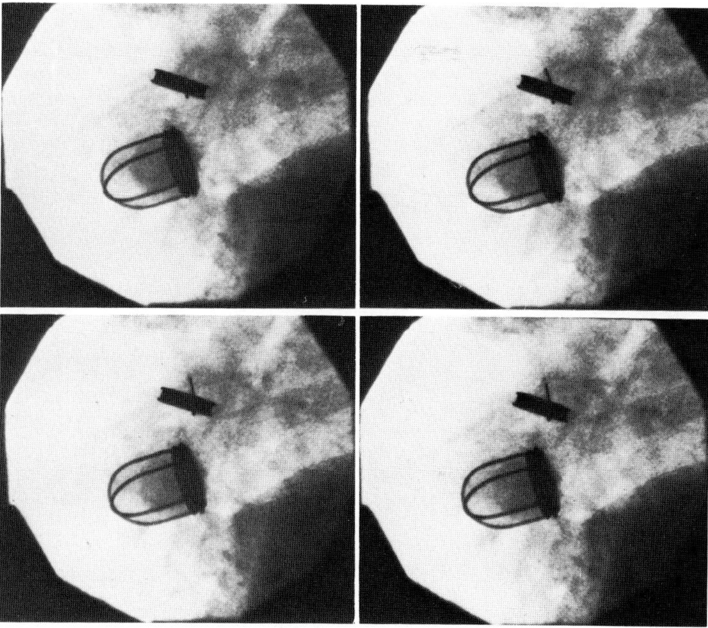

Fig. 12-7. Tilting-disc prosthesis. Frames from a cineradiograph in a patient with a Bjork-Shiley aortic prosthesis and a Starr-Edwards mitral valve. In the upper left frame the Bjork-Shiley valve is in the closed position. In the remaining frames the disc is in the open position with a normal angle of 60°. (Venkataraman K et al: Radiology 137:43–47, 1980, with permission)

a small ventricular chamber or in the aortic root. Since the cross-sectional area is large when in the open position, flow is relatively unimpeded and hemolysis is trivial.

The incidence of thromboemboli of Bjork-Shiley valves is less than 1.1% patient-years at the mitral level and 0.7% at the aortic level. Thrombosis of the valve has been reported (15), causing sticking of the tilting disc. Sticking is suggested when excursion in systole and diastole deviates from the usual 60° arc seen by fluoroscopy (17,18).

St. Jude Valve

A new mechanical prosthesis is the St. Jude valve, consisting of two semicircular discs which pivot into position, eliminating any supporting struts. Study of the St. Jude prosthesis demonstrates good hydraulic function and a low incidence of throm-boembolic complications. The half discs are visible by cinefluoroscopy, but there is no ideal predicted position and each patient must be individually evaluated (Fig. 12-8). In a tangential view, the valve leaflets traverse an arc of 50°–55° and lie at 30°–35° angles from each other when closed and at an 80° angle in the open position. En face, the discs open and close symmetrically. Asymmetric opening has been described in the mitral position with uncorrected aortic insufficiency (19).

Heterograft Valves

Heterograft tissue valves are in common use and include the Hancock porcine bioprosthesis (Fig. 12-9a), the Carpentier-Edwards porcine bioprosthesis (Fig. 12-9b), the Zerbini Duramater, the Angel-Shiley, and the Ionescu-Shiley (Fig. 12-9c) bovine pericardial valves.

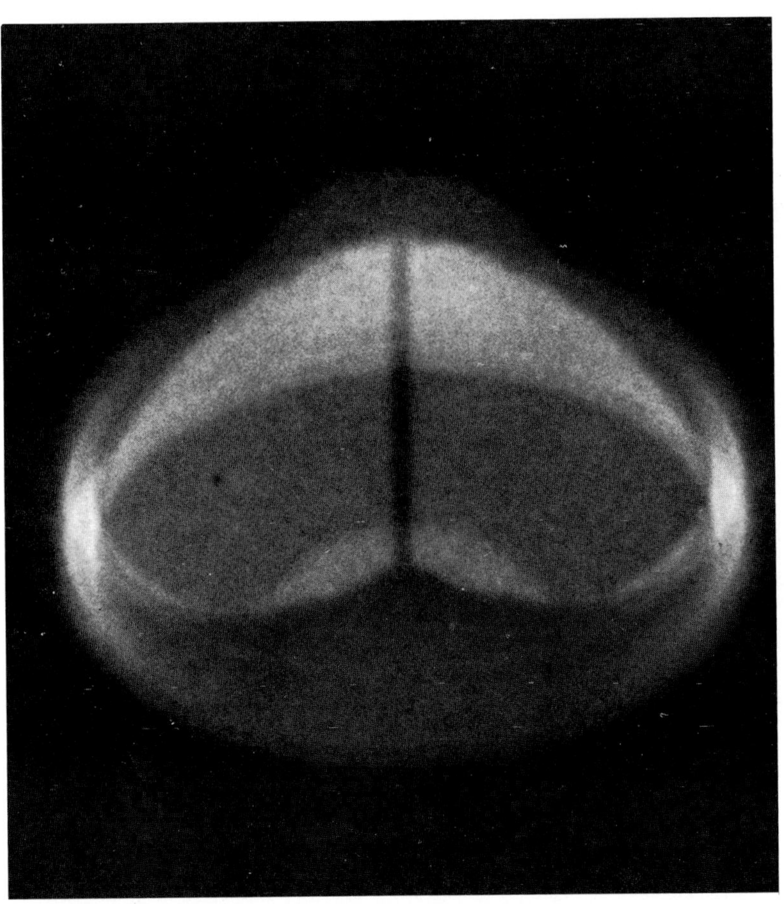

Fig. 12-8. Pivoting-leaflet prosthesis. AP radiograph of the St. Jude pivoting prosthesis.

                                                         R. M. Steiner and G. S. Mintz

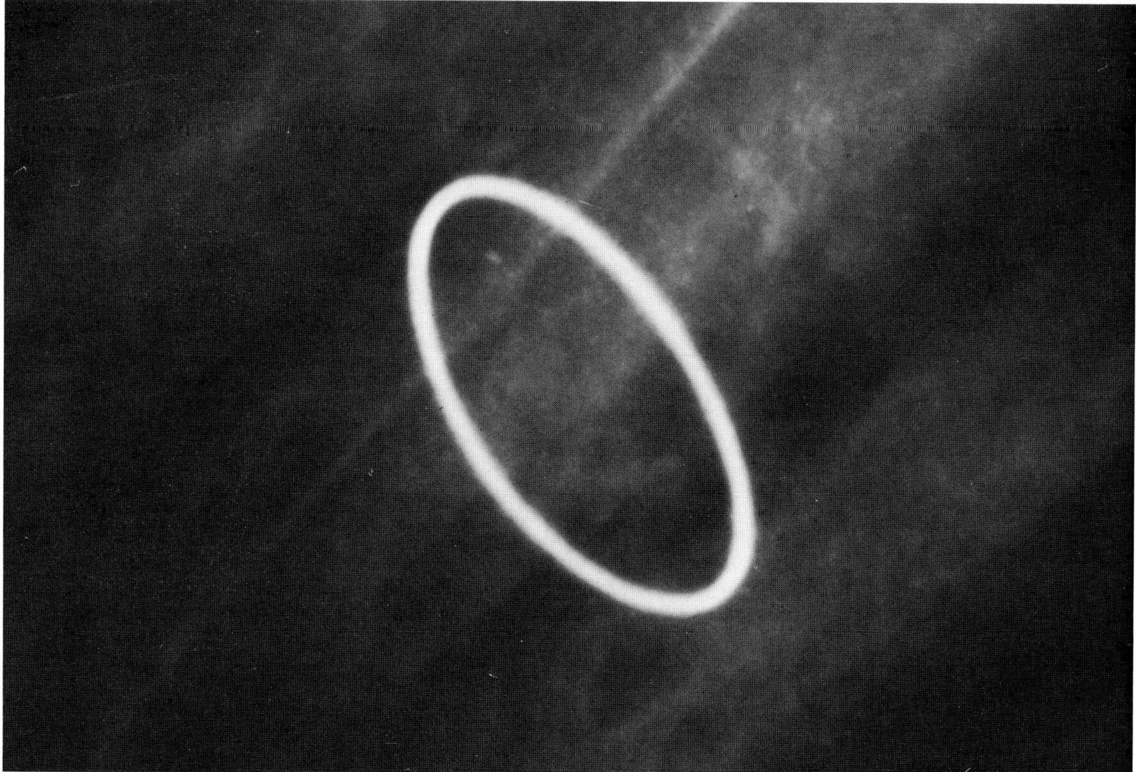

Fig. 12-9, a–c. Heterograft valves. a Hancock porcine valve. Only the metal supporting ring is radiopaque. **b** Carpentier-Edwards porcine mitral valve. The cobalt-nickel frame is radiopaque. Note the calcifications in the degenerating heterograft components. **c** Ionescu-Shiley calf pericardial tissue valve. The three-pronged stent with three holes in each stent and evenly spaced holes along the base is characteristic.

With the exception of the Angel-Shiley valve, all the tissue prostheses have radiopaque metal components.

Fluoroscopic Evaluation Following Valve Implantation

Fluoroscopy with cine or videotape recording is a valuable method to analyze the motion of the occluding leaflet or ball and the radiopaque elements of the cage and sewing ring. It is also useful to identify calcifications in tissue valves and in the native supporting structures.

"Normal" motion differs for each prosthetic model and for each individual patient. For this reason it is useful to perform fluoroscopy before the patient leaves the hospital to record the information in a videotape bank for future reference (3–5,20). The normal motion of several valves has been described, including the Starr-Edwards caged-ball valves, the Magovern-Cromie, the Bjork-Shiley, the Hall-Kaster, and the St. Jude valve (3–5,13,17,21,22). Gimenez (21) described the normal range of motion of the Starr-Edwards mitral prosthesis to be 0°–9°, with a mean of 3.2°. The Starr-Edwards aortic valve motion had the same range, with a mean of 3.5°.

White (5) found the range of tilt of the sewing ring in normal Starr-Edwards caged-ball aortic valves to be 2°–6° and the mitral valve range of tilt to be 5°–21°. Since much overlap exists between the normal and abnormal range of values, the importance of postoperative baseline studies is reinforced (Fig. 12-10a).

Table 12-1. Checklist for Evaluating Patients for Valve Replacement by Plain-Film Radiography and Fluoroscopy

1. The presence or absence of valve, chordae, or annulus calcification
2. The presence or absence of coronary artery or cardiac chamber wall calcification
3. Evidence of pulmonary arterial hypertension
4. Evidence of pulmonary venous hypertension
5. Abnormalities of cardiac contractility
6. Intrinsic pulmonary or pleural pathology
7. Diaphragmatic excursion
8. Aorta and hilar vessel motion

Method of Fluoroscopy

In order to examine the patient with a central occluding prosthesis, the patient is rotated so the base of the cage is parallel to the central beam. The patient is usually placed in the right anterior oblique position for the mitral prosthesis and in the left anterior oblique position for the aortic prosthesis to obtain optimal visualization of the valve in profile. The patient is then rotated toward the opposite oblique, and the base ring is positioned in an en face projection so that the occluder can be observed through the base ring. It is rare to be able to position the base ring symmetrically en face without angling the tube in a sagittal plane as well as in the axial plane. For proper localization a C-arm or other multiplane fluoroscopy unit is required. The observer should evaluate the fixed component of the valve for the rare strut fracture or deformity. The position of the base in relation to the mitral valve area is estimated by the fat line in the atrioventricular (AV) groove. In this position a partially dehisced mitral valve prosthesis may dislocate superiorly into the left atrium above the AV groove (15,22).

The axial alignment of the aortic valve is estimated by its relationship to the top of the ascending aorta. The aortic valve occluder tends to maintain a constant axial relationship with the top of the ascending aorta, so that deviations from this relationship will suggest tissue encroachment, aneurysm or dehiscence (22). In general, aortic valves are more stable than mitral valves with respect to their normal range of motion. This is because the normal native mitral valve motion is greater in both the long and short axes than the aortic valve motion, and there is greater variability in the amount of tissue left by the surgeon after implantation of a mitral prosthesis (5,15,22). In several series in which the angles of tilt of the mitral and aortic prosthesis have been measured, abnormal motion was suspected when the tilt in the base ring axis consistently exceeded 6°–9° in the aortic valve and 9°–12° in the mitral valve (5,21) (Fig. 12-10b).

Central Occluding Valves

Analysis of central occluding ball-cage valves includes careful observation of poppet configuration and motion with respect to the length and smooth-

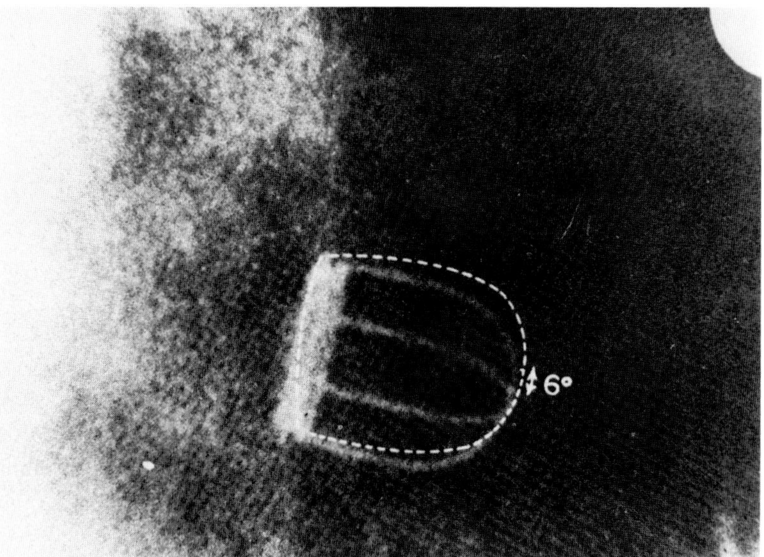

a

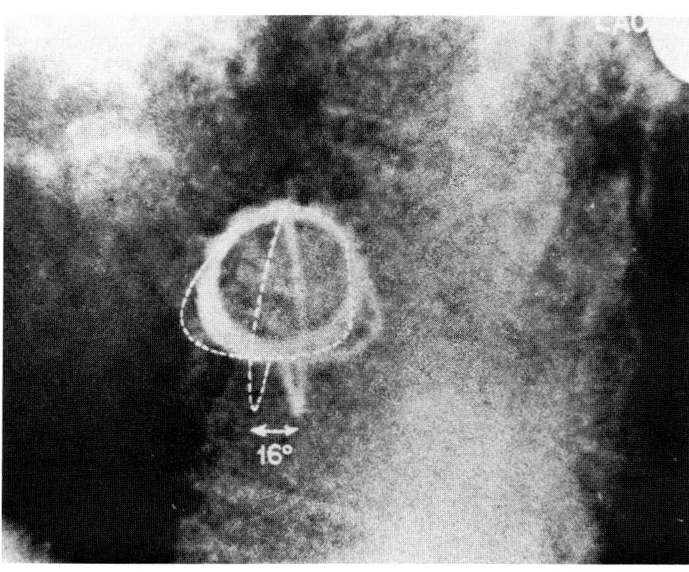

b

Fig. 12-10, a and b. Starr-Edwards mitral prosthesis. a Normal range of tilt in a Starr-Edwards mitral prosthesis. **b** A 16° tilt shown in systole compared with position in diastole (*dotted lines*). Left ventricular angiography demonstrated a paravalvular leak. (White A et al: Circulation 48:882–886, 1973, with permission)

ness of the stroke and clearance between the occluder and the cage struts or prongs. The ball of the Starr-Edwards mitral valve, for example, drops directly to the apex of the cage during left atrial systole, traveling along the dependent wall. During ventricular filling the ball moves listlessly. As ventricular systole is initiated, the ball rapidly approaches the base ring, striking the rim and jumping up to become firmly seated in the center of the cage base. This motion is called the *rim seat phenomenon,* noted by photocardiography. This is a cause of slight mitral insufficiency. The ball approaches the seat eccentrically because the struts have a greater diameter than the centrally placed seat which the ball occupies during ventricular systole (5,15,21).

The Cutter mitral valve has a shorter cage than the Starr-Edwards valve. It has open struts and is also slightly incompetent. The Cutter ball rolls in the left ventricular portion of the cage during systole, but it does not travel eccentrically and has no rim seat effect (3). The Starr-Edwards aortic ball seats centrally in diastole and does not demonstrate the rim seat effect, as the struts have the same diameter as the cage. During ventricular systole the ball goes directly to the top of the cage, where it vibrates forcibly as blood enters the aorta from the left ventricle.

Caged-Disc Prosthesis

The caged-disc prosthesis is exemplified by the Beall mitral valve. The disc travels in a constant motion from the base to the top of the struts. Transient cocking or delay may be seen under simulated high-pressure low-flow conditions and may be seen normally as well, except that the disc will complete a full excursion (23). Intermittent disc cocking occurs in the Cross-Jones mitral valve due to the impact of the regurgitant jet on one side of the disc during long systolic filling causing mild aortic incompetence (23).

Tilting-Disc Prosthesis

The most widely used mechanical valve is the Bjork-Shiley disc prosthesis first developed in 1969. The opaque components of this valve consist of a metal ring and plastic disc containing a radiopaque ring (since 1975) suspended between two metal struts opening in one direction. The flow pattern is laminar, and there is mild incompetence. The degree of tilting is nominally 60° in both aortic and mitral valves (17,24). In the aortic area the valve is placed in a subcoronary position, opening toward the noncoronary cusps (25).

Analysis of a Bjork-Shiley valve requires a multiplanar fluoroscope to visualize the base ring and disc in profile simultaneously (Fig. 12-11a,b). This can be done by first projecting the valve in the vertical axis of the C-arm fluoroscope, bringing the valve into a superior-inferior orientation, followed by rotation into the horizontal axis to view the valve in profile. A third 90° rotation in this same horizontal plane will bring the valve into an en face position. In this orientation the disc appears as a circle in ventricular systole and assumes an ellipsoid appearance when open in ventricular diastole (24). The result of using this man-

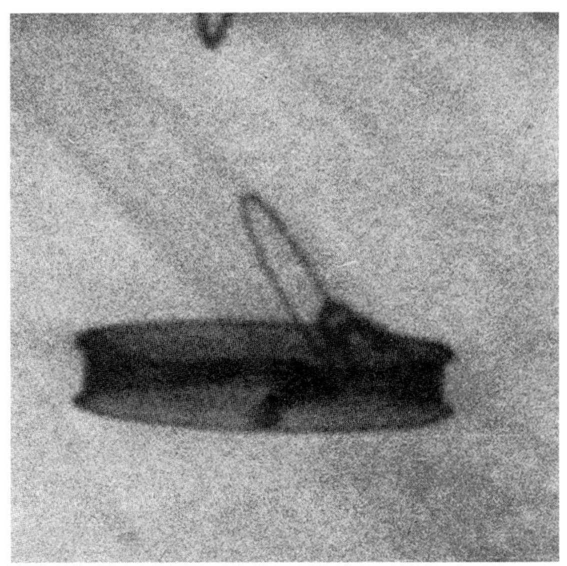

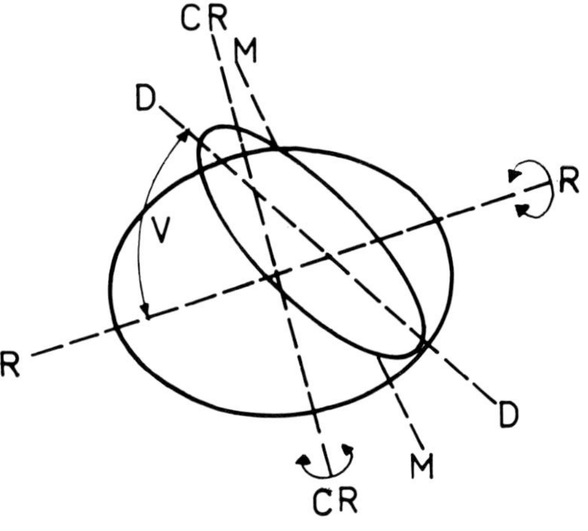

a   b

Fig. 12-11, a and b. Bjork-Shiley prosthesis. a Fluoroscopy of a Bjork-Shiley aortic tilting-disc valve in open position. **b** Bjork-Shiley prosthesis with the disc in open position. M, axis of motion; R, axis corresponding to the valve ring plane diameter perpendicular to M; D, axis of disc plane diameter perpendicular to M; CR, central perpendicular axis of the valve ring plane; V, prosthetic opening angle between D and R. (Bjork V et al: J Thorac Cardiovasc Surg 73:563–569, 1977, with permission)

uever shows that the Bjork-Shiley valve tilt angle varies normally from 50° to 68° (24).

Since thrombosis will interfere with disc closure (17), it is helpful to fluoroscope with the beam direction 20°–30° from the valve ring plane to confirm valve closure to best advantage. Complete opening will indicate free mobility of the disc without thrombotic obstruction or tissue encroachment.

Tissue Valves

Fluoroscopy is of limited value in detecting abnormalities of function of tissue valves, since the tissue components are radiolucent and motion of the leaflets cannot be appreciated by fluoroscopy or plain-film radiography. However, rocking of the radiopaque base ring will suggest dehiscence. Calcification of the tissue components will indicate degeneration (Fig. 12-9b).

Ultrasonic Evaluation of Prosthetic Valves

Cardiac ultrasound has the advantage of being noninvasive and free of radiation exposure. Thus, serial evaluation can be performed without discomfort or known hazard to the patient. Unlike conventional cinefluoroscopy or plain-film radiography, echocardiography can and should be related directly to auscultatory findings and phonocardiography (9,25). Echocardiography can detect both direct evidence of malfunction in mechanical and tissue valves and indirect evidence of malfunction, including increasing cardiac chamber enlargement, native valve malfunction secondary to prosthetic valve insufficiency, and objective evidence of thrombosis or vegetation not possible with cinefluoroscopy alone. Although normal values for specific valve models are available, the pattern recorded in each patient is sufficiently different so that a postoperative baseline study is important. M-mode echocardiography is most useful in the study of metal and plastic valves, whereas tissue valves require two-dimensional real-time echocardiography (9).

M-mode Echocardiography

A standardized technique is necessary to yield reproducible results. For ball or disc central occluder valves the transducer is placed at the cardiac apex and angled cephalad and medially. The ultrasound beam is parallel to the direction of the poppet motion in order to record maximum excursion. Mitral tilting-disc monocuspid valves are examined from the third and fourth left interspace next to the sternum, with the transducer tilted until maximum excursion is recorded. In a patient with an aortic prosthesis, the transducer is placed at the right supraclavicular fossa or the right parasternal area directed toward the aortic root. The tricuspid valve should be examined from the left fifth intercostal space (7).

In the normal prosthesis the anterior cage ring moves in parallel, with the annulus. The opening and closing velocities, the E-F slope, and the excursion of the poppet are measured. The posterior ball echo in hollow metal poppets may not be recorded, as most of the sound is reflected back from the interior ball surface. In the case of the older Silastic poppets, the posterior ball surface may be recorded and a diameter determined. However, since ultrasound travels more slowly through Silastic material than through soft tissue, the decreased velocity is reflected as an increase in the distance from the transducer, so that the posterior surface may appear to lie behind the base ring. Except for reduced motion reflecting less aortic annulus motion, the characteristics of the aortic valve are similar to those of the mitral valve (Fig. 12-12).

In a central occluder disc valve such as the Beall Valve, the anterior strut surface, the disc surface, and the suture ring can be seen. Opening and closing velocity and disc excursion can be determined (7) (Fig. 12-13). The disc opens briskly in early diastole, contacts the struts, and closes promptly in systole. This motion produces opening and closing clicks on phonocardiography.

The tilting-disc central-flow valve is exemplified by the Bjork-Shiley prosthesis. The characteristic echo pattern of a normal Bjork-Shiley mitral prosthesis is a brisk opening motion of 180 mm/sec, a sharp E point, and a prolonged E-F slope. Closing velocity is approximately 300 mm/sec. Rounding of the opening upstroke and then the downstroke, together with decreased amplitude, has been related to the presence of thrombus. Variation of this pattern is dependent on transducer

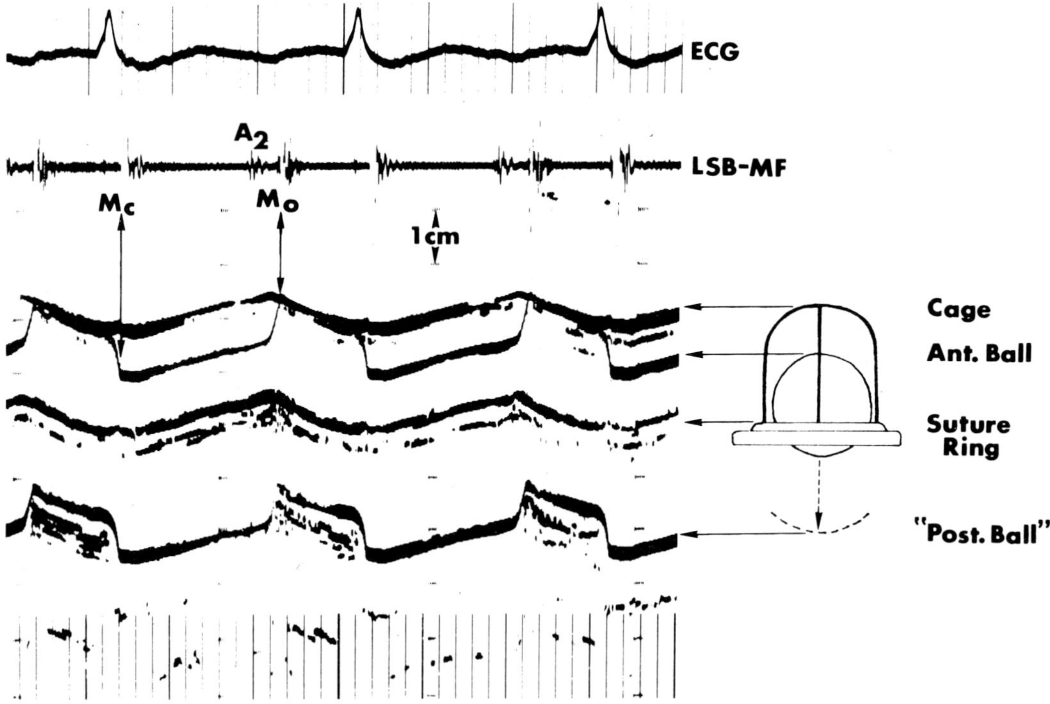

Fig. 12-12. Caged-ball valve. The anterior and posterior surfaces of a caged-ball mitral prosthesis with a Silastic ball. The motion of the anterior surface (anterior ball) resembles that of a caged-disc prosthesis. Failure of the anterior surface to contact the cage would suggest intervening thrombus. Because of slow transmission through the ball, the posterior surface (posterior ball) appears to be behind the sewing ring. This illusionary distance between the anterior and posterior surface recordings is material-dependent.

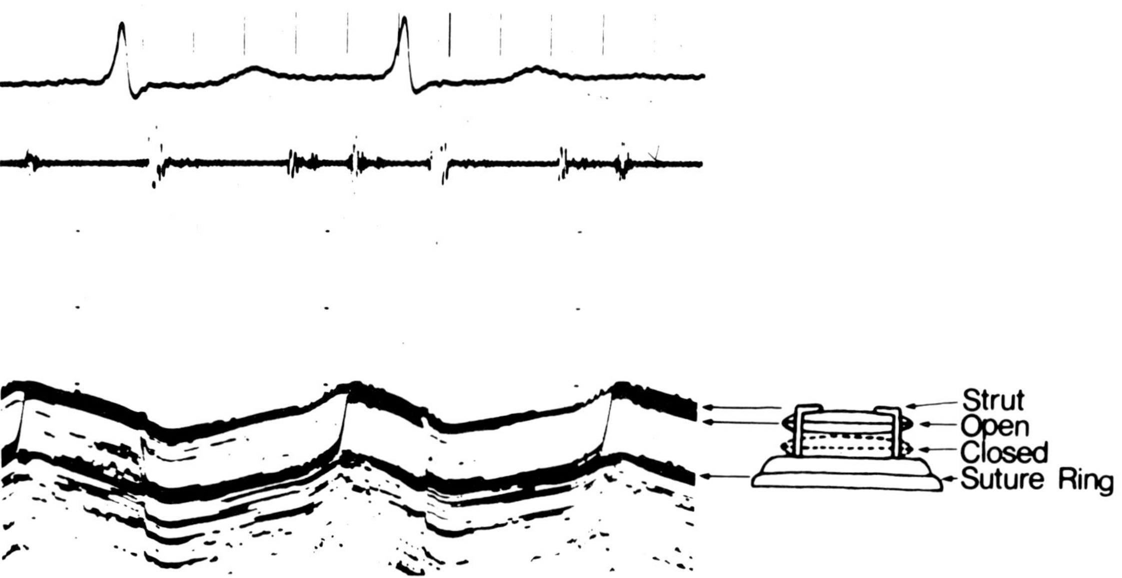

Fig. 12-13. Caged-disc valve. Phonocardiogram and echocardiogram of a normal Beall mitral valve. During diastole the disc moves anteriorly to collide with the struts. During systole, the disc moves posteriorly to collide with the suture ring. (Johnson ML: *In* Gramiak R, Wang R (eds): Cardiac Ultrasound. St Louis: CV Mosby Co., 1975, with permission)

position as well as transvalvular blood flow. A drastic change on a follow-up study may suggest malfunction. A hump seen in early diastole may be due to mitral insufficiency and has been associated with paravalvular leaks (8,26).

Aortic valve tilting-disc prostheses are more difficult to evaluate by echocardiography than mitral valves (9). Motion of the tilting disc is variable and the image is particularly related to transducer position and to the position of the valve in the aortic root. Here, again, serial echos are helpful.

Two-Dimensional Real-Time Echocardiography—Heterograft Valves

It is possible to study both the morphology and the function of the aortic and mitral tissue valve leaflets using echocardiography, since the normal heterograft has the structure and function of the normal valve. In tissue valves, two-dimensional real-time echocardiography is superior to M-mode (9) (Fig. 12-14). Valve motion reflects blood flow, and degeneration or stenosis causes a pattern of leaflet restriction, thickening, and unsharpness. Insufficiency may cause increased frequency of diastolic leaflet flutter. Calcifications and fenestrations of the ring or leaflet cusps can be detected (6,9,25).

Complications of Prosthetic Valves

Structural Failure

Ball or Disc Variance

Variance is defined as mechanical dysfunction resulting from alterations in the configuration of the occluder. Variance of the silicone rubber ball was

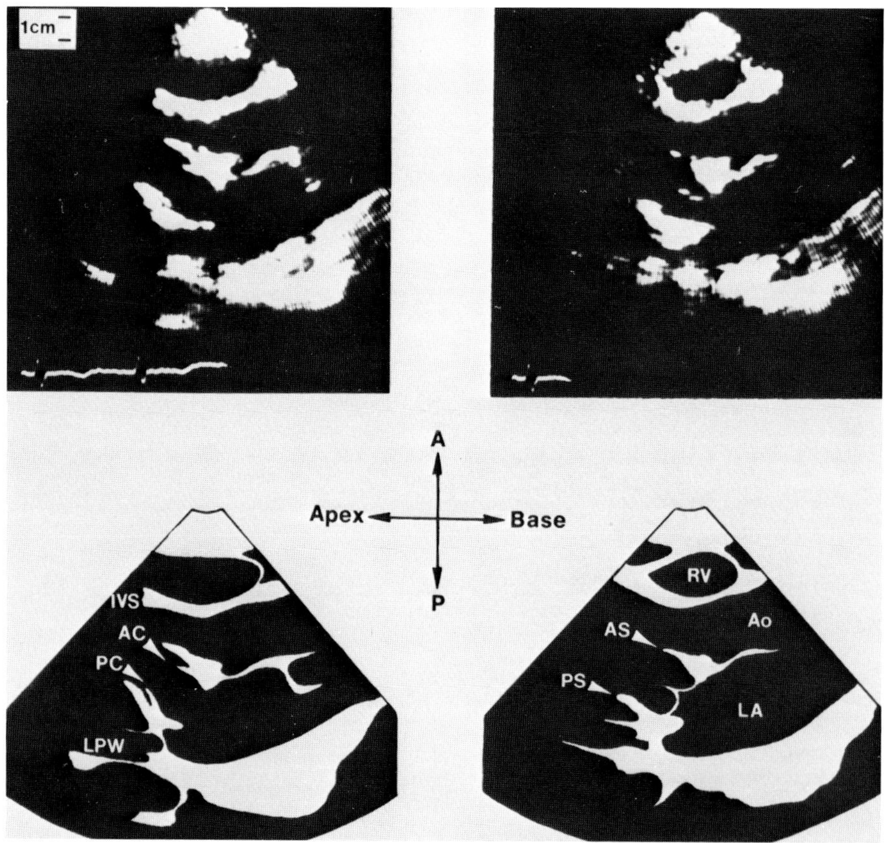

Fig. 12-14. Two-dimensional echocardiographic study of a heterograft prosthesis. The leaflets are thin and during diastole open fully to contact the stents. IVS, intraventricular septum; AC, anterior cusps; PC, posterior cusps; AS, anterior stent; PS, posterior stent; LPW, left ventricular posterior wall; RV, right ventricle; Ao, aorta; LA, left atrium. (Mintz G, Kotler M, Steiner RM, Walinsky P: CRC Crit Rev Diagn Imaging 14:243–279, 1981, with permission)

Table 12-2. Complications of Prosthetic Valves (3,27–29,16,43)

A. Occluder dysfunction
1. Poppet variance (14,15,22,29)
2. Disc embolization (30)
3. Disc wear (3)
4. Dislodgement (22)
5. Thrombus (15,18,22,31)
6. Poppet entrapment (4,35)

B. Cage and base ring dysfunction
1. Paravalvular leak (4,23,32–34)
2. Detachment (21)
3. Bacterial endocarditis (36,37)
4. Strut fracture (39)
5. Calcification (40,41)
6. Tissue encroachment (2)

C. Systemic effects
1. Gastrointestinal and pulmonary hemorrhage (3)
2. Hemolysis (38,43)
3. Cholelithiasis (42)

particularly common in the early Starr-Edwards (Model 1200) valves. Alterations in ball configuration include grooving, cracking, decreased or increased diameter, and fragmentation. Changes in the ball core with formation of fluid lakes due to lipid infiltration occur and cause increased diameter. This is related to microscopic disruption of the structure of the Silastic material. Embolization of poppet material, thrombi, or regurgitation may be due to sticking and/or impingement resulting from enlargement of the ball diameter with lipid infiltration. Fragmentation following grooving or fracture may result in embolization or thrombus (Figs. 12-15, 12-27, 12-28)

Aortic ball variance has occurred in Model 1000 and 1200 Starr-Edwards prostheses (29). Of the 189 patients studied at the University of Oregon Medical School who underwent aortic ball valve replacement from 1962 to 1966, 25% had ball variance at autopsy or reoperation. Approximately 200 cases of aortic ball variance have been reported with the Magovern SCDK-Cutter, Smelloff-Cutter, and Harken prostheses. Implicated in the development of ball variance are abnormalities of implantation causing increased stress. These include malalignment of the prosthesis in relation to the aortic axis and narrow aortic root and misplaced sutures. Tissue impinging on the aortic wall and thrombosis have also been implicated. Abrasion of the occluder by Teflon cloth reducing the diameter of the ball has been described with the Braunwald-Cutter aortic valve, causing regurgitation and poppet embolization. For this reason this

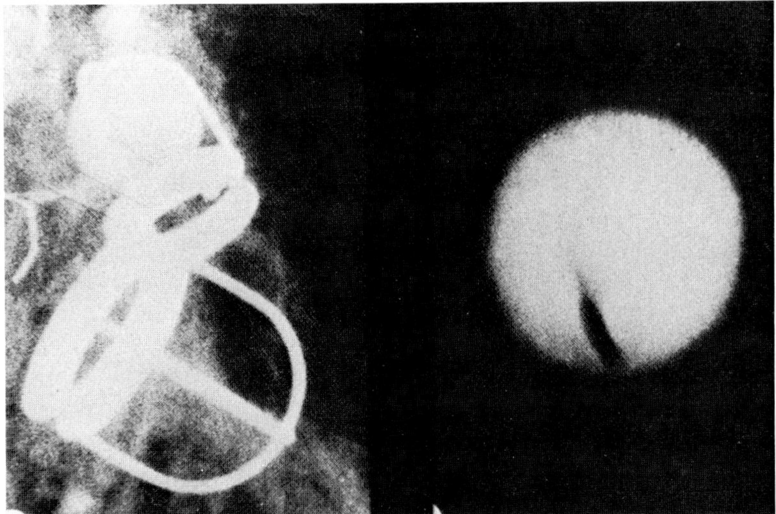

Fig. 12-15. Ball fracture. Cineradiograph shows a radiolucent defect in a Starr-Edwards aortic barium-impregnated ball due to cracking as a result of lipid infiltration. Following removal, irregularities of the edge of the Silastic ball are noted together with the crack. (Hylen J, Kloster F, Starr A: Ann Intern Med 72:1–8, 1970, with permission)

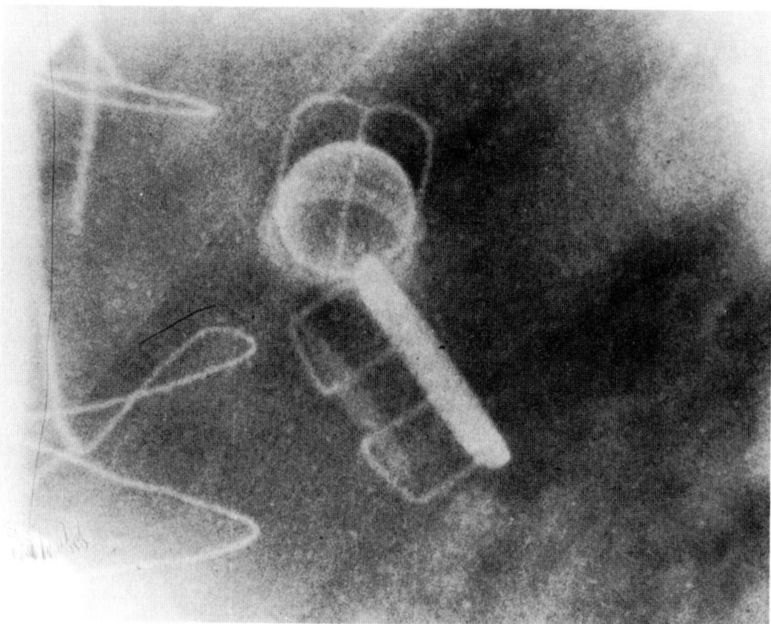

Fig. 12-16. Peripheral disc wear. Cineradiography shows marked wear of the edges of the disc of a Beall caged-disc mitral valve which was the cause of regurgitation in this patient. There is a hollow steel ball valve in the aortic area.

valve was withdrawn for use in 1974 (3). Disc variance is seen in the Beall low-profile mitral valve, with a reported incident of Teflon disc wear causing regurgitation (43). Recently, Carlson et al. found that the degree of peripheral disc wear in series 104 Beall valves, as measured by the ratio of the diameters of the disc and the sewing ring, could be correlated with the amount of mitral regurgitation. If the ratio was 0.75 or less, abnormal motion of the disc could be appreciated at fluoroscopy, and regurgitation could be predicted (44) (Fig. 12-16).

The diagnosis of variance has been made in part on the decrease in the intensity of the aortic opening sound on phonocardiography. Fluoroscopy is useful to detect the radiolucent line of fracture or fatty infiltration. Mitral poppet dysfunction due to variance is less common than aortic variance in the case of Starr-Edwards valves. Unlike aortic variance, which is often clinically silent, mitral valve variance is accompanied by signs of cardiac failure and arterial emboli because of the greater strut-poppet tolerance in the mitral valve. In caged-disc valves, uneven wear rapidly occurs in the edge of the Teflon disc during closure and opening. This increases stress on the edge of both

struts. This dysfunction due to disc wear has been reported in Hufnagle, Kay-Shiley, Kay-Suzuki, Cross-Jones, and Beall valves, among others (3,31). With the substitution of metal ball occluders and the replacement of caged-disc valves with tilting-disc prostheses and heterografts, poppet variance has become an unusual problem.

Strut Fracture

Strut fracture has been reported occasionally in many of the mechanical valves including the DeBakey (39) and in the Beall valve. This is thought to be due to structural wear of titanium struts, in the case of the DeBakey valve (Fig. 12-17), and the pyrolite struts of the Beall low-profile caged-disc valve. Potentially the disc may embolize because of strut breakage.

Poppet Embolization

Embolization of ball occluders has been reported following severe abrasion causing reduced diameter of the ball (15), and disc embolization has occurred following extensive wear of a Beall valve

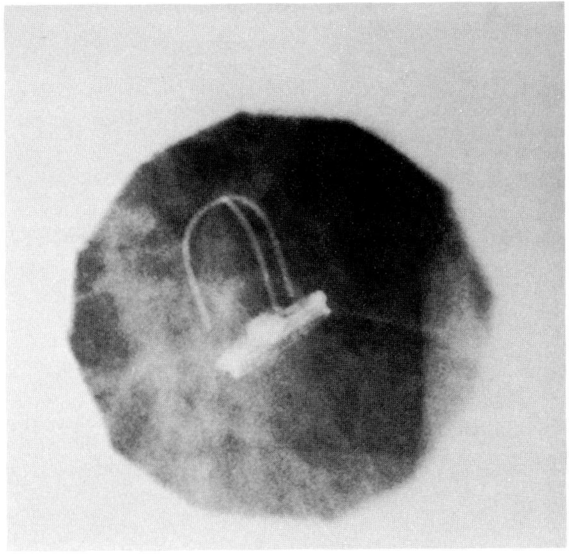

Fig. 12-17. Broken struts. Cinefluoroscopy demonstrates two broken struts in this DeBakey aortic valve with titanium metal struts. (Zumbro GL et al: J Thorac Cardiovasc Surg 74:469–470, 1977, with permission)

disc (30). Embolized poppets have also occurred with the Wada-Cutter mitral prosthesis. The higher incidence of disc embolization with the Beall valve is related to the severe grooving and wear occurring in the Teflon disc of the earlier Beall models. The Teflon flow properties are also such that gentle pressure over time can deform the original shape of these discs. Embolization can lead to severe regurgitation and distal arterial occlusion. Immediate surgery is the procedure of choice (Fig. 12-18a,b).

Infection

Prosthetic endocarditis may develop early or late in the postoperative period. The incidence of both early and late infective endocarditis averages about 2.3% (36). Early infective endocarditis is usually defined as endocarditis appearing within two months of surgery. It occurs in over 1% of patients (3,36,43). The incidence of infection of an aortic prosthesis is much higher than for a mitral prosthesis and is even higher if multiple valves are implanted.

Prior to the use of prophylactic antibiotics, as many as 12% of patients undergoing caged-ball valve replacement developed infection, but this has been reduced by improvement in surgical technique together with prophylactic antibiotics (3).

Source of Infection

The potential sources of infection include contaminated prepump and postpump blood, the heart-lung machine, contamination in the surgical field, preexisting infection of the mitral valve or annulus and of the prosthetic valve itself. Postoperative sources of infection include catheters, endotracheal tubes, pacemaker, and other invasive sources. Typical infecting organisms include *Pseudomonas aeruginosa, Serratia marcescens, Candida albicans, Staphylococcus aureus, epidermidis* and *diphtheroides* (36,37).

Vegetations developing at the coronary ostium, the ascending aorta, and the annulus are related to high-pressure regurgitant jets of blood which tend to destroy the valve attachments and cause local abscess formation. Aneurysms may develop at the site of infection. Vegetations obstruct flow through the valve orifice or limit the motion of the poppet or tilting disc. Mycotic sinus aneurysms or periannular aneurysms may develop (37) (Figs. 12-19 and 12-20). Paravalvular insufficiency may occur as tissue fragments and sutures loosen.

The diagnosis of regurgitation will be made by observing the motion of the prosthetic valve, searching for rocking of the sewing ring due to suture dehiscence or reduced excursion of the poppet due to vegetations or thrombus. Two-dimensional real-time ultrasound is particularly useful in demonstrating the site, form, and size of vegetations or thrombus, particularly in the case of diseased heterograft valves. Contrast angiography will record the presence of mycotic aneurysms. Infection may spread beyond the area of the valve to the right atrium and intraventricular septum to the posterior wall of the ascending aorta or the pulmonary outflow tract. The left atrium and mitral valve may be invaded from the left and posterior coronary cusps (3,36,46) (Figs. 12-19 and 12-20).

Regurgitation

Minor regurgitant flow occurs normally with many of the mechanical valves, but major regurgi-

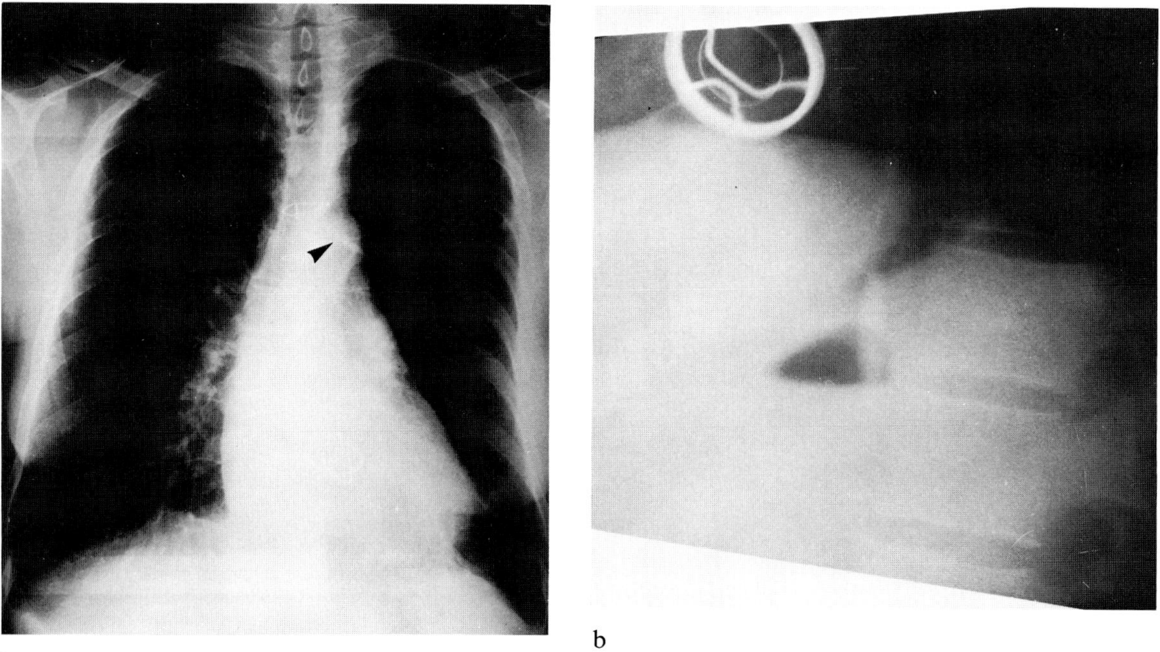

a

b

Fig. 12-18, a and **b. Embolized disc. a** An embolized disc from a Model 103 Beall mitral prosthesis in the aortic arch. There is no obstruction of blood flow. **b** Embolized disc in another patient from a Model 103 Beall mitral prosthesis in the upper abdominal aorta. The valve was replaced with a Bjork-Shiley prosthesis. (Gutierrez FR et al: J Thorac Cardiovasc Surg 81:758–761, 1981, with permission)

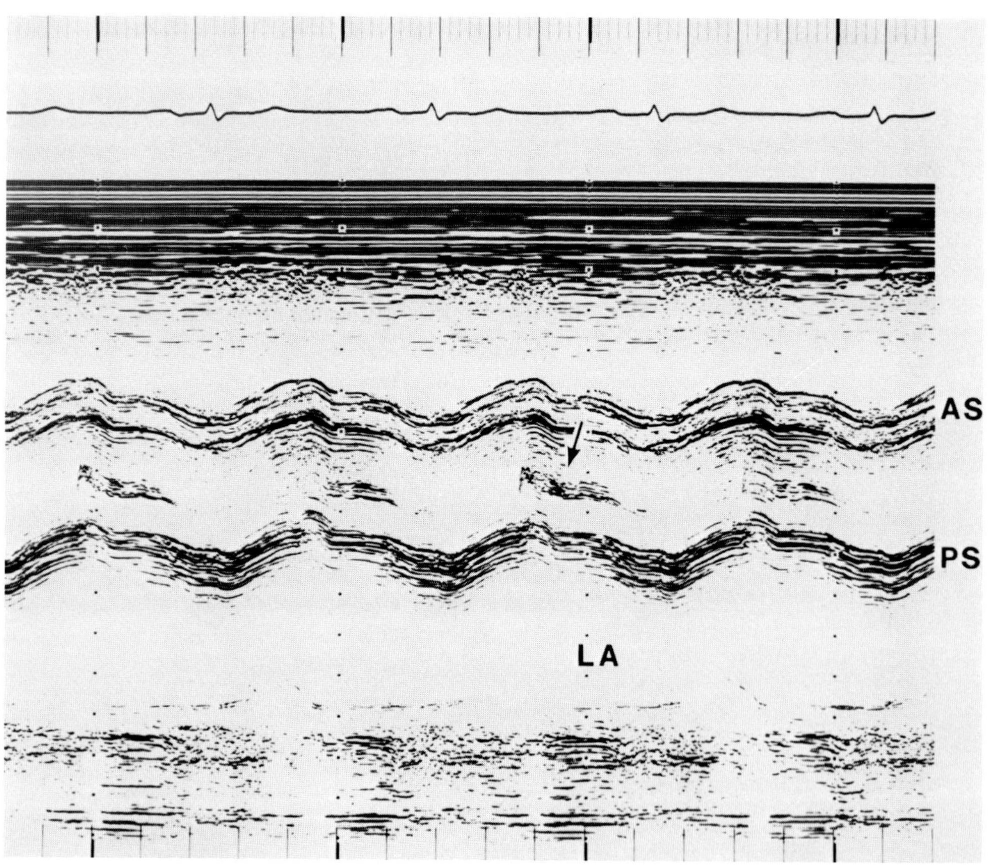

Fig. 12-19. Leaflet vegetations. The criteria for porcine heterograft leaflet vegetations are similar to those for native aortic valve endocarditis. In this patient with an aortic prosthesis, the new finding of a localized increased leaflet thickness (*arrow*) with unrestricted leaflet motion suggests the diagnosis. The presence of a vegetation was confirmed at surgery. AS, anterior stent; PS, posterior stent; LA, left atrium. (Mintz GS, Kotler MN, Steiner RM, Walinsky P: CRC Crit Rev Diagn Imaging 11:243–279, 1981, with permission)

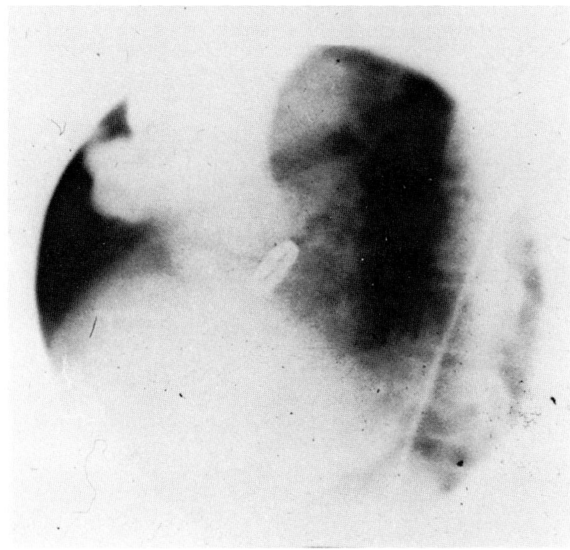

Fig. 12-20. Mycotic aneurysm at the site of aortic valve replacement. (Bjork VO, Henze A, Jareb M: Scand J Thorac Cardiovasc Surg 7:1–6, 1973, with permission)

tant flow usually occurs as a consequence of disc wear or ball variance or because of dehiscence between the sewing ring and the valve annulus (Fig. 12-21). Dehiscence often occurs when the annulus is heavily calcified or when there is defective tissue, as in the Marfan syndrome. Paravalvular leaking may also occur through the crevices of a heavily calcified valve between the prosthesis and the annulus (15). Detachment of the valve is a major cause of regurgitation and may be due to dehiscence of the suture ring as a result of infection, stress, or chest trauma (45). Dehiscence is caused by strain of the sutures in the anchoring tissue resulting from the force of the ventricular contraction. In the mitral position, normal motion of the prosthesis is anterior and posterior along the long axis and side-to-side on the vertical axis. Strain on the suture line is greatest at the medial and lateral aspects of the sewing ring. If the suture breaks at one of these locations, a strain is produced on adjacent sutures, causing continuous dehiscence and leading eventually to complete detachment and possible embolization.

Evaluating the Cause of Valve Insufficiency

Both fluoroscopy and echocardiography are helpful in evaluating valve dysfunction when regurgitation, thrombus, or vegetation is suspected because of sudden cardiac enlargement and when the signs,

symptoms, and radiographic findings of pulmonary edema are present. Fluoroscopy will demonstrate rocking and tilting of the base ring of the prosthesis. Tilting of more than 9°–10° is considered highly suspicious for dehiscence. There must be continuous interruption of at least 40% of the base ring sutures before abnormal rocking will occur. Therefore fluoroscopy without contrast media will be helpful in advanced cases only. Echocardiography, where aortic prosthetic regurgitation will cause native mitral valve flutter, will yield a more sensitive but less specific finding of abnormal function (Fig. 12-22a and b).

Mintz et al. evaluated 50 Beall and Bjork-Shiley mitral valves and 25 Bjork-Shiley aortic valves by means of cinefluoroscopy and echocardiography. They demonstrated abnormal valve motion using the following criteria: Cineradiography was considered abnormal when the degree of tilt was 10° or more. Echocardiography was considered abnormal when there was both abnormal aortic prosthetic disc motion and diastolic native mitral valve flutter. Abnormal disc motion was suggested when the A_2-MVO interval was less than .07 or above .16 (normal = .10). They found that, at the aortic level, sensitivity with echocardiography was 58% and with cinefluoroscopy 33%. Specificity at the aortic valve was 73% with echocardiography and 100% with fluoroscopy. At the mitral valve sensitivity was 79% with echocardiography and 86% with fluoroscopy. Specificity with echocardiography was 64% at the mitral valve level and fluoroscopy 89%. These findings suggest that fluoroscopy at the mitral valve level is more sensitive and more specific than echocardiography. At the aortic level, echocardiography was more sensitive but less specific. These findings suggest that echocardiography and fluoroscopy are complementary procedures in the evaluation of major mechanical valves in use today (47).

Both echocardiography and fluoroscopy are helpful in evaluating regurgitation secondary to disc wear. Echocardiography will demonstrate both intermittent and complete seating of the prosthetic disc valves. Abnormal seating or cocking is accompanied by shortening of the A_2-MVO interval. Since disc wear is common in the Beall 103 mitral valve prostheses, these valves should receive careful follow-up. The disc in the later 105 and 106 Beall valve series shows less evidence of disc wear. The A_2-MVO interval may also narrow due to left ventricular dysfunction, valve obstruc-

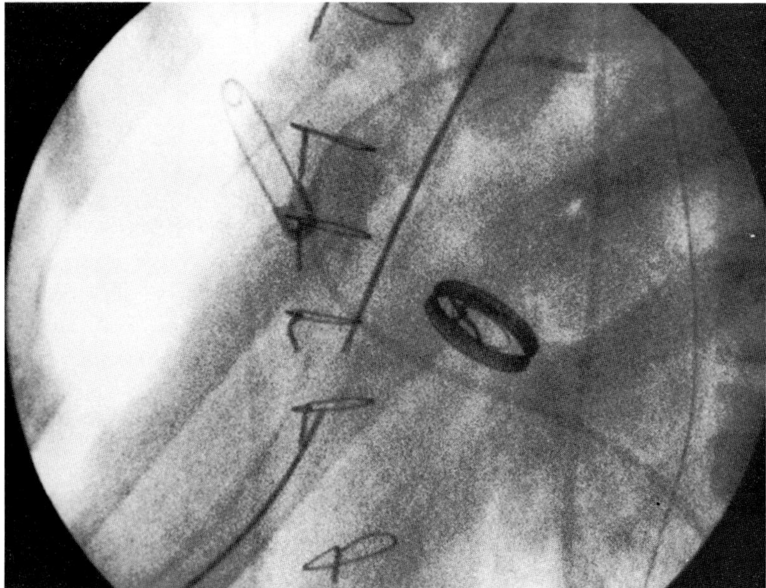

a

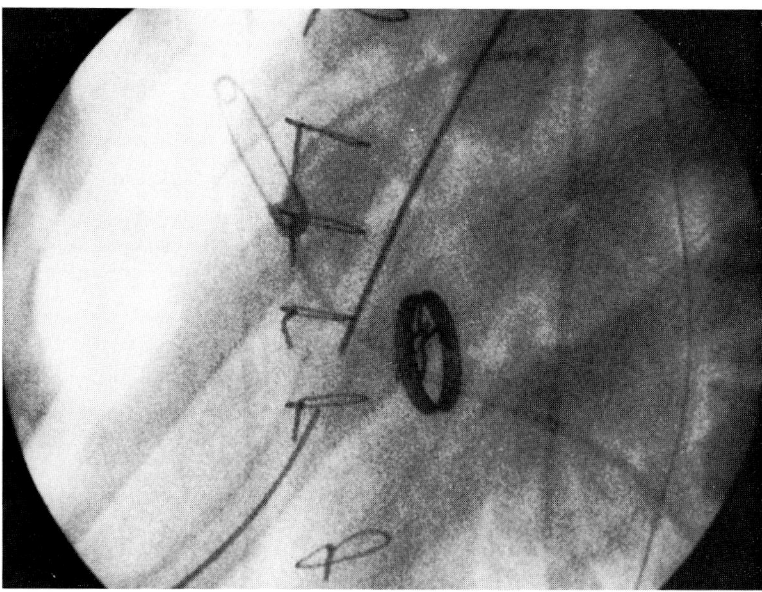

b

Fig. 12-21, a and **b. Paravalvular leak.** Fluoroscopic documentation of marked tilting of the Bjork-Shiley valve with excursion of 61° suggesting paravalvular leak and dehiscence. (Chun P et al: Am Heart J 99:230–234, 1980, with permission)

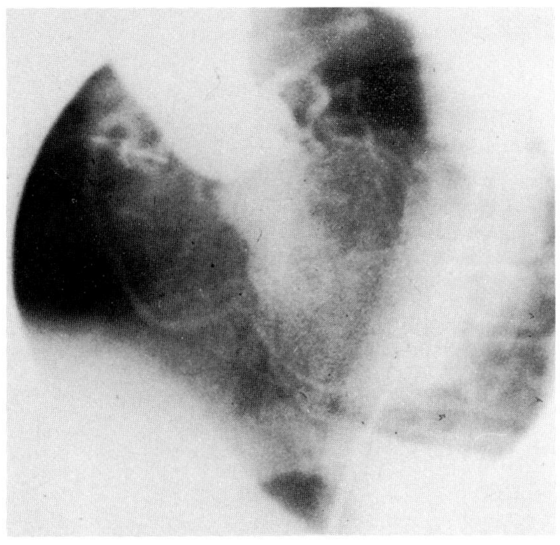

Fig. 21-22. Paravalvular leak. Aortography in the LAO projection demonstrates significant anterior paravalvular leak in a patient with an implanted Bjork-Shiley valve. (Reprinted from Bjork V et al: Scand J Thorac Cardiovasc Surg 7:1–6, 1973, with permission)

tion, or paravalvular insufficiency. Delayed opening may be present secondary to sticking of the disc due to thrombus, vegetation, or disc strut mismatch. Fluoroscopy will demonstrate cocking of the disc together with edge wear causing a decrease in the ratio of diameters of the disc and the base ring (Fig. 12-23a–d).

Prosthetic Valve Thrombosis

Thrombosis of a prosthetic valve may cause limitation of poppet motion or other moving parts. Thrombosis of aortic valves is uncommon and may be related to discontinuation of anticoagulant therapy. Reduction in the excursion of both the ball valve or the tilting-disc valve may be seen. Failure of the ball valve to reach the top of the cage or to seat well at the bottom of the cage may be due to either tissue encroachment or thrombosis. Mitral valve thrombosis has a greater incidence than aortic valve thrombosis. Acute thrombosis of the left atrium and the prosthetic valve in the early postoperative period is an uncommon but fatal complication of mitral valve replacement and

may be associated with reduced cardiac output postoperatively. Late thrombosis with mechanical malfunction is often accompanied by endocarditis.

Thromboembolism has remained a major hazard of prosthetic cardiac valves. With the early prosthetic valves, the frequency of thromboembolism was in the range of 24%–37%. Since the introduction of cloth-covered prostheses, the incidence has decreased to approximately 3%–5%. Risk of thromboembolism continues to diminish with time after implantation. The risk is similar for patients with aortic, mitral, or multiple valve replacements. Emboli usually occur within six months after implantation before the material covering the surface of the valve has completely organized to form a neointima, which resists thrombus formation (15).

Thrombosis tends to develop at the junction between the autogenous tissue and the metallic prosthesis. Thrombosis may be secondary in some patients to protrusion of the muscular interventricular septum or the aortic walls into the cage, preventing full descent of the ball during diastole and causing obstruction.

Early recognition of thrombus formation is vital in preventing the late sequelae of arterial embolism. This may best be done by fluoroscopy showing abnormal motion of the prosthetic occluder or identification of thrombus by means of two-dimensional real-time echocardiography (9,15).

Tissue Encroachment

Aortic root obstruction occurs when the prosthesis is large in relation to the size of the proximal ascending aorta. If the prosthetic base ring and cage are too large for the orifice, encroachment may occur, causing functional stenosis or limitation in occluder motion (15,35).

Aneurysm

False aortic aneurysms following aortic valve surgery may be mycotic or traumatic in origin. They may arise from the longitudinal incision made in the ascending aorta for valve repair or insertion of the prosthetic valve, or the aneurysms may arise because of infective endocarditis following aortic valve surgery (19,46) (Fig. 12-20).

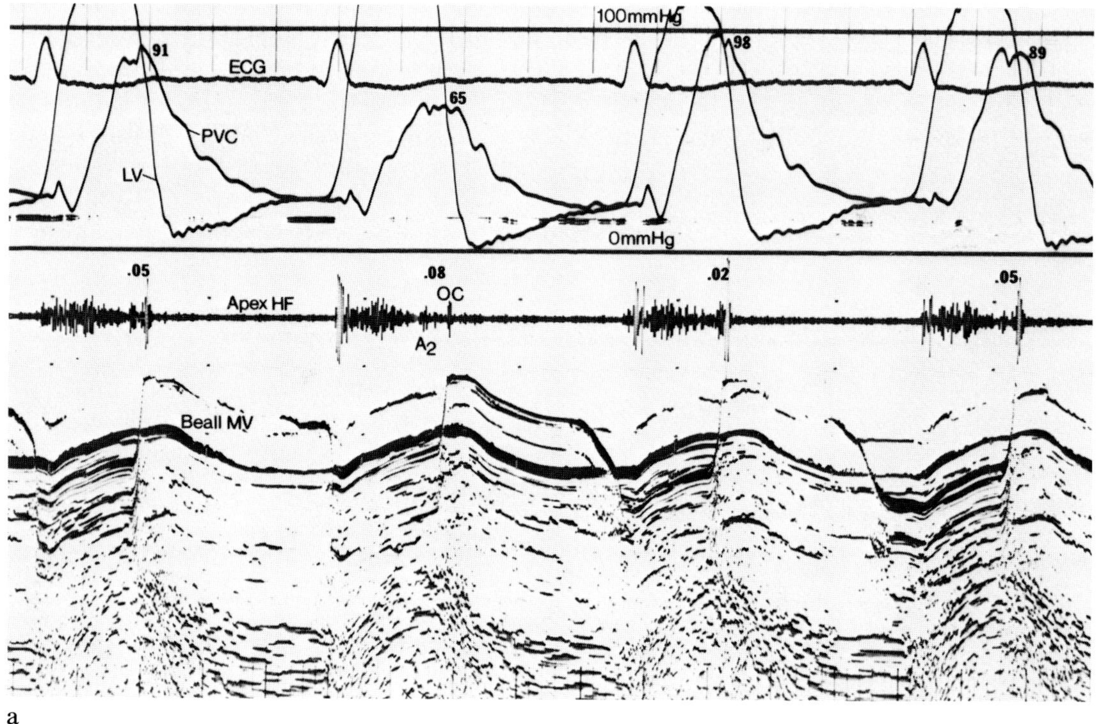

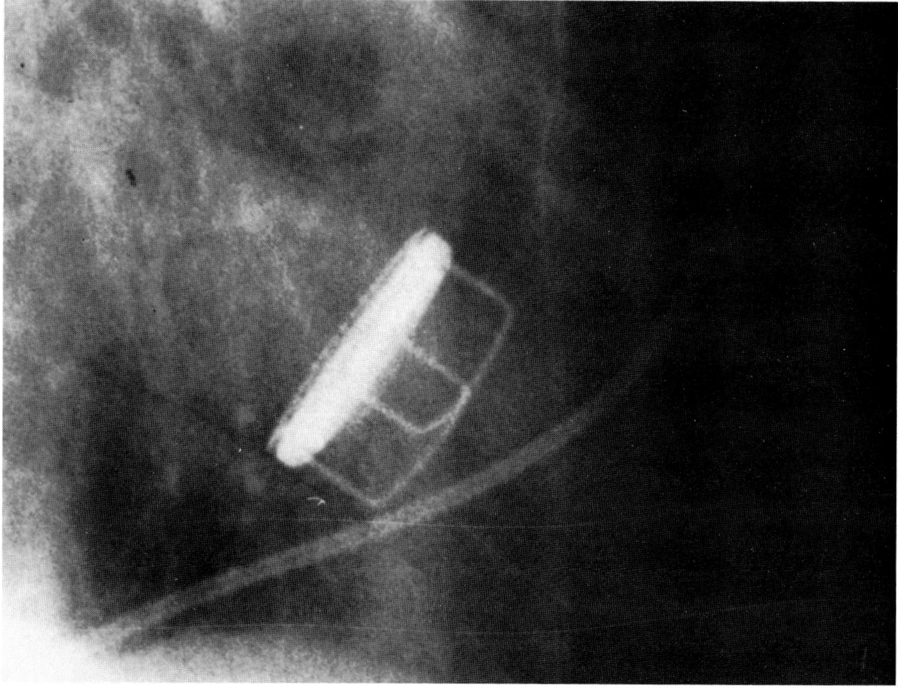

Fig. 12-23, a–d. Valve insufficiency. a Photocardiographic and echocardiographic tracings recorded during cardiac catheterization. Simultaneous left ventricular and pulmonary capillary wedge pressures are shown. The narrow A₂-OC interval is inversely related to the degree of mitral insufficiency as indicated by the height of the V wave in the PVC tracing. The consistency of the systolic murmur indicates that there is some mitral insufficiency with every beat. **a** Abnormal Beall mitral prosthesis studied fluoroscopically shows normal systolic position.

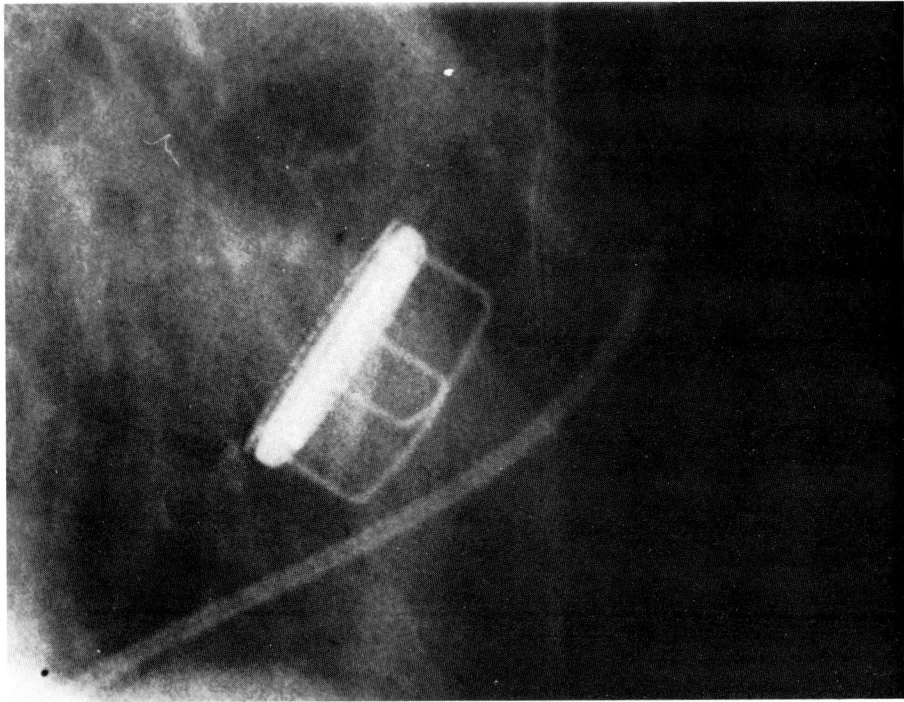

a

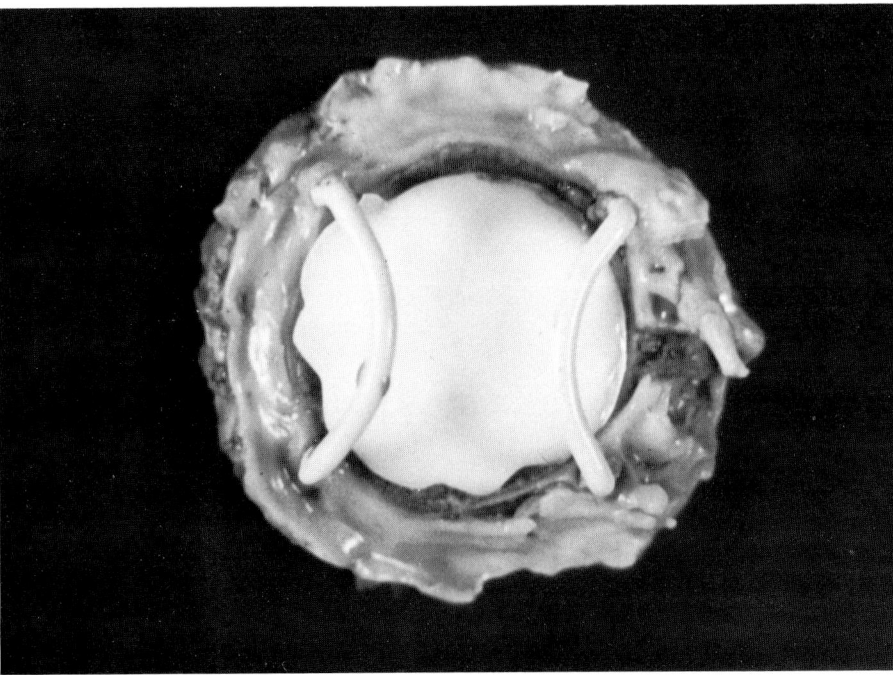

b

Fig. 12-23 (cont.) **c** Abnormal systolic frame showing cocking. Note the disc is smaller relative to the space between the struts. The small worn disc allows some insufficiency with left ventricular systole. **d** Abnormal mitral Beall prosthesis removed at surgery. The small notches resulted in intermittent systolic cocking of the valve. (Mintz G, Kotler M, Steiner RM, Walinsky P: CRC Crit Rev Diagn Imaging 14:243–279, 1981, with permission)

Summary

In this chapter, the radiologic findings associated with the complications of cardiac valve implantation are discussed. Emphasis is placed on the complementary roles of fluoroscopy, plain films, and echocardiography in the early recognition of the life-threatening problems associated with this surgical procedure.

References

1. Bonchek LI: Current status of cardiac valve replacement: selection of a prosthesis and indications for operation. Am Heart J 101:196–105, 1981.
2. Gulsham KS, Scott S, Takaro T: Iatrogenic coronary artery stenosis following aortic valve replacement. J Thorac Cardiovasc Surg 77:760–767, 1979.
3. Steiner RM: The radiology of cardiac valve replacement. In Morse D, Steiner RM: A Guide to Pacemaker and Valve Identification. Garden City, Long Island: Medical Examinations, Inc, 1978.
4. Sands MJ, Lachman AS, O'Reilly DJ, Leach CW, Sappington JB, Katz AM: Diagnostic value of cinefluoroscopy in the evaluation of prosthetic valve dysfunction (in press).
5. White AF, Dinsmore R, Buckley MJ: Cineradiographic evaluation of prosthetic cardiac valves. Circulation 48:882–890, 1973.
6. Ashok M, Kessler KM, Tamer D, Petkaros K, Kessler R, Myerburg R: Two-dimensional echographic observations in major detachment of a prosthetic aortic valve. Am Heart J 101:231–233, 1981.
7. Manus S, Walinsky P: Ultrasound of prosthetic heart valves. In Morse D, Steiner RM: A guide to Pacemaker and Valve Identification. Garden City, Long Island: Medical Examinations, Inc, 1978.
8. Cunha C, Giuliani E, Callahan J, Pluth J: Echophonocardiographic findings in patients with prosthetic heart valve. Mayo Clin Proc 55:231–242, 1980.
9. Mintz G, Kotler M, Steiner RM, Walinsky P: Ultrasonography of prosthetic cardiac valves. CRC Crit Rev Diagn Imaging 14:243–279, 1981.
10. Bream P, Tonkin I, Elliott L: Acquired valvular heart disease. In Teplick G, Haskins M (eds): Surgical Radiology. Philadelphia: WB Saunders Co, 1981, Vol II, pp 1769–1779.
11. Mehlman D, Resnekov L: A guide to the radiographic identification of prosthetic valves. Circulation 57:613–623, 1978.
12. Silver M, Datta B, Bowes V: A key to identify heart valve prostheses. Arch Pathol Lab Med 99:132–136, 1975.
13. Chun P, Nelson W: Common cardiac prosthetic valves. JAMA 238:401–403, 1977.
14. Hylen J, Kloster F, Starr A: Aortic ball variance: diagnosis and treatment. Ann Intern Med 72:1–8, 1970.
15. Hipona F, Petronio L, Santiago P: Radiologic diagnosis of late complications associated with cardiac valve surgery in acquired heart disease. Radiol Clin North Am 9:265–283, 1971.
16. Kloster FE: Diagnosis and management of the complications of prosthetic heart valves. Am J Cardiol 35:872–883, 1976.
17. Bjork HO, Hindmarsh T: Radiopaque marker in the tilting disc of the Bjork-Shiley heart valve. J Thorac Cardiovasc Surg 73:563–569, 1977.
18. Venkataraman K, Beer R, Matthews N, Carl J, Harrison E, Turner AF, Finck E: Thrombosis of Bjork-Shiley aortic valve prostheses. Radiology 137:43–47, 1980.
19. Castaneda-Zuniga W, Nicoloff D, Jorgeensen C, Nath PH, Zollikofer C, Amplatz K: In vivo radiographic appearance of the St. Jude valve prosthesis. Radiology 134:775–776, 1980.
20. Wilson W, Amplatz K, Everhart F: Cine fluorographic study of prosthetic cardiac valves. Radiology 88:779–783, 1967.
21. Gimenez J, Soulen R, Davila J: Prosthetic valve detachment; its roentgenographic recognition. Radiology 103:595–600, 1968.
22. Gabriel O: Postoperative radiography of aortic valve prostheses. J Thorac Cardiovasc Surg 58:248–249, 1969.
23. Oliva P, Johnson M, Pomerantz M, Levine A: Dysfunction of the Beall mitral prosthesis and its detection by cine fluoroscopy and echocardiography. Am J Cardiol 31:393–395, 1973.
24. Goodwin RJ: Cineradiographic assessment of Bjork-Shiley aortic and mitral prosthetic heart valves. Clin Radiol 28:355–360, 1977.
25. Fernandez J, Maranhao V, Gooch AS, Morse D, Nichols HT: The Bjork-Shiley prosthesis—a significant advance in aortic valve replacement. Ann Thorac Surg 14:527–538, 1960.
26. Bernal-Ramirez J, Phillips J: Echocardiographic study of malfunction of the Bjork-Shiley heart valve in the mitral position. Am J Cardiol 40:449–453, 1977.
27. Kittredge R, McCord C: Roentgenographic diagnosis of complications in heart valve replacement. AJR 107:392–399, 1969.
28. Humphries JO, O'Neal J, Gott V, Benson DW: Case of the patient undergoing valvular heart surgery. Prog Cardiovasc Dis 16:233–274, 1973.
29. Hylen J, Judkins M, Herr R, Starr A: Radiographic diagnosis of aortic-ball variance. JAMA 207:1120–1122, 1969.
30. Gutierrez F, McKnight R, Clark R, Bishop A, Ludbrook P, Nordlicht S: Chest film diagnosis of disc embolization in patients with Beall mitral valve prostheses. J Thorac Cardiovasc Surg 81:758–761, 1981.
31. Hylen J: Mechanical malfunction and thrombosis of prosthetic heart valves. Am J Cardiol 30:396–402, 1972.

32. Lansing A: Unusual radiographic sign of loose mitral valve prosthesis. Radiology 88:789–790, 1967.

33. Sands M, Kreulen T, McDonough M, Fadali M, Spann J: Pseudomalfunction of a Beall mitral valve prosthesis in the presence of paravalvular aortic regurgitation. Am J Cardiol 36:88–90, 1975.

34. Chun P, Rajfer S, Donohue D, Bowen T, Davia J: Bjork-Shiley mitral valvular dehiscence. Am Heart J 99:230–234, 1980.

35. Seningen R, Buckley B, Roberts WC: Prosthetic aortic stenosis. Circulation 49:921–924, 1974.

36. Watanakunakorn C: Prosthetic valve infective endocarditis. Prog Cardiovasc Dis 22:181–192, 1979.

37. Ellis K, Jaffe C, Malm J, Bowman F: Infective endocarditis. Radiol Clin North Am 11:415–442, 1973.

38. Frankl W: Selection of patients for prosthetic valve surgery. *In* Morse D, Steiner RM, Fernandez J: A Guide to Prosthetic Cardiac Valves. Philadelphia: FA Davis Co, (in preparation).

39. Zumbro GL, Cundey P, Fishback M, Galloway R: Strut fracture in DeBakey valve. J Thorac Cardiovasc Surg 74:469–470, 1977.

40. Gordon M, Walters M, Allen P, Burton J: Calcific stenosis of a glutaraldehyde-treated porcine bioprosthesis in the aortic position. J Thorac Cardiovasc Surg 80:788–791, 1980.

41. Freed M, Bernhard W: Prosthetic valve replacement in children. Prog Cardiovasc Dis 17:475–487, 1975.

42. Edmiston WA, Chan L, Tatter D, Lau FYK: Cholelithiasis: a frequent complication of artificial heart valve replacement. Am Heart J 95:483–488, 1978.

43. Morton M, Rahimtoola S: How to follow patients with prosthetic heart valves. J Cardiovasc Med 5:1–10, 1980.

44. Carlson EB, Mintz GS, Bemis CE: Hemodynamic significance of normal and abnormal fluoroscopic patterns of disc motion in the Beall mitral valve prosthesis. Radiology 141:335–339, 1981.

45. Arditi LI, Holswode GR, Steinberg I: Aortic regurgitation following trauma in a patient with Magovern valve prosthesis. AJR 104:420, 1968.

46. Bjork-V, Henze A, Jereb M: Aortographic follow-up in patients with the Bjork-Shiley aortic disc valve prosthesis. Scand J Thorac Cardiovasc Surg 7:1–6, 1973.

47. Mintz G, Carlson E, Kotler M: Comparison of noninvasive techniques in the evaluation of the nontissue cardiac valve prosthesis. Am J Cardiol 49:39–44, 1982.

Index

R

Index